Neuroethics

Neuroscience has dramatically increased understanding of how mental states and processes are realized by the brain, thereby opening doors for treating the multitude of ways in which minds become dysfunctional. This book explores questions such as: When is it permissible to alter a person's memories, influence personality traits or read minds? What can neuroscience tell us about free will, self-control, self-deception and the foundations of morality?

The view of neuroethics offered here argues that many of our new powers are continuous with much older abilities to alter minds. They have, however, expanded to include almost all our social, political and ethical decisions. Written primarily for graduate students, this book will appeal to anyone with an interest in the more philosophical and ethical aspects of the neurosciences.

NEIL LEVY is a Senior Research Fellow at the Centre for Applied Philosophy and Public Ethics, University of Melbourne, Australia, and a James Martin Research Fellow at the Program on Ethics of the New Biosciences, Oxford. He has published more than fifty articles in refereed journals, as well as four books previous to this one.

Neuroethics

NEIL LEVY

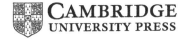

CAMBRIDGE
UNIVERSITY PRESS

CAMBRIDGE UNIVERSITY PRESS
Cambridge, New York, Melbourne, Madrid, Cape Town, Singapore, São Paulo, Delhi

Cambridge University Press
The Edinburgh Building, Cambridge CB2 8RU, UK

Published in the United States of America by Cambridge University Press, New York

www.cambridge.org
Information on this title: www.cambridge.org/9780521687263

First published 2007

A catalogue record for this publication is available from the British Library

ISBN 978-0-521-86782-5 hardback
ISBN 978-0-521-68726-3 paperback

Transferred to digital printing 2009

Contents

Preface

In the late 1960s, a new field of philosophical and moral enquiry came into existence. *Bioethics*, as it soon came to be called, quickly mushroomed: it developed its own journals, its own professional associations, its own conferences, degree programs and experts. It developed very rapidly for many reasons, but no doubt the main impetus was that it was needed. The problems and puzzles that bioethics treats were, and are, urgent. Bioethics developed at a time when medical technology, a kind of technology in which we are all – quite literally – vitally interested, was undergoing significant growth and developing unprecedented powers; powers that urgently needed to be regulated. The growth in life-saving ability, the development of means of artificial reproduction, the rapid accumulation of specialist knowledge, required new approaches, concentrated attention, new focuses and sustained development; in short, a new discipline. Bioethics was born out of new technical possibilities – new reproductive technologies, new abilities to intervene in the genetic substrate of traits, new means of extending life – and the pressing need to understand, to control and to channel these possibilities.

Predicting the future is a dangerous business. Nevertheless, it seems safe to predict that the relatively new field dubbed *neuroethics* will undergo a similarly explosive growth. Neuroethics seems a safe bet, for three reasons: first because the sciences of the mind are experiencing a growth spurt that is even more spectacular than the growth seen in medicine over the decades preceding the birth of bioethics. Second, because these sciences deal with issues which are every bit as personally gripping as the life sciences: our minds are, in some quite direct sense, *us*, so that understanding our mind, and increasing its power, gives us an unprecedented degree of control over ourselves. Third because, as Zeman (2003) points out, the neurosciences straddle a major fault line in our self-conception: they promise to link *mind* to *brain*, the private and subjective world of experience, feeling and thought with the public and objective world of hard physical data. Neuroscience (and the related sciences of the mind) does not simply hold out the promise, one day soon, of forestalling dementia or enhancing our cognition, and thereby raise urgent questions concerning our identities and the self; beyond this it offers us a window into what it means to be human. Our continuing existence as conscious beings depends upon our minds, and the medical technologies that can sustain or improve our minds are therefore vital to us, but we are also gripped by the deep philosophical questions raised by the possibility of finally coordinating dimensions of experience that so often seem incommensurable.

For these reasons, I suggest it is a safe bet that neuroethics will take off as a field; that it will take its place alongside bioethics as a semi-independent discipline, sheltering philosophers and scientists, legal scholars and policy analysts, and spawning specialists of its own. Hence, too, the need for this book. This book is not the very first to reflect upon the ethical issues raised by the neurosciences and by the technologies for intervening in the mind they offer us, though it is among the first.[1] It is, however, the first to offer a comprehensive framework for thinking about neuroethical issues; a vision of the relationship between mind and the world which (I claim) will enable us better to appreciate the extent to which the sciences of the mind present us with unique and unprecedented challenges. It is also the first to attempt to understand the ways in which the neurosciences alter or refine our conception of ourselves as moral agents. Since the neurosciences seem to penetrate deeply into the self, by offering us the chance of understanding the mind, subjectivity and consciousness, and because they require that we seek to understand the relationship between the subjective and the objective, a philosophical approach to neuroethics is necessary. I do not claim that it is the *only* approach that is necessary: obviously neuroscientists must contribute to neuroethics, but so must specialists in other fields. Neuroethics is, by its very nature, interdisciplinary. But the kind of approach that only philosophy can provide is indispensable, and, I believe, fascinating. Moreover, I shall claim, the broader philosophical perspective offered here will help illuminate the ethical issues, more narrowly construed. Only when we understand, philosophically, what the mind is and how it can be altered can we begin properly to engage in the *ethics* of neuroethics. Indeed, I shall claim that understanding the mind properly plays a significant role in motivating an important alteration in the way ethics is understood, and in what we come to see as the bearers of moral values. What might be called an *externalist ethics* gradually emerges from the pages that follow, an ethics in which the boundaries between agents, and between agents and their context, is taken to be much less significant than is traditionally thought.

Despite this insistence on the necessity for philosophy, I shall not assume any philosophical background. Since I believe that philosophical reflection will illuminate the ethical issues, and that these ethical issues are the concern of all reflective people, I shall attempt to provide necessary background, and to explain terminology and debates, as it becomes relevant. I do not aim here to produce a work of popular philosophy, which too often means philosophy over-simplified. Instead, I aim to produce genuine philosophy that is also accessible to non-philosophers. Since I am constructing a case for a novel view of neuroethics, I expect that professional philosophers will find a great deal of interest in what follows.

In this brief preface, I have added, in a small way, to the hype surrounding neuroscience and neuroethics. I have claimed that the sciences of the mind have the potential to help us understand the nature of the self, and of humanity, our very identity. These claims are, I believe, true. Yet this book defends a somewhat deflationary

thesis, so far as the ethics of neuroethics is concerned. I shall argue
for what I call the *parity thesis*: our new ways of altering the mind
are not, for all that, entirely unprecedented, and ought not to be
regarded, as a class, as qualitatively different in kind from the old.
They are, instead, on a par with older and more familiar ways of
altering the mind. New technologies are often treated with suspicion
simply because they are new; sometimes they are celebrated for
precisely the same reason. Neuroscientific technologies ought not be
celebrated or reviled for being new: in fact, they – typically – raise
much the same kinds of puzzles and problems as older, sometimes
far older, technologies. That is *not* to say that they do not present
us with genuine ethical dilemmas and with serious challenges; they
do. But, for the most part, these dilemmas and challenges are new
versions of old problems.

If the new sciences of the mind often pose serious challenges,
they also present us with opportunities: since the challenges they
pose are often new versions of old challenges, they present us with
the opportunity to revisit these challenges, and the older
technologies that provoke them, with fresh eyes. Sometimes we
accept older practices simply because they are well established, or
because we have ceased to see their problems; reflecting on the new
neurosciences gives us the opportunity to reassess older ways of
altering minds. I hasten to add, too, that the parity thesis defended
here concerns the new technologies of the mind as a *class*. Some
particular applications of these technologies do raise new, and
genuinely unprecedented, challenges for us. We must assess each on
its own merits, for the powers and perils it actually possesses and
promises.

I will defend the parity thesis, in large part, by way of reflection
on what it means to be human. Thus while the thesis is deflationary
in one sense – deflating the pretensions of the technologies of the
mind to offer entirely novel and unprecedented possibilities for
altering human beings – it is also exciting in another: it offers us a
perspective upon ourselves, as individuals and as a species that is,

if not entirely novel (for as I shall show the thesis, or something
rather like it, has its philosophical defenders) at least little
appreciated or understood. We are, I shall claim, animals of a peculiar
sort: we are self-creating and self-modifying animals. We alter our
own minds, and use technological means to do so. This is not
something new about *us*, here and now in the "postmodern" West
(for all that so much about us, here and now, *is* genuinely new). That
is the kind of animal we human beings are. We are distinctive
inasmuch as we have public and distributed minds: minds that
spread beyond the limits of individuals, but which include and are
built out of other minds and the scaffolding of culture. The sciences
of the mind offer us new opportunities for altering our minds and
increasing their powers, but in doing so they offer us new means of
doing what we have always done; the kind of thing that makes us the
beings that we are.

End note

1. The honor of publishing the very first *philosophical* monograph on
   neuroethics falls to Walter Glannon (Glannon 2006). The first monograph
   on neuroethics, appropriately enough, was written by the distinguished
   neuroscientist Michael Gazzaniga (Gazzaniga 2005). Several important
   collections of papers have also been published; see, in particular Illes
   (2006) and Garland (2004).

Acknowledgements

I have incurred many intellectual debts in the course of writing this book. Many of the ideas here owe their genesis to discussions and collaborations with Tim Bayne. Richard Ashcroft, Jill Craigie, Walter Glannon, Gert-Jan Lokhorst and Saskia Nagel read the entire manuscript and offered many useful comments. Many more people read parts of the manuscript, in various stages of composition, or listened to versions presented at conferences. Their comments saved me from many embarrassing errors. They include Piers Benn, David Chalmers, Randy Clark, George Graham Jeanette Kennett, Morten Kringelbach Al Mele, Dick Passingham Derk Pereboom, Julian Savulescu and Daniel Weiskopf. Finally, I want to thank Jo Tyszka for her efficient copy-editing.

The ideas here have developed over many years; earlier versions of some of them have previously been published. Chapter 6 contains ideas that previously appeared in "Addiction, autonomy and ego-depletion," *Bioethics*, **20** (2006): 16–20 and "Autonomy and addiction," *Canadian Journal of Philosophy*, **36** (2006): 427–47. Chapter 7 builds on "Libet's impossible demand," *Journal of Consciousness Studies*, **12** (2005): 67–76. Chapter 8 is a modified version of "Self-deception without thought experiments," to appear in J. Fernandez and T. Bayne, eds., *Delusions, Self-Deception and Affective Influences on Belief-formation*, New York: Psychology Press, and Chapter 9 builds on "The wisdom of the Pack," *Philosophical Explorations*, **9** (2006): 99–103 and "Cognitive Scientific Challenges to Morality" *Philosophical Psychology*, forthcoming. I thank the editors of all these journals and books for permission to reprint relevant sections.

I Introduction

Neuroethics is a new field. The term itself is commonly, though erroneously, believed to have been coined by William Safire (2002), writing in *The New York Times*. In fact, as Safire himself acknowledges, the term predates his usage.[1] The very fact that it is so widely believed that the term dates from 2002 is itself significant: it indicates the recency not of the term itself, but of widespread concern with the kinds of issues it embraces. Before 2002 most people saw no need for any such field, but so rapid have been the advances in the sciences of mind since, and so pressing have the ethical issues surrounding them become, that we cannot any longer dispense with the term or the field it names.

Neuroethics has two main branches; the *ethics of neuroscience* and the *neuroscience of ethics* (Roskies 2002). The *ethics of neuroscience* refers to the branch of neuroethics that seeks to develop an ethical framework for regulating the conduct of neuroscientific enquiry and the application of neuroscientific knowledge to human beings; *the neuroscience of ethics* refers to the impact of neuroscientific knowledge upon our understanding of ethics itself.

One branch of the "ethics of neuroscience" concerns the conduct of neuroscience itself; research protocols for neuroscientists, the ethics of withholding incidental findings, and so on. In this book I shall have little to say about this set of questions, at least directly (though much of what I shall say about other issues has implications for the conduct of neuroscience). Instead, I shall focus on questions to do with the *application* of our growing knowledge about the mind and the brain to people. Neuroscience and allied fields give us an apparently unprecedented, and rapidly growing, power to intervene in the brains of subjects – to alter personality traits, to enhance cognitive capacities, to reinforce or to weaken memories, perhaps, one day, to insert beliefs. Are these applications of neuroscience ethical? Under what conditions? Do they threaten important elements of human agency, of our self-understanding? Will neuroscientists soon be able to "read" our minds? Chapters 2 through 5 will focus on these and closely related questions.

The *neuroscience of ethics* embraces our growing knowledge about the neural bases of moral agency. Neuroscience seems to promise to illuminate, and perhaps to threaten, central elements of this agency: our freedom of the will, our ability to know our own minds, perhaps the very substance of morality itself. Its findings provide us with an opportunity to reassess what it means to be a responsible human being, apparently making free choices from among alternatives. It casts light on our ability to control our desires and our actions, and upon how and why we lose control. It offers advertisers and governments possible ways to channel our behavior; it may also offer us ways to fight back against these forces.

If the neuroscience of ethics produces significant results, that is, if it alters our understanding of moral agency, then neuroethics is importantly different from other branches of applied ethics. Unlike, say, bioethics or business ethics, neuroethics reacts back upon itself. The neuroscience of ethics will help us to forge the very tools we shall need to make progress on the ethics of neuroscience. Neuroethics is therefore not just one more branch of applied ethics. It occupies a pivotal position, casting light upon human agency, freedom and choice, and upon rationality. It will help us to reflect on what we are, and offer us guidance as we attempt to shape a future in which we can flourish. We might not have needed the term before 2002; today the issues it embraces are rightly seen as central to our political, moral and social aspirations.

NEUROETHICS: SOME CASE STUDIES

Neuroethics is not only important; it is also fascinating. The kinds of cases that fall within its purview include some of the most controversial and strange ethical issues confronting us today. In this section, I shall briefly review two such cases.

Body integrity identity disorder

Body integrity identity disorder (BIID) is a controversial new psychiatric diagnosis, the principal symptom of which is a persisting desire to have some part of the body – usually a limb – removed (First 2005). A few sufferers have been able to convince surgeons to accede to their requests (Scott 2000). However, following press coverage of the operations and a public outcry, no reputable surgeon offers the operation today. In the absence of access to such surgery, sufferers quite often go to extreme lengths to have their desire satisfied. For instance, they deliberately injure the affected limb, using dry ice, tourniquets or even chainsaws. Their aim is to remove the limb, or to damage it so badly that surgeons have no choice but to remove it (Elliott 2000).

A variety of explanations of the desire for amputation of a limb have been offered by psychiatrists and psychologists. It has been suggested that the desire is the product of a *paraphilia* – a psychosexual disorder. On this interpretation, the desire is explained by the sexual excitement that sufferers (supposedly) feel at the prospect of becoming an amputee (Money *et al.* 1977). Another possibility is that the desire is the product of body dysmorphic disorder (Phillips 1996), a disorder in which sufferers irrationally perceive a part of their body as ugly or diseased. The limited evidence available today, however, suggests that the desire has a quite different aetiology. BIID stems from a mismatch between the agent's body and their *experience* of their body, what we might call their *subjective body* (Bayne and Levy 2005). In this interpretation, BIID is analogous to what is now known as gender identity disorder, the disorder in which sufferers feel as though they have been born into a body of the wrong gender.

Whichever interpretation of the aetiology of the disorder is correct, however, BIID falls within the purview of neuroethics. BIID is a neuroethical issue because it raises *ethical* questions, and because answering those questions requires us to engage with the sciences of the mind. The major ethical issue raised by BIID focuses on the question of the permissibility of amputation as a means of treating the disorder. Now, while this question cannot be answered by the sciences of the mind alone, we cannot hope to assess it adequately unless we understand the disorder, and understanding it properly requires us to engage in the relevant sciences. Neuroscience, psychiatry and psychology all have their part to play in helping us to assess the ethical question. It might be, for instance, that BIID can be illuminated by neuroscientific work on phantom limbs. The experience of a phantom limb appears to be a near mirror image of BIID; whereas in the latter, subjects experience a desire for removal of a limb that is functioning normally, the experience of a phantom limb is the experience of the continued presence of a limb that has been amputated (or, occasionally, that is congenitally absent).

The experience of the phantom limb suggests that the experience of our bodies is mediated by a neural representation of a body schema, a schema that is modifiable by experience, but which resists modification (Ramachandran and Hirstein 1998). Phantom limbs are sometimes experienced as the site of excruciating pain; unfortunately, this pain is often resistant to all treatments. If BIID is explained by a similar mismatch between an unconscious body schema and the objective body, then there is every chance that it too will prove very resistant to treatment. If that's the case, then the prima facie case for the permissibility of surgery is quite strong: if BIID sufferers experience significant distress, and if the only way to relieve that distress is by way of surgery, the surgery is permissible (Bayne and Levy 2005).

On the other hand, if BIID has an origin that is very dissimilar to the origin of the phantom limb phenomenon, treatments less radical than surgery might be preferable. Surgery is a drastic course of action: it is irreversible, and it leaves the patient disabled. If BIID can be effectively treated by psychological means – psychotherapy, medication or a combination of the two – then surgery is impermissible. If BIID arises from a mismatch between cortical representations of the body and the objective body, then – at least given the present state of neuroscientific knowledge – there is little hope that psychological treatments will be successful. But if BIID has its origin in something we can address psychologically – a fall in certain types of neurotransmitters, in anxiety or in depression, for instance – then we can hope to treat it with means much less dramatic than surgery. BIID is therefore at once a question for the sciences of the mind and for ethics; it is a neuroethical question.

Automatism

Sometimes agents perform a complex series of actions in a state closely resembling unconsciousness. They sleepwalk, for instance: arising from sleep without, apparently, fully awaking, they may dress and leave the house. Or they may enter a closely analogous state, not by first falling asleep, but by way of an epileptic fit, a blow on the head, or (very rarely) psychosis. Usually, the kinds of actions that agents perform in this state are routine or stereotyped. Someone who enters the state of automatism while playing the piano may continue playing if they know the piece well; similarly, someone who enters into it while driving home may continue following the familiar route, safely driving into their own drive and then simply sitting in the car until they come to themselves (Searle 1994).

Occasionally, however, an agent will engage in morally significant actions while in this state. Consider the case of Ken Parks (Broughton, *et al.* 1994). In 1987, Parks drove the twenty-three kilometres to the home of his parents-in-law, where he stabbed them both. He then drove to the police station, where he told police that he thought he had killed someone. Only then, apparently, did he notice that his hands had been badly injured. Parks was taken to hospital where the severed tendons in both his arms were repaired. He was charged with the murder of his mother-in-law, and the attempted murder of his father-in-law. Parks did not deny the offences, but claimed that he had been sleepwalking at the time, and that therefore he was not responsible for them.

Assessing Parks' responsibility for his actions is a complex and difficult question, a question which falls squarely within the purview of neuroethics. Answering it requires both sophisticated philosophical analysis and neuroscientific expertise. Philosophically, it requires that we analyze the notions of "responsibility" and "voluntariness." Under what conditions are ordinary agents responsible for their actions? What does it mean to act voluntarily? We might hope to answer both questions by highlighting the role of *conscious intentions* in action; that is, we might say that agents are responsible for their actions only when, prior to acting, they form a conscious intention of acting. However, this response seems very implausible, once we realize how rarely we form a conscious intention. Many of our actions, including some of our praise- and blame-worthy actions, are performed too quickly for us to deliberate beforehand: a child runs in front of our car and we slam on the brakes; someone insults us and we take a swing at them; we see the flames and run into the burning building, heedless of our safety. The lack of a conscious intention does not seem to differentiate between these, apparently responsible, actions, and Parks' behavior.

Perhaps, then, there is no genuine difference between Parks' behavior and ours in those circumstances; perhaps once we have sufficient awareness of our environment to be able to navigate it (as Parks did, in driving his car), we are acting responsibly. Against this hypothesis we have the evidence that Parks was a gentle man, who had always got on well with his parents-in-law. The fact that the crime was out of character and apparently motiveless counts against the hypothesis that it should be considered an ordinary action.

If we are to understand when and why normal agents are responsible for their actions, we need to engage with the relevant sciences of the mind. These sciences supply us with essential data for consideration: data about the range of normal cases, and about various pathologies of agency. Investigating the mind of the acting subject teaches us important lessons. We learn, first, that our conscious access to our reasons for actions can be patchy and unreliable (Wegner 2002): ordinary subjects sometimes fail to recognize their own reasons for action, or even *that* they are acting. We learn how little *conscious* control we have over many, probably the majority, of our actions (Bargh and Chartrand 1999). But we also learn how these actions can nevertheless be intelligent and rational responses to our environment, responses that reflect our values (Dijksterhuis *et al.* 2006). The mere lack of conscious deliberation, we learn, cannot differentiate responsible actions from non-responsible ones, because it does not mark the division between the voluntary and the non-voluntary.

On the other hand, the sciences of the mind also provide us with good evidence that *some* kinds of automatic actions fail to reflect our values. Some brain-damaged subjects can no longer inhibit their automatic responses to stimuli. They compulsively engage in *utilization behavior*, in which they respond automatically to objects in the environment around them (Lhermitte *et al.* 1986). Under some conditions, entirely normal subjects find themselves prey to stereotyped responses that fail to reflect their consciously endorsed values. Fervent feminists may find themselves behaving in ways that apparently reflect a higher valuation of men than of women, for instance (Dasgupta 2004). Lack of opportunity to bring one's behavior under the control of one's values *can* excuse. Outlining the precise circumstances under which this is the case is a problem for neuroethics: for philosophical reflection informed by the sciences of the mind.

Parks was eventually acquitted by the Supreme Court of Canada. I shall not attempt, here, to assess whether the court was right in its finding (we shall return to related questions in Chapter 7). My purpose, in outlining his case, and the case of the sufferer from BIID, is instead to give the reader some sense of how fascinating, and how strange, the neuroethical landscape is, and how significant its findings can be. Doing neuroethics seriously is difficult: it requires a serious engagement in the sciences of the mind and in several branches of philosophy (philosophy of mind, applied ethics, moral psychology and meta-ethics). But the rewards for the hard work are considerable. We can only understand ourselves, the endlessly fascinating, endlessly strange, world of the human being, by understanding the ways in which our minds function and how they become dysfunctional.

THE MIND AND THE BRAIN

This is a book about the mind, and about the implications for our ethical thought of the increasing number of practical applications stemming from our growing knowledge of how it works. To begin our exploration of these ethical questions, it is important to have some basic grasp of what the mind is and how it is realized by the brain. If we are to evaluate interventions into the mind, if we are to understand how our brains make us the kinds of creatures we are, with our values and our goals, then we need to understand what exactly we are talking about when we talk about the mind and the brain. Fortunately, for our purposes, we do not need a very detailed understanding of the way in which the brain works. We shall not be exploring the world of neurons, with their dendrites and axons, nor the neuroanatomy of the brain, with its division into hemispheres and cortices (except in passing, as and when it becomes relevant).

All of this is fascinating, and much of it is of philosophical, and sometimes even ethical, relevance. But it is more important, for our purposes, to get a grip on how minds are constituted at much a higher level of abstraction, in order to shake ourselves free of an ancient and persistent view of the mind, the view with which almost all of us begin when we think about the mind, and from which few of us ever manage entirely to free ourselves: dualism. Shaking ourselves free of the grip of dualism will allow us to begin to frame a more realistic image of the mind and the brain; moreover, this more realistic image, of the mind as composed of mechanisms, will itself prove to be important when it comes time to turn to more narrowly neuroethical questions.

Dualism – or more precisely *substance* dualism (in order to distinguish it from the more respectable *property* dualism) – is the view that there are two kinds of basic and mutually irreducible substances in the universe. This is a very ancient view, one that is perhaps innate in the human mind (Bloom 2004). It is the view presupposed, or at least suggested by, all or, very nearly all, religious traditions; it was also the dominant view in philosophical thought for many centuries, at least as far back as the ancient Greeks. But it was given its most powerful and influential exposition by the seventeenth century philosopher René Descartes, as a result of which the view is often referred to as Cartesian dualism. According to Descartes, roughly, there are two fundamental kinds of substance: *matter*, out of which the entire physical world (including animals) is built, and *mind*. Human beings are composed of an amalgam of these two substances: mind (or soul) and matter.

It is fashionable, especially among cognitive scientists, to mock dualists, and to regard the view as motivated by nothing more than superstition. It is certainly true that dualism's attractions were partly due to the fact that it offered an explanation for the possibility of the immortality of the soul and therefore of resurrection and of eternal reward and punishment. If the soul is immaterial, then there is no reason to believe that it is damaged by the death and decay of the body; the soul is free, after death, to rejoin God and the heavenly hosts (themselves composed of nothing but soul-stuff). But dualism also had a more philosophical motivation. We can understand, to some extent at least, how mere matter could be cleverly arranged to create complex and apparently intelligent behavior in animals. Descartes himself used the analogy of clockwork mechanisms, which are capable of all sorts of useful and complex activities, but are built out of entirely mindless matter. Today, we are accustomed to getting responses magnitudes more complex from our machines, using electronics rather than clockwork. But even so, it remains difficult to see how mere matter could really *think*; be rational and intelligent, and not merely flexibly responsive. Equally, it remains difficult to see how matter could be *conscious*. How could a machine, no matter how complex or cleverly designed, be capable of experiencing the subtle taste of wine, the scent of roses or of garbage; how could there be something that it is *like* to be a creature built entirely out of matter? Dualism, with its postulation of a substance that is categorically different from mere matter, seems to hold out the hope of an answer.

Descartes thought that matter could never be conscious or rational, and it is easy to sympathize with him. Indeed, it is easy to agree with him (even today some philosophers embrace property dualism because, though they accept that matter could be intelligent, they argue that it could never be conscious). Matter is unconscious and irrational – or, better, *a*rational – and there is no way to make it conscious or rational simply by arranging it in increasingly complex ways (or so it seems). It is therefore very tempting to think that since we are manifestly rational and conscious, we cannot be built out of matter alone. The part of us that thinks and experiences, Descartes thought, must be built from a different substance. Animals and plants, like rocks and water, are built entirely out of matter, but we humans each have a thinking part as well. It follows from this view that animals are incapable not only of thought, but also of experience; notoriously, this doctrine was sometimes invoked to justify vivisection of animals. If they cannot feel, then their cries of pain must be merely mechanical responses to damage, rather than expressions of genuine suffering (Singer 1990).

It's easy to share Descartes' puzzlement as to how mere matter can think and experience. But the centuries since Descartes have witnessed a series of scientific advances that have made dualism increasingly incredible. First, the idea that there is a *categorical* distinction to be made between human beings and other animals no longer seems very plausible in light of the overwhelming evidence that we have all evolved from a common ancestor. Human beings have not always been around on planet Earth – indeed, we are a relatively young species – and both the fossil evidence and the morphological evidence indicate that we evolved from earlier primates. Our ancestors got along without souls or immaterial minds, so if we are composed, partially, of any such stuff, it must have been added to our lineage at some relatively recent point in time. But when? The evolutionary record is a story of continuous change; there are no obvious discontinuities in it which might be correlated with ensoulment.[2] Moreover, it is a story in which increasingly complicated life forms progressively appear: first simple self-replicating molecules, then single-celled organisms, then multicellular organisms, insects, reptiles and finally mammals. Each new life form is capable of more sophisticated, seemingly more intelligent, behavior: not merely responding to stimuli, but anticipating them, and altering its immediate environment to raise the probability that it'll get the stimuli it wants, and avoid those it doesn't. Our immediate ancestors and cousins, the other members of the primate family, are in fascinating – and, for some, disturbing – ways very close to us in behavior, and capable of feats of cognition of great sophistication. Gorillas and chimpanzees have been taught sign language, with, in some cases, quite spectacular success (Savage-Rumbaugh *et al.* 1999). Moreover, there is very strong evidence that other animals are conscious; chimpanzees (at least) also seem to be self-conscious (DeGrazia 1996; for a dissenting view see Carruthers 2005).

Surely it would be implausible to argue that the moment of ensoulment, the sudden and inexplicable acquisition by an organism of the immaterial mind-stuff that enables it to think and to feel, occurred prior to the evolution of humanity – that the first ensouled creatures were our primate ancestors, or perhaps even earlier ancestors? If souls are necessary for intelligent behavior – for tool use, for communication, for complex social systems, or even for morality (or perhaps, better, proto-morality) – then souls have been around much longer than we have: all these behaviors are exhibited by a variety of animals much less sophisticated than we are.[3] If souls are necessary only for consciousness, or even self-consciousness, then perhaps they are more recent, but they almost certainly still predate the existence of our species. It appears that mere matter, arranged ingeniously, had better be capable of allowing for all the kinds of behavior and experiences that mind-stuff was originally postulated to explain.

Evolutionary biology and ethology have therefore delivered a powerful blow to the dualist view. The sciences of the mind have delivered another, or rather a series of others. The cognitive sciences – the umbrella term for the disciplines devoted to the study of mental phenomena – have begun to answer the Cartesian challenge in the most direct and decisive way possible: by laying bare the mechanisms and pathways from sensory input to rational response and conscious awareness. We do not have space to review more than a tiny fraction of their results here. But it is worth pausing over a little of the evidence against dualism these sciences have accumulated.

Some of this evidence comes from the ways in which the mind can malfunction. When one part of the brain is damaged, due to trauma, tumor or stroke, the person or animal whose brain it is can often get along quite well (natural selection usually builds in quite a high degree of redundancy in complex systems, since organisms are constantly exposed to damage from one source or another). But they may exhibit strange, even bizarre, behavioral oddities, which give us an insight into what function the damaged portion of the brain served, and what function the preserved parts perform. From this kind of data, we can deduce the functional neuroanatomy of the brain, gradually mapping the distribution of functions across the lobes.

This data also constitutes powerful evidence against dualism. It seems to show that mind, the thinking substance, is actually dependent upon matter, in a manner that is hard to understand on the supposition that it is composed of an ontologically distinct substance. Why should mind be altered and its performance degraded by changes in matter, if it is a different *kind* of thing? Recall the attractions of the mind-stuff theory, for Cartesians. First, the theory was supposed to explain how the essence of the self, the mind or soul, could survive the destruction of the body. Second, it was supposed to explain how rationality and consciousness were possible, given that, supposedly, no arrangement of mere matter could ever realize these features. The evidence from brain damage suggests that soul-stuff does not in fact have these alleged advantages, if indeed it exists: it is itself too closely tied to the material to possess them. Unexpectedly – for the dualist – mind degrades when matter is damaged; the greater the damage, the greater the degradation. Given that cognition degrades when, and to the extent that, matter is damaged, it seems likely that any mind that could survive the wholesale decay of matter that occurs after death would be, at best, sadly truncated, incapable of genuine thought or memory, and entirely incapable of preserving the identity of the unique individual whose mind it is. Moreover, the fact that rationality degrades and consciousness fades or disappears when the underlying neural structures are damaged suggests that, contra the dualist, it is these neural structures that support and help to realize thought and consciousness, not immaterial mind – else the coincidental degradation of mind looks miraculous. Immaterial minds shouldn't fragment or degrade when matter is damaged, but *our* minds do.

Perhaps these points will seem more convincing if we have some actual cases of brain lesions and corresponding mind malfunction before us. Consider some of the agnosias: disorders of recognition. There are many different kinds of agnosias, giving rise to difficulty in recognizing different types of object. Sometimes the deficit is very specific, involving, for instance, an inability to identify animals, or varieties of fruit. One relatively common form is *prosopagnosia*, the inability to recognize faces, including the faces of people close to the sufferer. What's going on in these agnosias? The response that best fits with our common sense, dualist, view of the mind preserves dualism by relegating some apparently mental functions to a physical medium that can degrade. For instance, we might propose that sufferers have lost access to the store of information that represents the people or objects they fail to recognize. Perhaps the brain contains something like the hard drive of a computer on which memories and facts are stored, and perhaps the storage is divided up so that memories of different kinds of things are each stored separately. When the person perceives a face, she searches her "memory of faces" store, and comes up with the right answer. But in prosopagnosia, the store is corrupted, or access to it is disturbed. If something like this was right, then we might be able to preserve the view that mind is a spiritual substance, with the kinds of properties that such an indivisible substance is supposed to possess (such as an inability to fragment). We rescue mind by delegating some of its functions to non-mind: memories are stored in a physical medium, which can fragment, but mind soars above matter.

Unfortunately, it is clear that the hypothesis just sketched is false. The agnosias are far stranger than that. Sufferers have not simply lost the ability to recognize objects or people; they have lost a sense-specific ability: to recognize a certain class of objects *visually* (or tactilely, or aurally, and so on). The prosopagnosic who fails to recognize his wife when he looks at her knows immediately who she is when she speaks. Well, the dualist might reply, perhaps it is not his store of information that is damaged, but his visual system; there's nothing wrong with his mind at all, but merely with his eyes. But that's not right either: the sufferer from visual agnosia sees perfectly well. Indeed, he may be able to describe what he sees as well as you or I. Consider Dr. P., the eponymous "man who mistook his wife for a hat" of Oliver Sack's well-known book, and his attempts to identify an object handed to him by Sacks (here and elsewhere I quote at length, in order to convey the strangeness of many dysfunctions of the mind):

> 'About six inches in length,' he commented. 'A convoluted red form with a linear green attachment.'
> 'Yes,' I said encouragingly, and what do you think it *is*, Dr. P.?'
> 'Not easy to say.' He seemed perplexed. 'It lacks the simply symmetry of the Platonic solids, although it may have a higher symmetry of its own ... I think this could be an infloresence or flower.'

On Sack's suggestion, Dr P. smelt the object.

> Now, suddenly, he came to life. 'Beautiful!' he exclaimed. 'An
> early rose!'
>
> *(Sacks 1985: 12–13)*

Dr. P. is obviously a highly intelligent man, whose intellect is intact
despite his brain disorder. His visual system functions perfectly well,
allowing him to perceive and describe in detail the object with which
he is presented. But he is forced to try to infer, haltingly, what the
object is – even though he knows full well what a rose is and what it
looks like. Presented with a glove, which he described as a container
of some sort with "five outpouchings," Dr. P. did even worse at the
object-recognition task.

It appears that something very strange has happened to Dr. P.'s
mind. Its fabric has unravelled, in some way and at one corner, in a
manner that no spiritual substance could conceivably do. It is difficult to see how to reconcile what he experiences with our common
sense idea of what the mind is like. Perhaps a way might be found to
accommodate Dr. P.'s disorder within the dualist picture, but the
range of phenomena that needs to be explained is wide, and its
strangeness overwhelming; accommodating them all will, I suggest,
prove impossible without straining the limits of our credibility.

One more example: another agnosia. In *mirror agnosia*,
patients suffering from *neglect* mistake the reflections of objects for
the objects themselves, even though they know (in some sense) that
they are looking at a mirror image, and only when the mirror is
positioned in certain ways. First, a brief introduction to neglect,
which is itself a neurological disorder of great interest. Someone
suffering from neglect is profoundly indifferent to a portion of their
visual field, even though their visual system is undamaged. Usually,
it is the left side of the field that is affected: a neglect sufferer might
put makeup on or shave only the right side of their face; when asked
to draw a clock, they typically draw a complete circle, but then
stuff all the numbers from one to twelve on the right hand half.

Ramachandran and colleagues wondered how neglect sufferers would respond when presented with a mirror image of an object in their neglected left field. The experimenters tested the subjects' cognitive capacities and found them to be "mentally quite lucid," with no dementia, aphasia or amnesia (Ramachandran *et al.* 1997: 645). They also tested their patients' knowledge of mirrors and their uses, by placing an object just behind the patient's right shoulder, so that they could see the object in the mirror, and asking them to grab it. All four patients tested correctly reached behind them to grab the object, just as you and I would. But when the object reflected in the mirror was placed in the patient's left, neglected, field, they were not able to follow the instruction to grab it. Rather than reach behind them for the object, they reached *toward* the mirror. When asked where the object was, they replied that it was in, or behind, the mirror. They knew what a mirror was, and what it does, but when the object reflected was in their neglected field, this knowledge guided neither their verbal responses nor their actions.

A similar confusion concerning mirrors occurs in the delusion known as *mirror misidentification*. In this delusion, patients mistake their own reflection for another person: not the *reflection* of another person, but the very person. Presented with a mirror, the sufferer says that the person they see is a stranger; perhaps someone who has been following them about. But once again their knowledge concerning mirrors seems intact. Consider this exchange between an experimenter and a sufferer from mirror misidentification. The experimenter positions herself next to F.E., the sufferer, so that they are both reflected in the mirror which they face. She points to her own reflection, and asks who that person is. 'That's you,' F.E. replies; agreeing that what he sees in the mirror is the experimenter's reflection. And who is the person standing next to me, she asks? 'That's the strange man who has been following me,' F.E. replies (Breen *et al.* 2000: 84–5).

I won't advance any interpretation of what is occurring in this and related delusions (we shall return to some of them in later chapters). All I want to do, right now, is to draw your attention to how strange malfunctions of the mind can be – far stranger than we might have predicted from our armchairs – and also how (merely) physical dysfunction can disrupt the mind. The mind may not be a thing; it may not be best understood as a physical object that can be located in space. But it is entirely dependent, not just for its existence, but also for the details of its functioning, on mere things: neurons and the connections between them. Perhaps it is possible to reconcile these facts with the view that the mind is a spiritual substance, but it would seem an act of great desperation even to try.

PEERING INTO THE MIND

I introduced some of the disorders of the mind in order to show that substance dualism is false. Now I want to explore them a little further, in order to accomplish several things. First, and most simply, I want to demonstrate how strange and apparently paradoxical the mind can be, both when it breaks down and when it is functioning normally. This kind of exploration is fascinating in its own right, and raises a host of puzzles, some of which we shall explore further in this book. I also have a more directly philosophical purpose, however. I want to show to what extent, contra what the dualist would have us expect, unconscious processes guide intelligent behaviour: to a very large extent, we owe our abilities and our achievements to sub-personal mechanisms. Showing the ways in which mind is built, as it were, out of machines will lay the ground for the development of a rival view of the mind which I will urge we adopt. This rival view will guide us in our exploration of the neuroethical questions we shall confront in later chapters.

Let's begin this exploration of mind with a brief consideration of one method commonly utilized by cognitive scientists, as they seek to identify the functions of different parts of the brain. Typically, they infer function by seeking evidence of a *double dissociation* between abilities and neural structures; that is, they seek evidence that damage to one part of the brain produces a character-istic dysfunction, and that damage to another produces a com-plementary problem. Consider prosopagnosia once more. There is evidence that prosopagnosia is the inverse of another disorder, *Cap-gras delusion*. Prosopagnosics, recall, cannot identify faces, even very familiar faces; when their spouse or children are shown to them, they do not recognize them, unless and until they hear them talk. Capgras sufferers have no such problems; they immediately see that the face before them looks familiar, and they can see whose face it resembles. But, though they see that the face *looks exactly like* a familiar face, they deny that it *is* the person they know. Instead, they identify the person as an impostor.

What is going on, in Capgras delusion? An important clue is provided by studies of the autonomic system response of sufferers. The autonomic system is the set of control mechanisms which maintain homeostasis in the body, regulating blood pressure, heart rate, digestion and so on. We can get a read-out of the responses of the system by measuring heart rate, or, more commonly, *skin con-ductance*: the ability of the skin to conduct electricity. Skin con-ductance rises when we sweat (since sweat conducts electricity well); by attaching very low voltage electrodes to the skin, we can measure the skin conductance response (SCR), also known as the galvanic skin response. Normal subjects exhibit a surge in SCR in response to a range of stimuli: in response, for instance, to loud noises and other startling phenomena, but also to familiar faces. When you see the face of a friend or lover, your SCR surges, reflecting the emotional significance of that face for you. Capgras sufferers have normal autonomic systems: they experience a surge in SCR in response to loud noises, for instance. But their autonomic system does not dif-ferentiate between familiar and unfamiliar faces (Ellis *et al.* 1997); they *recognize* (in some sense), but do not autonomically *respond to*, familiar faces. Prosopagnosics exhibit the opposite profile: though they do not explicitly recognize familiar faces, they do have normal autonomic responses to them.

Thus, there is a double dissociation between the autonomic system and the face recognition system: human beings can recognize a face, in the sense that they can say who it resembles, without feeling the normal surge of familiarity associated with recognition, and they can feel that surge of familiarity without recognizing the face that causes it. We are now in a position to make a stab at identifying the roles that the autonomic system and the face recognition system play in normal recognition of familiar faces, and explaining how Capgras and prosopagnosia come about. One, currently influential, hypothesis is this: because Capgras sufferers recognize the faces they are presented with, but fail to experience normal feelings of familiarity, they think that there is something odd about the face. It *looks like* mom, but it doesn't *feel* like her. They therefore infer that it is *not* mom, but a replica. Capgras therefore arises when the autonomic system fails to play its normal role in response to outputs from the facial recognition system. Prosopagnosia, on the other hand, is a dysfunction of a separate facial recognition system; prosopagnosics have normal autonomic responses, but abnormal explicit recognition (Ellis and Young 1990).

On this account, normal facial recognition is a product of two elements, one of which is normally below the threshold of conscious awareness. Capgras sufferers are not aware of the lack of a feeling of familiarity; at most, they are consciously aware that something is odd about their experience. The inference from this oddity to its explanation – that the person is an impostor – is very probably not drawn explicitly, but is instead the product of mechanisms that work below the level of conscious experience. Cognitive scientists commonly call these mechanisms *subpersonal*, to emphasize that they are partial constituents, normally unconscious and automatic, of persons. Prosopagnosics usually cannot use their autonomic response to familiar faces to categorize them, since they – like all of us – have great difficulty in becoming aware of these responses.

The distinction between the personal level and the subpersonal level is very important here. If we are to understand ourselves, and how our brains and minds make us who, and what, we are, we need to understand the *very* large extent to which information processing takes place automatically, below the level of conscious awareness.

This is exactly what one would predict, on the basis of our evolutionary past. Evolution tends to preserve adaptations unless two conditions are met: keeping them becomes costly, and the costs of discarding them and redesigning are low. These conditions are very rarely met, for the simple reason that it would take too many steps to move from an organism that is relatively well-adapted to an environment, to another which is as well or better adapted, but which is quite different from the first. Since evolution proceeds in tiny steps, it cannot jump these distances; large-scale changes must occur via a series of very small alterations each of which is itself adaptive. Evolution therefore tends to preserve basic design features, and tinker with add-ons (thus, for instance, human beings share a basic body plan with all multicellular animals). Now, we know that most organisms in the history of life on this planet, indeed, most organisms alive today, got along fine without consciousness. They needed only a set of responses to stimuli that attracted and repelled them according to their adaptive significance. Unsurprisingly, we have inherited from our primitive ancestors a very large body of subpersonal mechanisms which can get along fine without our conscious interference.

Another double dissociation illustrates the extent to which our behavior can be guided and driven by subpersonal mechanisms. Vision in primates (including humans) is subserved by two distinct systems: a *dorsal* system which is concerned with the guidance of action, and a *ventral* system which is devoted to an internal representation of the world (Milner and Goodale 1995). These systems are functionally and anatomically distinct; probably the movement-guidance system is the more primitive, with the ventral system being a much later add-on (since guidance of action is something that all organisms capable of locomotion require, whereas the ability to form complex representations of the environment is only useful to creatures with fairly sophisticated cognitive abilities). Populations of neurons in the ventral stream are devoted to the task of object discrimination, with subsets dedicated to particular classes of objects. Studies of the abilities of primates with lesioned brains – experimental monkeys, whose lesions were deliberately produced, and of human beings who have suffered brain injury – have shown the extent to which these systems can dissociate. Monkeys who have lost the ability to discriminate visual patterns nevertheless retain the ability to catch gnats or track and catch an erratically moving peanut (Milner and Goodale 1998). Human beings exhibit the same kinds of dissociations: there are patients who are unable to grasp objects successfully but are nevertheless able to give accurate descriptions of them; conversely, there are patients who are unable to identify even simple geometric shapes but who are able to reach for and grasp them efficiently. Such patients are able to guide their movements using visual information *of which they are entirely unconscious* (Goodale and Milner 2004).

What's it like to guide one's behavior using information of which one is unconscious? Well, it's like everyday life: we're all doing it all the time. We all have dorsal systems which compute shape, size and trajectory for us, and which send the appropriate signals to our limbs. Sometimes we make the appropriate movements without even thinking about it; for instance, when we catch a ball unexpectedly thrown at us; sometimes we might remain unaware that we have moved at all (for instance when we brush away a fly while thinking about something else). Action guidance without consciousness is a normal feature of life. We can easily demonstrate unconscious action-guidance in normal subjects, using the right kind of experimental apparatus. Consider the Titchener illusion, produced by surrounding identical sized circles with others of different sizes. A circle surrounded by larger circles appears smaller than a circle surrounded by small circles. Aglioti and colleagues wondered whether the illusion fooled both dorsal and ventral visual systems. To test this, they replaced the circles with physical objects; by surrounding identical plastic discs with other discs of different sizes, they were able to replicate the illusion: the identical discs appeared different sizes to normal subjects. But when the subjects reached out to grasp the discs, their fingers formed exactly the same size aperture for each. The ventral system is taken in by the illusion, but the dorsal system is not fooled (Aglioti *et al*. 1995). Milner and Goodale suggest that the ventral system is taken in by visual illusions because its judgments are guided by stored knowledge about the world: knowledge about the effects of distance on perceived size, of the constancy of space and so on. Lacking access to such information, the dorsal system is not taken in (Milner and Goodale 1998).

If the grasping behavior of normal subjects in the laboratory is subserved by the dorsal system, which acts below the level of conscious awareness, then normal grasping behavior outside the laboratory must similarly be driven by the same unconscious processes. The dorsal system does not know that it is in the lab, after all, or that the ventral system is being taken in by an illusion. It just does its job, as it is designed to. Similarly for many other aspects of normal movement: calculating trajectory and distance, assessing the amount of force we need to apply to an object to move it, the movements required to balance a ball on the palm of a hand; all of this is calculated unconsciously. The unconscious does not consist, or at least it does not only consist, in the seething mass of repressed and primitive drives postulated by Freud; it is also the innumerable mechanisms, each devoted to a small number of tasks, which work together to produce the great mass of our everyday behavior. What proportion of our actions are produced by such mechanisms, with no direct input or guidance from consciousness? Certainly the majority, probably the overwhelming majority, of our actions are produced by automatic systems, which we normally do not consciously control and which we cannot interrupt (Bargh and Chartrand 1999). This should not be taken as a reason to disparage or devalue our consciously controlled and initiated actions. We routinely take consciousness to be the most significant element of the self, and it is indeed the feature of ourselves that is in many respects the most marvellous. The capacity for conscious experience is certainly the element that makes our lives worth living; indeed, makes our lives properly human. Consciousness is, however, a limited resource: it is available only for the control of a relatively small number of especially complex and demanding actions, and for the solution of difficult, and above all novel, problems. The great mass of our routine actions and mental processes, including most sophisticated behaviors once we have become skilful at their performance, are executed efficiently by unconscious mechanisms.

We have seen that the identification of the mind with an immaterial substance is entirely implausible, in light of our ever-increasing knowledge of how the mind functions and how it malfunctions. However, many people will find the argument up to this point somewhat mystifying. Why devote so much energy to refuting a thesis that no one, or at least no one with even a modicum of intellectual sophistication, any longer holds? It is true that people prepared to defend substance dualism are thin on the ground these days. Nevertheless, I suggest, the thesis continues to exert a significant influence despite this fact, both on the kinds of conceptions of selves that guide everyday thought, and in some of the seductive notions that even cognitive scientists find themselves employing.

The everyday conception of the self that identifies it with consciousness is, I suspect, a distant descendant of the Cartesian view. On this everyday conception, *I* am the set of thoughts that cross my mind. This conception of the self might offer some comfort, in the face of all the evidence about the ways in which minds can break down, and unconsciously processed information guides behavior. But for exactly these reasons, it won't work: if we try to identify the self with consciousness, we shall find ourselves spectators of a great deal of what we do. Our conscious thoughts are produced, *at least* in very important part, by unconscious mechanisms, which send to consciousness only that subset of information which needs further processing by resource-intensive and slow, but somehow clever, consciousness.[4] Consciousness is reliant on these mechanisms, though it can also act upon and shape them. Many of our actions, too, including some of our most important, are products of unconscious mechanisms. The striker's shot at goal happens too fast to be initiated by consciousness; similarly, the improvising musician plays without consciously deciding how the piece will unfold. Think, finally, of the magic of ordinary speech: we speak, and we make sense, but we learn precisely what we are going to say only when we say it (as E. M. Forster put it, "How can I tell what I think till I see what I say?"). Our cleverest arguments and wittiest remarks are not first vetted by consciousness; they come to consciousness at precisely the same time they are heard by others. (Sometimes we wonder whether a joke or a pun was intentional or inadvertent. Clearly, there are cases which fit both descriptions: when someone makes a remark that is interpreted by others as especially witty, but he is himself bewildered by their response, we are probably dealing with inadvertent humor, while the person who stores up a witty riposte for the right occasion is engaging in intentional action. Often, though, there may be no fact of the matter whether the pun I make and notice as I make it counts as intentional or inadvertent.)

Identifying the self with consciousness therefore seems to be hopeless; it would shrink the self down to a practically extensionless, and probably helpless, point. Few sophisticated thinkers would be tempted by this mistake. But an analogous mistake tempts even very clear thinkers, a last legacy of the Cartesian picture. This mistake is the postulation of a control centre, a CPU in the brain, where everything comes together and where the orders are issued.

One reason for thinking that this is a mistake is that the idea of a control centre in the brain seems to run into what philosophers of mind call the *homunculus fallacy*: the fallacy of explaining the capacities of the mind by postulating a little person (a homunculus) inside the head. The classic example of the homunculus fallacy involves vision. How do we come to have visual experience; how, that is, are the incoming wavelengths of light translated into the rich visual world we enjoy? Well, perhaps it works something like a camera obscura: the lenses of the eyes project an image onto the retina inside the head, and there, seated comfortably and perhaps eating popcorn, is a homunculus who views the image. The reason that the homunculus fallacy is a fallacy is that it fails to explain *anything*. We wanted to know how visual experience is possible, but we answered the question by postulating a little person who *looks* at the image in the head, using a visual system that is presumably much like ours. How is the homunculus' own visual experience to be explained? Postulating the homunculus merely delays answering the question; it does not answer it at all.

The moral of the homunculus fallacy is this: we explain the capacities of our mind only by postulating mechanisms that have powers that are simpler and dumber than the powers they are invoked to explain. We cannot explain intelligence by postulating intelligent mechanisms, because then we will need to explain *their* intelligence; similarly, we cannot explain consciousness by postulating conscious mechanisms. Now, one possible objection to the postulation of a control centre in the brain is that the suggestion necessarily commits the homunculus fallacy: perhaps it "explains" control by postulating a controller. It is not obvious, to me at any rate, that postulating a controller *must* commit the homunculus fallacy. However, recognition of the fallacy takes away much of the incentive for postulating a control centre. We do not succeed in explaining how we become capable of rational and flexible behavior by postulating a rational and flexible CPU, since we are still required to explain how the CPU came to have these qualities. Sooner or later we have to explain how we come to have our most prized qualities by reference to simpler and much less impressive mechanisms; once we recognize that this is so, the temptation to think there is a controller at all is much smaller. We needn't fear that giving up on a central controller requires us to give up on agency, rationality or morality. We rightly want our actions and thoughts to be controlled by an agent, by our*selves*, and we want ourselves to have the qualities we prize. But the only thing in the mind/brain that answers to the description of an agent is the *entire* ensemble: built up out of various modules and subpersonal mechanisms. And it is indeed the entire agent that is the controller of controlled processes.

In principle, there could be a CPU inside the head (though, as we have seen, this CPU would have to be a much less impressive mechanism than is generally hoped). As a matter of fact, however, the brain doesn't have a CPU, and for good reason. Central controllers constitute bottlenecks in decision-making machines; all the relevant information must get to the controller and be processed by it. Naturally, this is a relatively slow process, even at the speeds of today's computers. CPUs are *serial* processors; they deal with one task at a time. Because computers are very fast serial processors, they easily outrun human brains at serial tasks: they can perform long series of mathematical calculations that would take human beings hours in mere seconds. But long series of mathematical calculations do not represent the kinds of tasks that human brains are evolved to perform. Brains are much better than any computer at solving the incredibly complex information-processing problems that confront the organism as it navigates it way around its environment – catching a ball, keeping track of social networks, reading subtle clues in a glance or making a tool. How do they do it, when they run at a slower clock speed than today's computers? Rather than confronting problems in a serial fashion, brains are massively *parallel* processors: they process many pieces of information simultaneously. When the brain is confronted with a processing task – that is, all the time, even when the organism is asleep – that task is performed by many, many different brain circuits and mechanisms, working simultaneously. Moreover, these circuits might be widely distributed across the brain; hence, the kind of thinking the brain performs is often described as a kind of *parallel distributed processing*.

Catching a ball, for instance, requires that a number of different problems be solved simultaneously. We must track the ball's trajectory with our eyes, and calculate where it will be when it falls to a catchable height. We must get our bodies near that point, which involves coordinating leg muscles and distributing our weight to maintain balance. Then we must move our hands to exactly the right point in space to snatch the ball out of the air. Naturally, some of us are better at this kind of task than are others. But with a little practice most fit human beings can learn to perform this task pretty well. It's a task that remains well beyond today's robots, not for mechanical reasons, but because the computations are beyond their onboard computers. It all happens too fast for serial processors to handle the thousands of calculations necessary. Yet humans – and other animals – do it with ease.

To appreciate how difficult, in computational terms, catching a ball is, we must recognize that it is not three tasks in parallel – tracking the ball, moving the body, moving the hands – but (at least) dozens. Each one of these tasks can itself be subdivided into many other, parallel, processes. There are, for instance, separate systems for motion detection in the visual system, for calculating trajectories and for guiding our actions. All of this computational work is carried out subpersonally. We become aware only of the results of the calculations, if we become aware of anything at all. Where do all these distributed processes come together? Nowhere. There is no place in the brain, no CPU equivalent, which takes all the various sources of information into account and makes a decision. Or (to put the same point differently), the only place where all the distributed processes come together consists in the entire agent herself. The agent just *is* this set of processes and mechanisms, not something over and above them.

Human beings, like all complex organisms, are communities of mechanisms. The unity of the agent is an achievement, a temporary and unstable coalition forged out of persisting diversity. Under the right conditions, the diversity of mechanisms can be revealed: we can provoke conflict between parts of the agent, which reveal the extent to which they are a patchwork of systems and processes, sometimes with inconsistent interests. Indeed, this kind of conflict is also a striking feature of everyday life. Consider *weakness of the will*, the everyday phenomenon in which we find ourselves doing things of which we do not rationally approve. We have a second drink when we know we should stop at one; we resolve to skip dessert but our resolve crumbles when we glance at the menu, we continue smoking in spite of our New Year's resolution to stop. As Plato noticed 2500 years ago, these kinds of incidents seem to indicate the presence within the single agent of different centres of volition and desire: parts of the self with their own preferences, each of which battles for control of the agent so as to satisfy its desires.

This is not to say that our everyday view of ourselves as unified agents, as a single person with a character and with (relatively) consistent goals, is false. Rather, the unified agent is an achievement: we unify ourselves as we mature. If we do not manage to impose a relatively high degree of unity on ourselves, we shall always be at odds with ourselves, and our ability to pursue any goal which requires planning will be severely curtailed. Unification is a necessary condition of planning, for without a relatively high degree of unity we shall always be undermining our own goals. Lack of unity is observed in young children, and undermines their ability to achieve the goals they themselves regard as desirable. Longitudinal studies show that children who do not acquire the skills to delay gratification generally do worse on a range of indicators throughout their lives, but delaying gratification requires the imposition of unity. In order to become rational agents, capable of long-term planning and carrying out our plans, we need to turn diversity into unity. We achieve this not by eliminating diversity, but by forging coalitions between the disparate elements of ourselves. These coalitions remain forever vulnerable to disruption, short and long term. One way to understand drug addiction, for instance, is as a result of a disruption of the imposed unity of the agent. The drug-addicted agent might genuinely desire to give up his drug, but because he cannot extend his will across time and across all the relevant subagents which constitute him, he is subject to regular preference reversals. When he consumes his drug, he does so because he temporarily prefers to consume; when he sincerely asserts that he wishes to be free of his drug, his assertion reflects his genuine, but equally temporary, preference. (We shall explore the ways in which agents unify themselves, and the ways in which this unity can be disrupted, in a later chapter.)

THE EXTENDED MIND

The image of the mind we have been exploring so far is relatively uncontroversial, at least within cognitive science. There is widespread agreement that the mind contains, or even consists in, a plethora of relatively independent systems, that most of these systems operate, most or all of the time, below the level of conscious awareness, that these systems can conflict and that they guide the behavior of the organism as a whole by forming temporary coalitions. All of these claims conflict with our everyday conception of ourselves, but they are all well established. The claim to which we shall now turn, however, is far from uncontroversial. It is, I shall argue, nevertheless true. It will provide us with our framework for understanding neuroethics. The thesis is known as the *extended mind* hypothesis.

The extended mind hypothesis, stated simply, is this: the mind is not wholly contained within the skull, or even within the body, but instead spills out into the world. The mind, its proponents claim, should be understood as the set of mechanisms and resources with which we think, and that set is not limited to the internal resources made up of neurons and neurotransmitters. Instead, it includes the set of tools we have developed for ourselves – our calculators, our books, even our fingers when we use them to count – and the very environment itself insofar as it supports cognition.

A case intermediary between brain-based cognition and externalized cognition might help make the idea more intuitive. The idea that cognition is a "cool" – that is, unemotional – process is deeply entrenched in Western thought. Emotions, we think, ought to be kept out of reasoning: they'll only interfere with our thought processes. There is no doubt that emotions *can* interfere with rational cognition, but there is also increasing evidence, thanks in large part to the work of Antonio Damasio, that having the right feelings at the right time is indispensable to good decision-making. Moreover, in establishing an essential role for emotion in decision-making, Damasio establishes that non-brain-based elements are essential for reliable cognition.

Damasio's evidence comes from studies of patients with damage to the ventromedial prefrontal cortex. These patients, such as the famous Phineas Gage, injured in a railroad accident which sent a tamping iron through his skull, can recover remarkably well. They show little sign of cognitive impairment in standard tests. However, their lives typically go badly wrong after the damage. Gage himself underwent a dramatic personality change: formerly a hardworking and conscientious railway foreman, he became dissolute and incapable of carrying out long term plans. In these respects, his behavior was quite typical of patients with ventromedial damage. Long-term and short-term decision-making is significantly impaired in such people.

How does damage to the ventromedial prefrontal cortex impair decision-making? Interestingly, it seems that its effects are not *directly* upon rationality, but upon the relationship between the brain and the rest of the body. A well-known experiment conducted in Antonio Damasio's laboratory (Bechara, *et al.* 1997) provides a fascinating insight into what has gone wrong with subjects like Gage. In the experiment, subjects were asked to draw cards from four decks, in whatever order they liked. Every time they drew a card, they were rewarded: decks A and B yielded $100 each, and decks C and D yielded $50 each. But there were also punishments associated with some of the cards, and the penalties associated with decks A and B were (on average) much larger than those associated with C and D. The game was rigged so that drawing cards mainly from decks A and B led to an overall loss of money, whereas drawing cards mainly from C and D led to an overall gain. Bechara and colleagues tested normal subjects as well as people who had suffered bilateral ventromedial damage, to see how their decision-making compared on this task.

Both groups of subjects began in the same way: drawing cards pretty much at random from each of the decks. Soon they all began to gravitate toward decks A and B; understandably, because these decks had bigger rewards associated with them. However, as they encountered more punishments, normal subjects gradually came to favor the low gain, but lower punishment, decks. These subjects accumulated money as the game went on. Ventromedial patients, however, continued to favor A and B, and continued to lose money.

The remarkable finding was not that patients with ventromedial damage made disadvantageous decisions. We already knew that they did. What is fascinating is how normal subjects went about making their decisions. Bechara, *et al.* tracked the responses of participants in several ways. They asked them, at various points in the experiment, about their decision-making, and they also measured their skin conductance responses. By around card ten, normal subjects were generating anticipatory SCRs when they reached toward decks A and B. Yet it wasn't until around card fifty that they reported a "hunch" that A and B were riskier. By around card eighty, normal subjects knew at least roughly how the decks differed from one another. But normal subjects did not have to wait until they had explicit knowledge of how the decks were arranged before they began to choose advantageously; indeed, they did not even have to wait until they had an articulable hunch about the decks. Even before the hunch, they began to favor decks C and D. What explains their advantageous choices? Bechara, *et al.* suggest that the anticipatory SCRs, which preceded the hunch, are an important clue: though the bodily responses measured by the SCRs are usually too subtle to reach conscious awareness, they nevertheless help guide behavior. Because normal subjects generated anticipatory SCRs when considering drawing cards from decks A and B, they begin to favor C and D. Their *somatic* responses bias subjects toward certain choices and away from others.[5]

But the behavior of ventromedial patients was quite different. There is nothing wrong with these patients' autonomic system: they experience SCRs in response to punishment, in just the same way as do normal subjects (Damasio 1994). But they do not generate *anticipatory* SCRs. They do not get the "warning signals" which, unconsciously, bias normal subjects against certain actions (because the ventromedial prefrontal cortex stores dispositional knowledge which activates the relevant parts of the brain which in turn cause autonomic system response, Bechara *et al.* (1997) speculate). Ventromedial patients, because they lack this vital source of information, find it much more difficult to work out how the decks are arranged. They are, we might say, thrown back on pure, brain-based, rationality. But pure rationality, all on its own, is a relatively meagre resource. Indeed, even when it is sufficient for the production of knowledge, it may be insufficient to guide rational behavior: though some ventromedial patients did eventually work out how the decks were arranged, their behavior continued to differ from that of normal subjects. These patients remained more likely to risk the large punishment in order to secure the bigger rewards of decks A and B. Not only is the ability to generate anticipatory SCRs beneficial to cognition; it also proves to be an indispensable guide to prudent action. Pure – that is, brain-based – rationality cannot compensate for its absence.

We shall return to Damasio's theory, the so-called *somatic-marker hypothesis* (SMH), according to which bodily responses are an indispensable guide in beneficial decision-making and action, in later chapters. For the moment, what matters is the way in which the SMH expands our view of the resources needed for rational decision-making. Without bodily responses, cognition is impaired. It is, in important part, by referring to our bodily feelings, when we contemplate different courses of action, that we make good decisions. If the mind should be understood to consist of all the resources we use in assessing different courses of action, then the mind includes (parts of) the body, at least for some purposes and in some contexts. While he does not endorse the thesis of extended cognition, Damasio himself comes rather close to it:

> Mind derives from the entire organism as an ensemble [...] the body contributes more than life support and modulatory effects to the brain. It contributes a *content* that is part and parcel of the workings of the normal mind.
>
> *(Damasio 1994: 225–6)*

But if we are forced to admit that mind can extend beyond the skull and into the body, there is little – except prejudice – preventing us from extending it still further. If mind does not have to be entirely an affair of neurons and neurotransmitters, if it can encompass muscular tension or heart rate, then why not electronic pulses or marks on paper as well? When these things are coupled, in the right kinds of ways, to the brain, we think better, *much* better. Why not say that our mind can sometimes, in some contexts and for some purposes, encompass environmental resources?

In fact, reliance upon environmental resources is ubiquitous. Consider different possible ways of visually representing the world. On the one hand, the organism might survey the scene around it, and on this basis form an inner representation which it stores in short-term memory. To some extent, real organisms do exactly that. If you close your eyes *now*, you will be able to represent the room in which you are sitting, at least to some degree. You can, to some extent, recreate the scene in imagination. But the extent to which we actually have such internal representations is in fact much smaller than we tend to believe. In fact, our inner representations are extremely impoverished, as many studies have now shown. For instance, you probably think that as you read these words you possess a stable representation of the entire page in front of you. It seems to you as if you have some kind of inner representation not only of the words you are currently reading, but also of those that are not currently the focus of your attention. In fact, if the words alter dramatically after you have read them, you probably won't be aware of any change at all. In a well-known experiment, subjects read text on a computer screen. They had the experience of reading a stable, unchanging screen; exactly the same experience you have now. In fact, the screen was changing constantly, with junk characters replacing the words as soon as they were read. The only real words on the screen at any time were those the subject was actually reading. So long as the appearance of those words was timed to coordinate with the speed of the subject's eye movements, they remained totally unaware of the instability of the page (Rayner 1998). The experience we seem to have, of possessing a rich internal representation of the page, and of the world we survey, is in fact an illusion.

Our visual experience is *as of* a world that is internally represented. But the world is not internally represented, at least not in any great detail. There is nevertheless a sense in which we do possess a rich representation of the world. We represent the world to ourselves not by way of an internal image, but by using an external model: the world *itself*. Rather than take a snapshot of the scene and store it internally, we rely upon the actual stability of the world. We store our representation *outside* us. We are not aware of the fact that we do this, because we are not aware of the way in which our internal representations are constantly updated by our eye movements. The human eye has a very small area of high resolution vision; less than 0.01 percent of the entire visual field. But our eyes constantly dart about, moving this window of high resolution across the visual scene. These movements, called *saccades*, are intelligent; they are not random, but instead gather information relevant to the tasks currently confronting the person. They are also very fast, averaging about three per second. Our frequent and repeated saccades allow us to inspect the world and update our picture of it, so that it seems to us that we have a rich representation of it. And so we do, but it is not an internal representation. In a sense, this is unsurprising: why build a model of something when the original is there to be used as its own best model (Clark 1997)?

The phenomenon of *change blindness*, which Rayner's experiment demonstrates, is evidence of the extent to which we offload representational duties to the environment (Rowlands 2003). Since we have no internal model to compare to the visual scene, the latter can change dramatically without our noticing. Building an internal model would be costly, in terms of the resources required; why do it when we get the real thing for free? By exploiting the consistency of the environment, we avoid having to represent it to ourselves, and thereby lighten the cognitive load on our shoulders. This is an adaptive strategy for an organism to pursue, since evolution is very sensitive to even small increments in costs, and the alternative of forming internal representations is likely to be very costly. It is adaptive even if it occasionally has costs of its own: the conditions under which we are blind to change are relatively rare (we have mechanisms specially attuned to detecting external changes; we are change blind only when these mechanisms are fooled). Nevertheless, change blindness can be extremely dramatic, under the right conditions.

One striking demonstration of change blindness showed that we can even fail to notice the replacement of the person we are talking with by another person. Simons and Levin (1998) had experimenters approach unsuspecting passers-by and ask for directions. While the subject was replying, confederates carried a door between her and her interlocutor, who took advantage of the diversion to slip away and allow another person to take his place. Most subjects failed to notice the substitution, neither expressing surprise at it, nor even reporting anything unusual when asked directly. Interestingly, subjects who detected the change tended to be those who differed from the experimental interlocutors in some salient way (age or occupation); apparently we attend to features of people when we experience them as members of an out-group far more than when we don't. Attention is cognitively expensive: we use it to form an internal representation only when it seems necessary. For most purposes, most of the time, we save our cognitive resources by forming only the sketchiest of representations of the visual scene.

The important point, for our purposes, is this: though we could have had a rich internal representation of the world, we don't; instead, we store our representation of the world *outside* us. Now, suppose that, contrary to fact, we did form rich internal representations of the visual scene. We would have had no hesitation in concluding that these representations were parts of our minds. Cognitive scientists might have located the "visual scene module" where the representation was stored, studied the manner in which it represented and how it guided action, and the ways in which it broke down. As it turns out, the representing role is played less by parts of our brains and more by parts of the world, interacting with our brain. But if a representation would have been part of our minds had it been internal, why should we think that it is *not* part of our minds, just because it is external? Since it plays an important part in guiding cognition, isn't it sheer prejudice to conclude that it isn't part of the mind?

These considerations can motivate the extended mind thesis. The thesis consists, essentially, in two claims: one philosophical and one empirical. The philosophical claim is an answer to the question we have just asked: it would indeed be sheer prejudice to think that a cognitive resource is not mental just because it is external. Thus defenders of the extended mind advance the following principle:

> If something plays a role in cognitive activity, such that, were it internal we would have no difficulty in concluding that it was part of the mind, it should be counted as part of the mind whether it is internal or not.
>
> *(Clark and Chalmers 1998)*

The empirical claim is about the nature of actual human (especially, but not exclusively, human) cognition: as a matter of fact elements external to the brain and to the body play a role in cognitive activity such that, were these elements internal, we would have no hesitation in concluding that they were mental. Putting these two claims together, we get the extended mind thesis: the mind extends beyond the limits of the brain and body.

The first claim, that if we would count something as cognitive were it internal, we should count it as cognitive whether or not it is internal, has been the focus of most of the attention in the debate so far. I shall argue that this is a mistake: the so-called parity thesis ought to play no more than a heuristic role. It does not, as both defenders and detractors think, provide us with a criterion by which to distinguish the mental from the non-mental. Failure to play precisely the same role in cognition as internal structures is not a good reason to exclude external representations and resources from the domain of the mental. Nevertheless, the parity thesis is a useful heuristic device, inasmuch as it allows us to appreciate the extent to which external resources *can* play the same kinds of roles as internal, and therefore in appreciating the extent to which mere prejudice motivates the way the boundaries of the mind are usually drawn. Seeing how far the parity thesis will take us is, as it were, a way of expanding our minds.

The parity thesis

What kind of role must something play in cognitive activity such that were it internal we should have no hesitation in counting it as mental? It is not enough that I use it in thinking, Clark and Chalmers concede. In addition to use in cognition, several other conditions must be satisfied for a source of information to count as properly mental: the resource must be constantly available, the information it contains must be directly and easily accessible, it must be automatically endorsed and it must have been consciously endorsed at some time in the past (Clark and Chalmers 1998: 17). When these conditions are satisfied, they argue, the information store counts as mental, whether it is within or without the skull. Closely related views have been defended by Daniel Dennett (1996), Haugeland (1998), Donald (1991), Rowlands (1999) and Wilson (2004).

Clark and Chalmers argue, for instance, that when these conditions are satisfied by a store of information, that store counts as part of a person's memory. These conditions have generally been taken, by both defenders and proponents of the extended mind, to be necessary, such that failing to satisfy them disqualifies an information store from being mental. Even in terms of the parity thesis, however, this is a mistake: these conditions are merely *sufficient*, and not *necessary*. That is, something might count as part of memory even if it failed to meet one or more of the conditions outlined. Constant availability cannot be a necessary condition for counting as part of the mind, since the contents of our short-term memories are, by definition, only available for a brief period (no more than thirty seconds), and our longer-term memory is (notoriously) not always available for instant recall. Moreover, people suffering from dementia might have rather unreliable access to their memories; so long as they are able to recall memories sometimes, they seem not (yet) to have lost those elements of their minds. Because the constantly availability criterion is not necessary, I think there is a good case (from parity) to be made for regarding the visual scene before us as the place where our representation of the immediate environment is stored. Nor can easy accessibility be a necessary condition of the mental, as the example of the demented individual, or indeed even ordinary cases of failure of memory retrieval (such as the tip of the tongue phenomenon) show. Memories are not always easily accessible, yet they count as part of the mind; so do all the unconscious mechanisms that figure in information processing.

Given the similarities, in functional terms, of the role that external representations can play in cognition to the role played by internal, it seems mere prejudice to insist that they are not mental just because they are external. Moreover, it is not just external *representations* that should be counted as part of the mind, on the basis that they are an integral part of cognition. As well as external representations, we use external *tools* to enhance our thought. These tools for thinking are almost as old as human beings; indeed, perhaps we only became truly human when we developed them (Sterelny 2005). The most basic and obvious of these tools is speech. Speech does not merely allow us to articulate thoughts that we would have had in any case. Instead, it allows us to externalize our thoughts and thereby to treat them as objects for contemplation and for manipulation. Externalized thoughts can be worked over, criticized and improved. They can also be shared, and the mental resources of two, or many, people brought to bear on them. Once we take the further step of developing the capacity to write down our thoughts, the extent to which they can be manipulated, publicly criticized and thereby improved, increases exponentially. All kinds of ways of thinking become accessible for the first time with the invention of ways of keeping track of our thoughts by representing them externally; paradigmatically (but not only) by writing them down.

Think of mathematics, for instance. Even arithmetic, beyond a certain level of complexity, requires pen and paper – or a computer screen, or clay tablets, or what have you – if it is to be performed at all. Multiply 23 789 by 54 553. Without pen and paper, the calculation is beyond me. Perhaps you can perform it; there are short cuts that can be learned (though I suspect that these short cuts themselves rely on ways of extending cognition beyond the boundaries of skin and skull). For almost all of us, however, the calculation is impossible without some kind of tool, and as the complexity of the sum grows, the proportion of those unable to perform it without tools reaches 100 percent (divide the result of the above multiplication by 0.0034). Without some kind of means of making external representations, even arithmetic quickly exceeds our abilities. In fact, multiplication is multiply extended, across time and across space, across physical elements and across agents. How do you go about doing a three-digit multiplication (say 365×412), in the absence of a calculator? You probably use the method most of us learned at school: converting the sum into a series of single-digit multiplication tasks, remembering to carry the one, writing the results down sequentially, then moving to the next line, and repeating the process, until you have a series of numbers which can simply be added to get the right result. In other words, you use a simple algorithm you learned long ago. You did not develop the algorithm for yourself; you probably just accepted, on faith, that it worked. If that's right, your cognitive process is reliant not only on pencil and paper, but also on the intellectual products of previous agents, the agents, long since dead, who developed the algorithm (as well as the chain of agents who handed it down across the generations).

Of course, computers make available much greater calculating power than mere pen and paper, and thereby make possible entire new branches of mathematics, such as the mathematics of many-dimensional spaces and of chaos. Computers, too, are the embodiments of the knowledge of many agents, distributed across time and space. I rely upon my computer to translate my key strokes into sentences on the screen, without giving a thought to the thousands of calculations a second needed for the alchemy to work, or for the many thousands of people whose intellectual work is frozen in the hardware and software I use. I can think about neuroethics and the extended mind without the need to solve the intellectual problems whose ingenious solutions I use, without even properly understanding the nature of these problems. I think *with* the computer, and I can do so because many people have previously thought *about* computers. Their work simplified my cognitive landscape.

Human beings seem specially well equipped to integrate with tools for thinking. Indeed, maybe that's precisely the kind of creature we are; perhaps that's what makes us human. But extending into the environment is characteristic of many organisms. Richard Dawkins has introduced a notion into evolutionary biology that is in many ways analogous to the notion of the extended mind in the philosophy of mind. Dawkins claims that we cannot understand the adaptive biology of (at least) many organisms simply by considering them only from the skin in. Instead, we need to consider the *extended phenotype* of the organism, where the extended phenotype includes all the ways in which organisms modify their environment in adaptive ways (Dawkins 1983). Dawkins' argument for the extended phenotype is, like Clark and Chalmers' argument for the extended mind, an argument from parity.[6] If we would count something as part of the phenotype – that is, the set of observable characteristics constituting the organism – were it contiguous with, and growing out of, the organism, then we ought to count it as part of the phenotype even if it doesn't meet these conditions. Consider: some organisms grow shells by secreting minerals sourced from their food; clearly, these shells are part of their phenotype. Hermit crabs find their shells instead of growing them, but their shells play the same role in their life cycles as the shells of other crustaceans play in theirs. So hermit crab shells are part of their phenotype. Beavers' dams, spiders' webs, birds' nests: all of these count as part of their extended phenotype, on the same sorts of grounds. By the same parity argument, there is a strong case for considering our cognitive tools part of our phenotype: we are animals that owe our adaptive success to our ability easily to integrate external tools into our cognition.

Human beings are, by nature, the kind of creature that most easily extends its mind into the environment and into shared social space. We are, for instance, the animal most given to and adept at *imitation*, a capacity that allows us to learn far more flexible and complex behaviors than other animals, and therefore allows for the accumulation of innovative survival strategies far faster than would be possible if we were reliant on genetic coding of the information (Sterelny 2007). Adaptation via changes in gene frequency is a slow process, usually taking many generations to produce a noticeable effect; changes in behavior by learning, in contrast, can be dramatic, even within the space of a single generation. But though we are especially accomplished at it, human beings are not the only animals capable of using external tools for thinking. One of the most dramatic examples of the ways in which tools can expand the range and power of thought comes from studies of chimpanzees. The unadorned chimp brain is able to learn to categorize pairs of objects on the basis of their similarity or difference from one another. So, for instance, they can be trained to put any pair of identical objects – two cups, say, or two bananas – into one box, while placing any pair of dissimilar objects (say one cup and one banana) into another. But without external aids, they cannot sort *pairs of pairs* by similarity or difference. Two pairs of pairs are identical when they share their first-order properties: they are either both identical, or they are both dissimilar. Otherwise, they are dissimilar. So the pair (of pairs) apple–banana and cup–shoe is identical, while the pair cup–cup and apple–banana is different. This higher-order task is difficult enough for the human brain. Chimps can learn to accomplish it by, in effect, turning it into a first-order task. They do this by learning to associate tokens with the first-order pairs. For instance, they might learn to associate a plastic triangle with a pair of objects that are identical to one another, and a plastic square with a pair of objects that are dissimilar. Once they have accomplished that task, the higher-order task is simple. If you want to know whether a pair of pairs is similar or dissimilar, simply compare the tokens associated with them: if they are identical, so is the higher-order pair, if not, they are dissimilar (Thompson, *et al.* 1997).

It is very likely that human beings use closely analogous techniques to expand the power of our cognition (Clark 2003). We, too, associate tokens with concepts. The tokens we use are *words*; inside our skulls, or outside in the world. We are then able to keep track and manipulate our ideas far better than we could without the tokens. What chimps can do a little, we do far more efficiently and effectively, going far beyond them in the complexity and sophistication of the tokens we manipulate, and constantly inventing new ones as we feel the need. I do much of my thinking on paper: I write down my ideas, as fully as possible. When they are physically expressed, I am able to follow the links between them far more clearly and effectively than I could if they remained in the privacy of my head. I think with tools, not just with my biological brain. But if I use such tools to think with, we have good reason to count them as part of my mind.

If symbol use is an extended resource the use of which we share with other animals, another way in which we extend our minds seems uniquely human. We extend our minds not only using tools, but also using social structures and communities. This is a feature of the extended mind that has been little stressed in the debate so far, yet it may be the one feature that, more than any other, makes human thought so powerful. *Homo sapiens* is (as the name suggests) a pretty clever beast. But in order to be able to engage in systematic science, and to develop technology, from cooking to writing, from steam engines to computers, from water treatment plants to fMRI machines – we must be able to *accumulate* knowledge, and hand it on from generation to generation. If each generation had to start afresh, we would not still be in the Dark Ages; we could never have got anywhere near as advanced as the Dark Ages. Moreover, progress in knowledge requires a *distributed* approach: many people must tackle a problem, from many different directions at once, and the results of their work must be available to others for criticism. This, too, requires that results and techniques be made available in a publicly accessible, and long-lived, medium. For these reasons, both because we need a way of accumulating knowledge, and because great knowledge can be produced only by a community of enquirers, we need a means of expressing our ideas, our results, our findings and our failings, a means that is in principle relatively easy to access. We need external representations: a system of writing at very minimum. Obviously writing has its limitations, which makes it unsuitable for certain kinds of knowledge: for these we need specialized systems of representations, such as mathematical or chemical symbols.

Knowledge acquisition must be a public endeavor, if it is to be successful. The lone scientist, for all the mythology of the Dr. Frankenstein alone in his lab, doesn't get very far (even the scientists of earlier ages, who sometimes worked alone, generally required access to a library). Moreover, even for the individual cognizer, the advancement of knowledge requires that the cognitive environment is structured in a way that takes the load off their brains: they need, for instance, to be able to write down their calculations so as to ensure that they free up mental resources that would otherwise be drained by the effort of memory. One way we take the load off our brains is by developing tools that embody our knowledge; they preserve previous results for us, and suggest ways in which we could tackle new problems. We extend our cognitive capacities by building external tools and representations, and we are able to do *that* only because we already have minds that make use of external representations – for instance, by relying on the stability of the environment to spare us the effort of representing it – thus freeing cognitive resources for the building of new tools.

THE DEBATE OVER THE EXTENDED MIND

The extended mind hypothesis is very controversial. Many cognitive scientists and philosophers have rushed to defend the view that the mind, and with it all properly cognitive processes, is entirely contained within the skull. It's worth pausing for a moment over these debates. As I've already pointed out, these debates have generally focused on the parity thesis; this is, I think (as I've also already mentioned), a mistake. Nevertheless, I have also said that the parity thesis is a useful heuristic for expanding minds; for this reason it's worth seeing just how far it can take us. Seeing just how difficult it is to defend the claim that the mind is inside the head, even when we accept the parity thesis, will help to shake us free from this last legacy of Cartesianism.

The most influential criticisms of the extended mind hypothesis have been those advanced by Adams and Aizawa (2001) and Rupert (2004). Adams and Aizawa argue that in order to assess the claim that something counts as properly part of the mind, we need an account of what cognition consists in: we need to identify "the mark of the mental." They do not attempt to advance anything like a full theory of what cognition is; instead they argue for two necessary conditions which any process or state must satisfy in order to count as cognitive. First, it must involve *intrinsic content*. Second, cognitive processes must be *causally individuated*.

The notion of intrinsic content is best understood by contrast to its opposite, *derived content*. Roughly, a representation has derived content if it refers in virtue of a convention. The letters CAT refer to the animal "cat" in virtue of a set of nested conventions: the convention, on the part of speakers of English, of using the sounds represented by those letters to refer to cats, and the convention of using the letters CAT to refer to those sounds. Our world is full of representations that have derived content: words of natural languages, mathematical symbols, traffic signs, and so on. But if a sign refers in virtue of a convention, its referential power is derivative from the referential power of the human mind. Now, how do the paradigm mental states of human beings come to refer? If we are to avoid an infinite regress, Adams and Aizawa argue, we must recognize that human minds are capable of states that are *intrinsically* referential. When I read CAT, I have a mental state that refers to cats, but my mental state itself refers to cats in virtue of its *nature*, not in virtue of any convention. If this were false, if my mental state referred only in virtue of a convention, we would need to ask how that convention, in turn, came to be meaningful: eventually, we must stop at a representation that is intrinsically meaningful, or representation could never get off the ground in the first place.

Now for the second of Adams' and Aizawa's conditions, a condition also emphasized by Rupert. Why think that genuine cognitive processes must be causally individuated; that is, distinguished from each other and from anything else in terms of their physical causes? The motivation for this claim seems to be this: if a science of cognition is to be possible, then there had better be a discoverable set of causal regularities or laws for that science to capture. And the available evidence suggests that there are indeed such laws. The processes that occur in human minds are somewhat diverse, but they are nevertheless relatively unified, inasmuch as they can be described by a relatively small set of laws. Within more narrowly circumscribed domains, the degree of unification is even higher: thus, there is a set of rough, *ceteris paribus*, laws that describe a wide range of human memory systems, short and long term (Rupert 2004); hence, the domain of the mental should be expected to be causally individuated.[7]

Now, let's consider the case for the extended mind in the light of these (putative) necessary conditions. Most of the critics of the extended mind hypothesis have focused on one of Clark's and Chalmers' (1998) examples; we shall do likewise.

The example compares two agents, Inga and Otto. Both of them hear that there is a new exhibition on at the Museum of Modern Art (MOMA) in New York, and decide to visit it. After a moment's though, Inga recalls that the museum is on 53rd Street, so she sets out for 53rd Street. Otto, though, suffers from Alzheimer's disease. He carries a notebook around with him, in which he writes information he thinks he may need. Otto consults his notebook, where he reads that MOMA is on 53rd Street. Accordingly, he sets off in that direction. Clark and Chalmers argue that there is no reason to treat these cases differently. Both agents recalled the relevant information from their store of information; if, prior to the act of recall, we should say that Inga believed that MOMA was on 53rd Street (where a belief is a *mental* state), then we should say the same of Otto. Of course, Otto did not consciously entertain the thought that MOMA is on 53rd Street before he looked in his notebook. But neither did Inga. Her belief was *dispositional*: she was disposed to recall the information under the right circumstances. Since Otto, too, was disposed to recall the same belief, we should say that he, like Inga, dispositionally believed that MOMA is on 53rd Street, even *before* he recalled the information.

It should be obvious how Adams and Aizawa will respond. They claim that Inga's representational state has intrinsic content, whereas the scribbles in Otto's notebook merely have derived content. The scribbles mean what they mean in virtue of a convention. They therefore ought not to be counted as genuinely *mental* states.

However, this argument seems to me flawed. Adams and Aizawa insist that cognitive states must involve intrinsic content (2001: 48). Some philosophers deny this (e.g. Dennett 1990). I do not intend even to attempt to adjudicate this dispute. Instead, let's grant the assumption that properly cognitive states must *involve* intrinsic content, and ask whether such states must consist *only* of such content? Adams and Aizawa are unsure (2001: 50), and as Clark sees, this opens the way for admitting derived content within the purview of the mental. Clark asks us to consider the mental manipulation of Venn diagrams. Suppose that Otto sees that some Xs are also Ys by picturing Venn diagrams to himself. Is he not thereby engaged in cognition? Yet clearly Venn diagrams get their content from a convention (Clark 2005). Similarly, some ordinary human thought seems to be conducted in a natural language. We have no reason to exclude such thought from the domain of the cognitive.[8]

Clark also asks us to consider a thought experiment. Imagine alien beings capable of storing bit-mapped images of text. These aliens would have representations *of text* in their minds, not representations of the meaning of the text. When they wanted to know what the text meant, they would picture it and read it in the privacy of their heads. Clark asks us to think about the stretch of time prior to their reading the text. Wouldn't we count the *content* of the text as (dispositionally) part of their mind at that time? If so, then it is simply the prejudice that mind is within the skull that prevents us from counting Otto's similarly poised notebook as part of his mind.

In reply, Adams and Aizawa (forthcoming) insist that they have no inclination to count alien bit-mapped texts as part of alien minds. Such texts have no intrinsic content, prior to recall, and therefore fail to be cognitive. I wonder, though, whether they might not feel some pull toward Clark's view of the case if they compared it to actual cases of mental recall here on Earth. Some people – mainly children, but some adults as well – have what is known as *eidetic recall*. In certain circumstances, and with varying degrees of reliability, they are able to "picture," in their "mind's eye," a scene that is no longer before them. Of course, we are all capable of mental imagery, but eidetikers seem capable of something beyond most of us, in most circumstances: they are able to extract information from their mental image of which they were not previously aware.[9] They can, for instance, do exactly what Clark's imagined aliens do: see the individual letters of texts they have briefly scanned and later read them. One woman was even able to see the 3D image hidden in a stereogram, by committing one random dot pattern to memory, and then merging it with a second, visually presented, dot pattern to form the image (Bourtchouladze 2002: 110–11). Now, Adams and Aizawa do not claim that mental states are *necessarily* internal to the skull. Instead, they argue, as *a matter of fact* all actual mental states of human beings are internal (Adams and Aizawa, forthcoming). They therefore deny the relevance of Clark's thought experiments: no matter how things stand with the alien residents of possible worlds, here on earth mental states have the features they claim. But eidetikers, here and now, seem to be capable of representations with the features that Clark imagines. Moreover, it seems to me that some of *my* representations of texts are closely analogous to the representations of Clark's aliens. I know some songs and other texts "off by heart", a legacy of school assemblies. If you ask me what these songs are about, I would have to rehearse them, aloud or mentally, in order to discover the answer. If that's right, I have representations *inside my head* that do not (right now) have intrinsic content. If we should count these representations as mental, then even if I am only capable of thought at all because some of my representations have intrinsic content, and even if all my mental states must *involve* intrinsic content, such content is not "the mark of the mental" at all – and nothing stands in the way of our treating states which include *external* representations and artefacts as mental states.[10]

Causal regularities
Turn, now, to Adams' and Aizawa's second necessary condition of the cognitive, a condition also stressed by Rupert (2004). Here on Earth, all three philosophers argue, "mind" refers to the object of certain, rapidly progressing, sciences. But there is no science of the brain-plus-tools, and there is no prospect that there ever will be. The set of tools which might be taken to constitute the extended mind is

just too large and too disparate to ever form the object of a science. Whereas even now cognitive scientists are discovering the causal regularities governing the mind, traditionally conceived, there is no chance that they will discover an interesting set of regularities which circumscribes the domain of brains-plus-notebooks, brains-plus-calculators, brains-plus-marks-in-the-sand, and so on.

In response, Clark stresses that we ought not to try to second-guess the progress of science (Clark 2006). We cannot infer, from our current inability to unify extended cognition under a set of laws, that future science will not succeed where we fail. I think, however, that we ought to concede to Clark's critics that the probability of future unification is low. The set of processes and objects already supposed to extend our minds into the world – marks in clay, tattoos on the body, digitally encoded information, and many more besides – is already very disparate, and we have every reason to think that the current technological explosion will deliver us many more, and different, ways of manipulating and storing information. Of course we shall discover – are already in the process of discovering – laws that apply to all these resources, as well as to the brain. But that's not the question at issue; the question is, will we be able to delineate laws which uniquely circumscribe the domain of thought, where "thinking" is an activity distributed across brains and tools? The fact that the laws of physics (for instance) will apply to all these elements is neither here nor there: the laws of physics apply *everywhere*, and therefore cannot be used to delineate the subject matter of a special science. I think we ought to concede, then, that Adams, Aizawa and Rupert are on solid ground when they argue that we are unlikely to be able to develop a science of the extended mind, at least a science which is as well unified as the science of the mind/brain.

Why should this matter? Adams, Aizawa and Rupert are somewhat unclear on this point. Here is one reason to think that the contours of the science of mind ought to be taken seriously in these debates. Science, one may believe, is such a powerful means of gaining knowledge in part because each science "carves nature at its joints" (in Plato's phrase). In other words, scientific theories might be so powerful because they describe or pick out parts of the universe that are genuinely unified. If that's the case, then science may be a good guide to ontology, to the nature of reality: if a relatively discrete part of the universe can be captured by a set of scientific general-izations, then we have good reason to think that that part of the universe constitutes a natural kind. If this line of argument is right, then the fact (if it is a fact) that there is a set of causal regularities which applies to the brain/mind, and no such set that applies to the brain/mind plus its various add-ons gives us reason to think that the brain/mind constitutes a discrete entity, and the extended mind does not. If that's right, then the mind is identical to an entity circum-scribed at the relatively low level of causal regularities, and not at the functional level.

Critics of the extended mind could invoke this argument in an effort to confine mind to the skull. It is not, they can claim, mere prejudice that prevents us from extending the mind, but arguments, and a respect for the power of science. However, the critics adopt this line at their own peril. It will not vindicate the traditional conception of mind; instead it will undermine it.

The mind/brain, as we saw in the first chapter, contains a number of quite different mechanisms, which are sufficiently diverse to cast doubt on the claim that they form a single domain. Consider, for instance, the distinction often made between *controlled* and *automatic* processes (Bargh and Chartrand 1999; Wegner 2005). Both processes issue in complex behavior in human beings. But there are significant differences between them. Controlled processes are gen-erally conscious; they are also very demanding of cognitive resources, such that performance at them degrades significantly under cognitive load (we place subjects under cognitive load by requiring them to do two tasks at once: the controlled task we want to study and another, loading, task, such as counting backwards from 1000 in threes). Automatic processes are not consciously initiated, and do not degrade under cognitive load; they are also ballistic, which is to say that they cannot be interrupted once they are begun. Controlled processes are slow, automatic processes are fast. Now, if it is true that causal regularities pick out natural kinds, then the mind is not a natural kind: it is a compound entity, composed of at least two (and probably many) natural kinds. Either the critics of the extended mind should give up their commitment to the mind/brain, in favor of many brain modules and processes, or they should accept that functional similarity is sufficient to circumscribe a domain. Of course if they take the latter route, they no longer have a reason to resist the extended mind hypothesis.

Of course, a science of the extended mind will likely consist of processes even more disparate than those which fall in the purview of the traditional cognitive sciences. But there is no reason to think that such a science will be especially disunified. There are already a number of other sciences with a domain circumscribed on the basis of high-level similarities between phenomena, in the absence of lower-level unification. One of Adams' and Aizawa's (2001) own examples illustrates the point. The science of animal communication includes causal processes as disparate as communication by the use of pheremones, threat displays, the dance of honey bees and territory marking by birds, as well as natural language in human beings. There are few general laws which circumscribe all and only these phenomena: instead they are unified only by their functional similarities. Why think that the subject matter of the science of mind should be any more unified?

Adams and Aizawa reply to this kind of objection by repeating the claim that "in contrast to intracranial processes, transcranial processes are not likely to give rise to interesting scientific regularities" (2001: 61). But as it stands this reply is inadequate and question-begging. At the very least, Adams and Aizawa owe us much more. If they concede, as they seem to, that the science of animal communication does not give rise to interesting scientific regularities which pick it out as a unified domain, they must show us why it is entitled to call itself a science, whereas the future science of the extended mind would not be so entitled.

Here is one possible argument that might be advanced on their behalf. They might claim that so far as the science of animal communication is concerned, high-level unification is the best we can do. Unlike the sciences of the mind, they might argue, there are no low-level laws to be had here: whereas the science of the mind/brain can be circumscribed by a set of causal laws, none of the elements of the science of animal communication is internally unified, and therefore high-level unification is the only kind of unification to be had. But this claim seems to be simply false: the different elements of the science of animal communication *could* each form the domain of a separate science, understood in the way Adams and Aizawa want to.

Far from lamenting the loss of a unified science of the mind/brain, Wilson (forthcoming) looks forward to the day when representational practices are the object not of a single science, but of "an interdisciplinary, pluralistic motley," with input not only from psychology and neuroscience, but also from sociology, anthropology and evolutionary biology. It is worth pointing out the extent to which some of these sciences *already* play an ineliminable role in the study of the mind, even as it is currently – and narrowly – conceived.

Hypotheses are formulated, for instance, on the basis of evolutionary considerations, such as considerations concerning the environment in which cognitive adaptations developed; information concerning the size of typical groups of early hominids from anthropology has also guided research in psychology (Dunbar 1996). In any case, there is no need to choose between the sciences of the mind, traditionally conceived, and the interdisciplinary endeavour envisaged by Wilson. They can co-exist, and cross-fertilize one another. But specialists in the traditional sciences of the mind should not deceive themselves into thinking that the mind they study will be unaffected by external resources; even when it is abstracted from environmental props it will likely prove to have somewhat different characteristics for having been embedded.[11]

Informational integration

Let's consider one more objection. Weiskopf (submitted) notes the extent to which the extended mind hypothesis is motivated by functionalist premises. Functionalists are philosophers who hold, roughly, that mental state is as mental state does: thus (for instance) whatever occupies the functional role played by beliefs in our behavior ought to be regarded as a belief. For Clark, Dennett, Haugeland and other proponents of the extended mind hypothesis, we ought to regard certain external props and stores as beliefs, because the information contained in them guides behavior in the way in which beliefs paradigmatically do: for instance, by interacting with desires to produce actions. But, Weiskopf argues, they have overlooked certain important functions of beliefs in making their case. Beliefs are *informationally integrated*. But only brain-based beliefs have this feature. Therefore, external information sources do not contain beliefs.

Informational integration, as Weiskopf uses the phrase, refers to the holistic manner in which beliefs are updated. Consider Inga and Otto once more. Inga knows that George W. Bush is president of the United States, because she has this information encoded in her brain in the usual way. Otto knows (supposedly) that George W. Bush is president of the United States because he has written it down in his notebook. But now fast-forward to 2009, when, thanks to term limits, the United States will have a new president. Inga will at this time acquire the belief that, say, Hilary Clinton is president of the United States. Otto, let us suppose, learns of the election result as soon as Inga, and writes down the information, crossing out "George W. Bush,' and writing in "Hilary Clinton." So far so good. But now think of how Inga's beliefs are updated, when she learns that Hilary Clinton is president of the United States. She also immediately and automatically acquires the belief that Hilary Clinton is the occupant of the White House, is commander-in-chief of the armed forces; that Karl Rove is no longer political advisor to the president of the United States, that the president is of a different political party to the House majority leader and many other beliefs besides. All her relevantly related beliefs are automatically updated. But Otto's relevantly related beliefs are not automatically updated. Suppose he has written in his diary "Karl Rove is political advisor to the president." The act of crossing out "George W. Bush" and replacing it with "Hilary Clinton" does not automatically alter what is contained in his diary about Karl Rove. His beliefs are not informationally integrated, in the manner in which Inga's are.

As Weiskopf points out, informational integration is not a marginal feature of ordinary belief. The concept of belief plays an essential role in explaining and in enabling the prediction of human behavior, but only relatively integrated beliefs can guide behavior. The agent who believes p and that p entails q, but who believes not-q, is an irrational agent and it is difficult to know how they will act. It is only because normal agents who believe p and that if p then q also automatically go on to believe q that we can reliably predict and explain human behavior.[12]

It might be pointed out that the degree of informational integration of beliefs is variable, and that some perfectly ordinary beliefs are isolated, so that updating them has little or no effect on the texture of our web of belief. But this observation is of little help to the proponent of the extended mind hypothesis, since beliefs with a low degree of integration are also, at least typically, trivial beliefs. Their insignificance both explains and is explained by their isolation: they are isolated, in part, because we do not connect them to the ongoing narrative of our lives, and we do not connect them to this narrative because we perceive them as isolated (I have in mind such prima facie trivial beliefs as: I saw a man wearing a green coat on the train yesterday; three people living in my street own red cars, and so on). I take it that proponents of the extended mind hypothesis do not want to hang their hat on the claim that only trivial beliefs can leak out of skulls and into the world; the hypothesis loses all interest if that's what it amounts to.

I think we ought to concede that paradigm beliefs are normally informationally integrated, and that this is an important fact about them. The information stored in the environmental resources and props upon which we lean so heavily is not informationally integrated to anything like the same extent, or with anything like the same degree of automaticity (at least, not yet: perhaps databases constructed so that changes in one element ramify throughout the system in the appropriate manner will one day exist), and this is a significant difference between internal and external information stores. However, is this difference significant enough to require us to reserve the term "belief" only for internal representations? The answer to this question is not clear.

Informational integration is a feature of paradigm beliefs, and it is not a feature of extended information stores, not, at least, to anything like the same extent. So extended information differs from paradigm beliefs. But it does not differ in this manner from some internal mental states that many people are disposed to call beliefs. Consider the representational content of some delusions. Deluded patients sometimes present with delusions that are not merely impossible but contradictory. Sufferers from Cotard's delusion, for instance, claim to be dead, which is a claim that seems to be pragmatically self-defeating. Breen et al. (2000) report the case of a woman who believed (correctly) that her husband had died four years earlier, and had been cremated, and also that he was currently a patient in the same hospital she found herself in. Clearly, in both the case of the Cotard's sufferer, and in the case of the delusional woman, there is an extreme failure of informational integration: if one believes that one is dead, one also ought to give up the belief that one (say) needs to, or indeed is able to, eat, but Cotard's sufferers usually (though not always) continue to eat. If one believes that one's husband is in the next ward, one ought to give up the belief that he is dead and has been cremated. Ought we to conclude that delusional patients, or at least some of them, do not actually believe the content of their delusion?

Philosophers and neuroscientists are divided on this question. Delusions are bizarre, relatively unconnected to evidence, inconsistent and, we might add, lack informational integration; delusional patients often fail to act upon them as it seems they ought, given that they believe them (for instance, sufferers from Capgras' delusion, the delusion that familiar people have been replaced by replicas, do not usually report their relatives missing to police or seem concerned about their welfare). Pointing to these differences between delusions and ordinary beliefs, some philosophers maintain that, at least in the more florid delusions, the deluded do not actually believe what they say (Currie 2000; Hamilton forthcoming). But if there are reasons to refuse to attribute belief to the deluded, there are countervailing reasons pulling in the opposite direction. It is true that the deluded deviate from what Eric Schwitzgebel (2002) calls the *dispositional stereotype* of the belief: the set of dispositions we are apt to associate with it (behavioral dispositions, such as the disposition sincerely to assert *p* or to act as if *p*, phenomenal dispositions, such as the disposition to be surprised if not-*p*, and cognitive dispositions, such as the disposition to draw conclusions entailed by the belief *p*). But ordinary people fail to exhibit perfect conformity with dispositional stereotypes all the time, without us doubting that they believe what they profess. Dispositional stereotypes offer us some room for manoeuvre; we need not conform to them in every particular to count as believing. So the question is not: do the deluded depart from the dispositional stereotype associated with the belief they profess? But, is the degree to which they depart so great that we cannot attribute the belief to them? The deluded conform to the dispositional stereotype to *some* extent, and it may be that the degree of conformity is sufficient for us to attribute the belief to them (Bayne and Pacherie 2005).

Delusions are puzzling because they depart from the dispositional stereotype associated with the associated belief in some ways, often ways that seem central to the stereotype, and conform to the stereotype in others. The deluded do not *clearly* count as believing what they say, yet do not clearly count as disbelieving it either. Their mental state hovers somewhere between belief and disbelief, close enough to both to make its status contentious, and perhaps variable across time and across contexts. In some ways and in some contexts, however, external representations like Otto's representation of the address of MOMA are more clearly beliefs than are delusions. They lack informational integration, and to that extent they are capable of causing behavior that is inconsistent across time. But the deluded can exhibit this sort of inconsistency almost *simultaneously.* Consider the delusional patient referred to earlier, who believed that her husband was dead *and* that he was in another ward of the same hospital she found herself in:

Examiner:	I believe your husband died some years ago.
DB:	Four years ago.
[...]	
Examiner:	And he was cremated, you said?
DB:	Yes.
Examiner:	You were telling me your husband was also at this hospital. Is that right?
DB:	Yes, yes.
Examiner:	What's he doing in this hospital?
DB:	I don't know, I still can't find out.

(Breen, et al. 2000: 92)

DB goes on to agree with the examiner that her husband's presence in the hospital is odd – "Death is final isn't it, as a rule," she says – but insists that she's not mistaken: despite his dying and being cremated, her husband is being treated at the hospital. Compared to this dramatic deviation from the dispositional stereotype associated with believing that someone has died, the deviations that arise from the lack of informational integration of external representations are relatively mild.[13] If it is an open question whether the deluded count as believing what they say, then surely there is at least some pressure to count external representations as beliefs? At very least, we cannot settle the matter simply by pointing to the lack of informational integration associated with such representations.[14]

The parity thesis again

As we have seen, the debate over the extended mind has focused almost exclusively on the parity thesis. The parity thesis has generally been understood by both sides of the debate as providing a criterion by reference to which the mental can be distinguished from the non-mental. Now, though I think it is useful to examine the parity thesis, it is a mistake to place too much weight on it. Focusing on the parity thesis, and seeing just how far it takes us, has, I hope, shaken us free of the seductive view that whatever matters, mentally, must be internal to the skull. But I intend the thesis to serve only as a heuristic device, or (to change the metaphor), a ladder that can be kicked away once it is climbed. We ought to focus on the resources, internal and external, that enable thought, without worrying whether they pass this particular test. The argument for the extended mind is functionalist: something counts as cognitive if it plays a role in processes that are, intuitively, mental (that is, processes that allow agents to process information and thereby to achieve their goals). But analogy between internal mental processes and extended processes is sufficient for the functional claim to go through: the degree of similarity need not be as great as is suggested by the parity thesis.[15]

Indeed, I would go further: I think that to the extent to which the parity thesis is true, *the extended mind thesis loses its interest.* It is precisely *because* the external scaffolding has different properties from the internal resources that it is *worth* extending – or embedding – our minds. Consider, for instance, Rupert's (2004) claim that we ought to distinguish between the mind, on the one hand, and the set of external resources for thinking, on the other, on the basis that there is a set of empirical generalizations that characterize internal cognitive processes only, including characteristic ways in which they go wrong (e.g., interference effects typical of forgetting across all kinds of learning situations). If we obscure the difference between the internal and the external, he argues, we shall not be able to answer important questions, such as why these "learning curves, interference patterns, and so forth, are unavoidable when we rely on internal storage, while entirely optional [...] in the case of external storage" (2004: 418). Maybe so; maybe that is a reason to retain a science of the naked brain. But pointing to this difference between the internal and the external *cannot* be a refutation of an interesting externality thesis. Indeed, it is more like a *confirmation* of it. Why extend your mind if there's nothing to gain by doing so? It is because extending our mind extends our cognitive powers that it is worth doing, and extending our cognitive powers requires that the extended resources have *different* properties to the unadorned brain. You can't refute the extended mind hypothesis by pointing out that it's interesting.

In the end, it doesn't matter what we call the external scaffolding. If we are interested in our capacities for thought, in what makes human thought distinctive, and what enables the products of human cognition of which we are, rightly, proud (science, art, architecture, literature), then we must focus on the entire ensemble of tools, information stores and other resources, and this ensemble crosses the boundary between the inner and the outer. We might decide to reserve the name "mind" for the object of the science of the naked brain, or we may decide, instead, to use it for the object of the science(s) of extended cognition. Nothing turns on this terminological matter. What matters is that we acknowledge that it is the combination of our brains and the tools and props upon which we lean that makes us so smart. This much, at least, is or ought to be uncontroversial: high-level cognition, the kinds of thinking that makes us the kind of species we are, is heavily dependent on the environment. As Rupert (2004) concedes, even if the mind is not *extended* it is *embedded*, inasmuch as cognition "depends *very* heavily, in hitherto unexpected ways, on organismically external props and devices, and on the structure of the external environment in which cognition takes place" (2004: 393). Whatever we decide to use the term "mind" to refer to, we need to rethink the *significance* of the boundary between inner and outer – including, perhaps especially, its *ethical* significance.

Consider an analogy. Adams and Aizawa (2001) argue that it is very important to distinguish between inheritance of traits by organisms and their mere acquisition, and that inheritance properly understood can be defined sharply: "Inheritance involves genetic material in sex cells of a parent being passed on to offspring" (2001: 52). Everything else is mere acquisition. We can define inheritance as Adams and Aizawa suggest, if we like, but if we want to understand the adaptation of organisms to their environment, we would do well to work with a much looser definition. If parents passed on only their genes to their offspring, then for very many species offspring would be ill-equipped to cope with the demands of their world. Luckily for these organisms, they do not inherit just their genes from their parents: they also inherit nests and burrows, behavior and even, in some cases, the micro-organisms they will need to digest their food. In some animals, these micro-organisms are passed on in feeding, but in some species the micro-organisms are actually contained within the shell of the egg (Sterelny and Griffiths 1999: 69). Why should we refuse to call this inheritance? If we want to understand animals and their adaptations, we should think in terms of extended phenotypes and extended mechanisms of inheritance; if we want to understand human cognition, we should think in terms of extended cognition. No matter where we finally resolve to locate the mind, the boundary between inner and outer must be seen as having less significance, *much* less significance, than is generally thought.

Whether the mind is merely embedded, or actually extends into the environment, doesn't much matter, in the end – not once we see the extent to which thought, wherever it is located, depends upon the world. Clark and Chalmers (1998) argue for the extended mind on the basis of a parity principle: if some part of the external world functions in a manner that, were it internal to the skull, we should have no hesitation in calling cognitive, we should regard that external resource as part of the mind. Analogously, I suggest *an ethical parity principle* (EPP). The EPP comes in two versions, a strong and a weak version, corresponding to the hypotheses of extended and embedded cognition respectively:

EPP (strong): Since the mind extends into the external environment, alterations of external props used for thinking are (*ceteris paribus*) ethically on a par with alterations of the brain.

EPP (weak): Alterations of external props are (*ceteris paribus*) ethically on a par with alterations of the brain, to the precise extent to which our *reasons* for finding alterations of the brain problematic are transferable to alterations of the environment in which it is embedded.

EPP (strong) claims that our ethical responses to interventions into the cognitive environment ought to be consistent with our ethical responses to interventions into the brain. If we worry, say, that enhancing the brain pharmacologically is (for whatever reason) wrong, or that transforming it using, say, magnetic stimulation or surgery risks inauthenticity, then we should worry equally about analogous interventions into the extended mind. If Otto were to replace his notebook with a PDA, we might want to claim that he is cheating, just as some people claim that agents who take Ritalin to improve their cognitive perfomance are cheating. More plausibly perhaps, if interventions into the extended mind are not ethically problematic – if Otto's replacing his notebook with a PDA raises no ethical questions at all – then we ought not to regard analogous interventions into the brain as ethically problematic (other things equal; that is, not wrong simply *because* they are interventions into the brain). What counts as analogous is, however, a difficult question, and it is to this and related issues that the *ceteris paribus* (other things being equal) qualification directs us. There are often differences between brain-based and external resources, and some of these differences are ethically relevant. Most obviously, at our present level of technology, external resources have a much higher degree of fungibility than internal. Otto's notebook is far more easily replaced than his hippocampus (which, like his notebook, plays an important role in his memory); therefore damaging his notebook *might* not be as serious as damaging his hippocampus. However, if the information inside his notebook is irreplaceable, then the same amount of damage to it might be equally as serious.

Suppose, however, you remain unconvinced by my case for the extended mind. EPP (weak) is designed to be acceptable to those who hold that the mind is (merely) embedded in the external environment. It is common ground between the contending parties that the kinds of cognition we prize depends very heavily on environmental scaffolding. EPP (weak) asks us to examine the (rational) reasons we find some interventions into or alterations of the (narrowly construed) mind ethically impermissible or problematic. If we find that these reasons apply equally strongly to actual or possible interventions into the environmental scaffolding that supports the mind, then we ought to hold that internal and external interventions are (*ceteris paribus*) equally problematic. Thus, if it would be wrong to read someone's mind because it would be an invasion of their privacy, then it might be equally wrong, for the same reason, to read their diary; if it would be wrong to allow someone access to drugs that enhance memory because it would give them an unfair advantage over others, then it might be equally wrong to give them access to a PDA that would enhance memory (conversely, if it is unproblematic to give someone access to a PDA that would enhance their memory, we need to point to a relevant difference between giving them a PDA and giving them drugs to enhance memory, before we can condemn the latter). Unless we can identify *ethically relevant* differences between internal and external interventions and alterations, we ought to treat them on a par. Weak EPP simply insists that *the mere fact* that one kind of intervention is internal is not a ground for objection, no matter whether the mind is extended or – merely – embedded.

I have argued that the extended mind thesis hypothesis is true. Accordingly, I urge the reader to accept EPP in its strong form. I recognize, however, that many people will remain unconvinced. Though I suspect that resistance to the extended mind thesis reflects nothing so much as prejudice, this is a prejudice that it is difficult to overcome. Given the level of resistance I expect to encounter, it would be foolish to require EPP (strong) to do much work in what follows. Accordingly, I shall avoid invoking it. Instead, my arguments will turn only on EPP (weak), a principle that does not antecedently commit those who appeal to it to any particular view of the mind. In assessing interventions into the mind, I shall persistently return to the question whether there are actual or possible external interventions that raise precisely the same problems as the new neuroscientific techniques. Of course, asking this question is simply the first step in assessing new techniques. That there are, for instance, existing techniques that are ethically analogous to new technologies does not show that the new technologies are permissible. It might show that *neither* is permissible: to that extent assessing the new technologies affords us the opportunity to reassess the old. In any case, in the absence of relevant moral differences between the cases, we ought to treat them alike. The weak parity principle is important not because it provides us with the answers to our ethical questions, but because it allows us to set aside one bad, but tempting, response: that a neuroscientific technology is especially bad (or especially good) *just because* it is an intervention into the mind, narrowly construed. If, as I shall claim, the parallels between new, internal, interventions and older external techniques run deep, approaching neuroethics with the weak parity principle in mind serves to deflate the hype surrounding the new technologies, and encourages sober reflection on the ethical issues that are genuinely significant.[16]

I will not often have cause to invoke the extended, or, indeed, the embedded, mind hypothesis explicitly in what follows. Instead, I shall go directly to consideration of relevant differences between kinds of interventions. I take the very fact that EPP, in its weak form, can do so much ethical work in guiding our deliberations about permissibility without our invoking the extended or the embedded mind hypothesis as itself indirect evidence for the thesis: were it not true, it would not be able to guide us so reliably.

It is now time to turn directly to the neuroethical issues. New neurotechnologies offer us unprecedented powers to alter brains, and thereby thoughts; these technologies promise much, but for many people they are also profoundly troubling. Are there good reasons to find these technologies troubling, and if so, should we find some environmental interventions equally troubling? Or are the horrified responses to neurotechnologies a reflection of the prejudice that would confine mind to skull?

End notes

1. Safire acknowledged that the term predates his use in discussion with two leading neuroethicists, the neuroscientist Michael Gazzaniga and the legal scholar Henry Greely, at the Library of Congress in May 2005. A transcript of that discussion is available at http://www.nyas.org/snc/readersReport.asp?articleID=34&page=2. Safire suggests, however, that the earliest usage predated his by only a few months. In fact, "neuroethics," and cognates like "neuroethical" and "neuroethicist" date back more than a decade earlier. Illes (2003) records uses, from the scientific literature, from 1989 and 1991. I thank Morten Kringelbach for correcting my misapprehension that the term originated with Safire.
2. Readers who have a passing familiarity with Steven Jay Gould's theory of *punctuated equilibrium* might dispute the claim that evolution is a story of continuous change. Gould argues that evolution is characterized by long periods of stasis interrupted by sudden change. But Gould's claim does not in fact conflict with the view I'm putting forward here: speciation is sudden, in Gould's view, only on the geological timescale upon which evolution is normally measured.
3. On primate proto-morality, see de Waal (1996), and my own (2004).
4. In a later chapter, I shall argue that we cannot even take a great deal of comfort from the fact that consciousness is clever. This cleverness is *itself* a product of unconscious mechanisms: consciously processed problems get better solutions because consciousness allows more and better informed *unconscious* mechanisms to work on these problems.
5. More recent work suggests that Bechara *et al.* may have underestimated subjects' conscious knowledge of the payoff structure in the Iowa Gambling Task. Maia and McClelland (2004) repeated the experiment on

normal subjects, this time asking them more detailed questions about the game. They found that conscious awareness of the payoff structure was highly correlated with advantageous choice. Bechara *et al.* (2005) argue that these results are compatible with the somatic marker hypothesis, which aims to explain divergences between knowledge of the advantageous strategy and actual behavior: without the appropriate responses ventromedial patients choose badly *even when* they ascertain the payoff structure of the game. The work of Batson *et al.* (1999) on somatic markers in moral judgment appears to support this view: the researchers found that providing subjects with false feedback had no effect on their ranking of values – that is, upon their declarative knowledge – but did influence their decision-making concerning these very same values. It may also be suspected that Maia and McClelland's method was not merely a more sensitive measure of subjects' knowledge of the payoff structure, but actually was responsible for subjects' better understanding of the game: by continually probing their knowledge, asking them detailed questions that explicitly addressed gains, losses and net outcomes, they may have encouraged their subjects to make greater efforts to recall deck-by-deck outcomes and thereby to acquire knowledge of the payoff structure sooner than in the earlier experiment.

6. Wilson and Clark (forthcoming; Wilson forthcoming) have stressed the extent of the parallels between recent developments in philosophy of biology and the extended mind thesis: not only the idea of the extended phenotype, but also the rise of developmental systems theory (DST) and niche construction theory. DST holds that genes are just one, albeit an especially important, developmental resource that helps to build phenotypes; to that extent DST reorients biology away from the genetic, just as radical externalism reorients cognitive science away from the mental, narrowly conceived. Like niche construction theory, DST also emphasises the role of the environment in adaptation and development; to that extent, the boundary between inner and outer is shown by these approaches to be lacking in significance.

7. Interestingly, this argument seems to be a new version of an older argument, originally levelled by Jerry Fodor against the much less radical Burge-Putnam kind of externalism. For discussion of this kind of externalism see Wilson (2004) pp. 77–99; for Fodor's objection from scientific taxonomy, see pp. 96f.

8. In reply to Clark, Adams and Aizawa (forthcoming) claim that though Venn diagrams are meaningful in virtue of a convention, it doesn't follow that an agent's representation of Venn diagrams have representational content in virtue of that same convention. So far as I can see, however, they don't give us any reason to think that representations of Venn diagrams in the head do not get their content in virtue of the convention. Don't we manipulate symbols in our heads, quite directly, without translating those symbols into special mental representations in the language of thought? There is good evidence that mental rotation involves exactly that: the mental manipulation of a representation, and not the translation of that representation into something more basic or intrinsically meaningful (Pinker 1994). My *experience* when I contemplate Clark's thought experiment seems to be as of manipulating mental representations of physical objects, much like my experience of mental rotation; Adams and Aizawa therefore seem to owe us some argument for their claim that this experience is not veridical.

9. Earlier we noted that change blindness seems to be the price we pay for offloading the job of representing the world onto the environment. Eidetikers are not a counterexample to this claim; people with prodigious memories generally suffer from a range of problem solving difficulties (Farah 2002).

10. Dennett seems to suggest that far from intrinsic content being basic, there is a sense in which *derived* content is basic to the mind. How so? Dennett argues that *our* kind of consciousness – which, as Clark (2002) points out, is at least sometimes taken by Dennett to be the only kind of consciousness there is – emerges from culture: we become capable of self-consciousness, the ability to knowingly represent representations, only as a result of having first created external representations, such as words. As Clark (2002) puts it, these external representations position us to acquire the *idea* of representation. On this view, only because there were first derived representations could there be minds at all.

11. Wilson (forthcoming) gives the example of short-term memory; typical capacity may have been diminished by the transition from an oral to a literate culture (a fear expressed by Plato in the *Phaedrus*).

12. At least, this is the case where p and q are ordinary, empirical propositions, and not names of sceptical hypotheses, for instance.

13. In correspondence, Weiskopf has argued that we ought to refuse the status of beliefs to the extended states of an agent like Otto, because there is no explanatory payoff in doing so. I find this reply mystifying. Recall that the basic argument for the extended mind thesis is functionalist: we ought to regard extended processes and stores as mental because they play a similar role in guiding cognitive processes (that is, roughly, processes that allow us to solve problems in navigating the external world and in satisfying our needs and desires) as do internal structures and processes. It is explanatory payoff that motivates the entire project. Unless the opponent of the extended mind has the resources to dispute the very many cases cited in support of the functionalist claim, it seems foolhardy for them to contest the claim on these grounds. Moreover, even with regard to Otto's extended states it seems that the extended mind has an explanatory payoff. We shall best explain the inconsistencies in Otto's behavior that might arise from a lack of informational integration by attributing to him a quasi-belief state, one that guides his behavior when it is on-line, but which goes off-line whenever Otto is not accessing it.

14. Let me mention just one more objection sometimes voiced to the extended mind thesis. Some philosophers take the conditions advanced by Clark and Chalmers (1998) to be necessary for a resource to count as mental, and have objected that we do not automatically endorse external representations. Thus, they claim, there is a difference between internal and external resources, sufficient to ensure that the only first count as mental. Once again, I do not believe that the demonstration that internal and external resources differ amounts to a refutation of the thesis; however (once again) it is worth pointing out that it is more difficult than the critics believe to demonstrate such differences. In fact, there is ample evidence that endorsement of propositions, external as well as internal, is the automatic default response: only subsequently – if we have the time, the attentional resources and the motivation – do we come to doubt them (Gilbert 1991; 1993).

15. Menary (2006) is similarly critical of the parity thesis.

16. David Chalmers has suggested that something like the weak parity principle is all I need, and all I am entitled to. He argues that the neuroethical issues can all be understood parsimoniously in terms of differing causal routes whereby we can alter the mind, where "mind" is

conceived of traditionally. Pointing out, as I will do at length, that causal routes that are largely external to the mind are not, in any ethically relevant way, different from causal routes that are largely internal does not require us to subscribe to the extended mind hypothesis (Gert-Jan Lokhorst has offered a very similar criticism independently). I find this a surprising line of argument. Its similarity to defences of internalism against Chalmers himself should make us suspicious of it. We can, if we like, reserve the term "mind" for processes, states and mechanisms that are internal to the skull, but there is no explanatory gain in doing so; insofar as we want to understand cognition, we shall be forced to take into consideration the environmental scaffolding of cognition, as well as internal resources. Similarly, if we want to understand what is permissible and what impermissible, there is no explanatory gain in understanding the bearer of value in the traditional manner. Here's an illustration: some philosophers argue that to the extent to which an agent is reliant upon others, especially, but not only, cognitively, they are non-autonomous (Weithman 2005). But if we take the embedding of the agent in the social world seriously (and once we grasp the extent to which the agent shrinks to an extensionless, and powerless, point if we take the internalist view to its logical conclusion), this view loses its force. A responsible doxastic agent trusts others, rather than relying upon their own cognitive resources; similarly, a self-controlled agent allows the environment, including the social environment, to carry much of the load in controlling their behavior in the manner she wants (we shall explore the issue of autonomy more fully in a later chapter). Just as importantly, the extended mind hypothesis plays a significant heuristic role, enabling us to recognize the degree to which the intuition that external means of altering minds – means which impact on the mind by way of impacting on the environment – are less problematic than internal manipulations is the product of the prejudice that confines mind to skull. Finally, though this is not the place to develop the view, the extended mind hypothesis might play an important role in motivating an externalist meta-ethics. As Rowlands (2003) has pointed out, if we take externalism seriously, the traditional options for the location of value – either entirely in the world, or entirely in the minds of agents – no longer seem exhaustive. If mind extends into the world, then value can *depend* upon mind without being *located* only in the skulls of agents.

2 Changing our minds

There are two basic ways to go about changing someone's mind. What we might call the traditional way involves the presentation of evidence and argument. This way of going about things raises ethical problems of its own, all of which are familiar: Under what circumstances is it permissible to present *false* evidence? If it's in the person's own interests to come to have a false belief, must we nevertheless present them with the truth? What if we know that the available evidence is misleading? Can we hide the evidence in the interests of the truth? These questions and others like them constitute a small part of the traditional turf of moral philosophy.

Traditional psychotherapy is, in many ways, an extension of this familiar method of changing minds. The goal of the earliest fully developed method of psychotherapy, Freudian psychoanalysis, is truth, and the concomitant extension of the power of rational thought over libidinal impulse. "Where id was, there ego shall be," Freud famously wrote: the powerful unconscious drives of the id, the forces that tyrannize the neurotic patient, shall be replaced by the conscious forces of the rational ego, the *I*. To be sure, psychoanalysis does not take a direct route to truth. It does not seek to change minds by argument, or at least not by argument alone. Freud thought that it was not sufficient for the patient simply to be told the truth regarding his or her neuroses and their origins. Instead, the patient had to "work through" traumatic events, reliving them under the guidance of the analyst, in order for the cure to be successful. The truth has to be accepted emotionally, and not merely intellectually, if it is to have its curative effects.

Psychoanalysis and related psychotherapies raise ethical questions of their own, some of which concern the extent to which their departures from the pure form of the traditional way of changing minds – presenting reasons and arguments – are permissible. But the degree to which psychoanalysis departs from tradition pales into insignificance compared to the second way in which we might go about changing someone's mind (putting concerns about extended cognition to one side for the moment, and assuming that the mind is wholly bounded by the skull): by direct manipulation of the brain.

Of course, there is a sense in which presenting evidence is a kind of (indirect) manipulation of the brain – it alters connections between neurons, and might contribute, in a very small way, to changing the morphology of the brain (enough evidence, presented over a long enough period of time, can produce alterations which are large enough to be visible to the naked eye: a study of London taxi drivers demonstrated that the posterior hippocampus, which stores spatial information, was larger in drivers than in controls [Maguire *et al.* 2000]). But direct manipulation of the brain differs from indirect in an extremely significant way: whereas the presentation of evidence and argument manipulates the brain via the rational capacities of the mind, direct manipulation bypasses the agent's rational capacities altogether. It works directly on the neurons or on the larger structures of the brain. There are many different kinds of direct manipulation in use today: electroconvulsive therapy (ECT), in which a current is passed through the brain, inducing seizures; psychosurgery, which may involve the severing of connections in the brain surgically, or may involve the creation of lesions using radio frequency; transcranial magnetic stimulation of superficial structures of the brain; and deep brain stimulation.[1] But the most widely used kind of direct manipulation is, of course, pharmacological. Many millions of people have taken one or another drug designed to alter brain function: antipsychotics, lithium for manic-depression, Ritalin for attention-deficit/hyperactivity disorder (ADHD) and, most commonly, antidepressants. Here we shall focus, mainly, on psychopharmacological treatment of depression; the issues raised by this kind of intervention overlap significantly with those raised by other forms of direct manipulation.

People are much more reluctant to countenance medication as a treatment for depression than for psychosis. In part, no doubt, this is due to the perception that psychosis is more severe than depression; there is a corresponding greater acceptance of psychopharmacology to treat major depression – which is a life-threatening condition, as well as one that causes great suffering – than for the treatment of "mere" anxiety. But even with regard to major depression, perhaps even psychosis, there seems to be a widespread *presumption* in favor of the traditional way of changing minds, other things being equal (that is, if the costs, risks and benefits do not favor, or perhaps if they do not decisively favor, direct manipulation). If we *can* use the traditional means, we should, or so many people believe. In some cases psychotherapy will prove too expensive, or too costly, or too slow, and we will be forced to use psychopharmacology. Nevertheless, many people believe, this is a necessity to be regretted: direct means of changing minds are always ethically dubious.

Why is this intuition so widely shared? There are many reasons, I suggest, for the presumption against direct manipulation, some rational and some irrational. Some of these I wish to set aside here, though they are nonetheless worthy of respect. First, there are understandable safety concerns associated with the use of new technologies: direct stimulation of the brain or the use of psychoactive medications might have unforeseen, and potentially very serious, side effects. Deliberate lesioning of the brain will often produce deficits in cognition and memory (there are some tragic cases of people with complete anterograde amnesia – the inability to form new memories – following neurosurgery for intractable epilepsy). Second, many people are – once again, perfectly understandably – reluctant to support with their custom a pharmaceutical industry widely seen as having engaged in unethical practices: withholding research findings detrimental to their products, preventing or delaying the availability of generic drugs in the Third World, and so on

(Angell 2004). These are very serious objections to the use of psychopharmaceuticals, but I set them aside here in order to focus better on the *philosophical* issues, relatively narrowly construed. The question I want to examine is not whether, given the current state of the art, use of these drugs is advisable; rather I want to concentrate upon *in principle* objections to direct manipulations. In principle objections are objections that remain sound no matter how much the technologies improve, and no matter what the political and social context in which they are developed, prescribed and taken. I therefore set aside these objections, and assume that the products concerned are safe, or at least safe enough (inasmuch as their expected benefits to patients outweigh their risks), and ignore concerns about the industries that create and distribute them.

It might be objected that in setting these matters aside, we set aside the *ethics* of neuroethics: the very heart and soul of the questions. There is some justice in this accusation: of course, it will be necessary to factor these concerns back into the equation in coming to an all-things-considered judgment of the advisability of using or promoting these drugs in actual circumstances. But clarity demands that we treat the issues raised by direct manipulation one by one, and that requires isolating them from one another, not conflating them. Moreover, in a book defending a conception of the mind as extended and knowledge acquisition as distributed, it is not special pleading to note that others – policy specialists, lawyers, sociologists and many kinds of medical professionals – are better placed than philosophers to analyze the issues set aside here. By focusing on the questions where I can best contribute, I hope thereby to advance the entire neuroethical agenda all the more effectively.

What remains, once we set these concerns aside? No doubt some of the opposition to psychopharmacology that remains is simply irrational. In part, it seems to be an expression of a deep-seated prejudice against technologies regarded as "unnatural." When we investigate the roots of this kind of objection, we frequently find that by "unnatural" people tend to mean no more than "unfamiliar" (few people regard the use of vitamin tablets as unnatural; fewer still object to clothes). But there are also rational arguments against the use of direct means of changing minds.

There is an important and much discussed distinction between the *treatment* of disease, and the *enhancement* of traits that already fall within the normal range. Treatment is widely seen as more permissible than mere enhancement. In the next chapter, I shall argue that the treatment/enhancement distinction cannot be drawn in any defensible manner and is therefore morally irrelevant. For the moment, however, I shall focus on changing minds where it is least controversial: in the treatment of diagnosable illness. It is uncontroversial that when someone is undergoing a significant degree of suffering, and we have the means of alleviating that suffering, we ought to do so (other things being equal). If the only means, or by far the best means (in terms of the balance of benefits over risks and harms), involves direct manipulation, then we have a powerful reason in favor of direct manipulation. Nevertheless, many people think, it would be better if we could avoid direct manipulation, in favor of more traditional means of changing minds, even in cases involving treatment of serious illness. Why this presumption in favor of the traditional means? In what follows, I shall set out a number of considerations that have been, or might be, advanced in favor of the presumption. Only once they are all before us shall I proceed, in the next chapter, to evaluate them.

AUTHENTICITY

One worry focuses on the *authenticity* of the agent. Authenticity is one of the definitive values of modernity; it is a good highly valued by most of the citizens of – at least – most of the countries in the developed world. Authenticity, at least in the sense at issue in these debates, consists, roughly, in *being true to oneself*. The authentic individual finds their own way to live, a way that is truly theirs. They do not passively accept social roles imposed upon them. They do not simply select between the conventional ways of living that their society makes available. Instead, they look for and actively create their *own* way, by reference to who they, truly and deeply, are. Authenticity is a modern ideal. It could not exist in premodern societies, in which social roles were relatively few, and people had little freedom to move between them. A medieval peasant had few options available to him or her, and little leeway to choose between them. Authenticity requires the growth of cities, and the consequent decrease in the social surveillance and mutual policing characteristic of village life. In the anonymity of the city, people were free to remake themselves. They could, if they wished, break free (at least somewhat) from the expectations of their family, their church, their friends and even of social conventions, and remake themselves in their own image.[2]

Authenticity, the search for a way of life that is truly one's own, has gradually gone from a mere possibility to an ideal. Today, most of us feel stung by the charge of inauthenticity. Conformism, going along with the crowd, the herd mentality – all of these are, if not quite vices, at least imperfections to be avoided. Of course, we may authentically choose to do what most everyone else is doing, but to choose it authentically is to choose it because it is right for *us*, and not because it is what everyone else does.

Authenticity, as Charles Taylor (1991) has argued, exists in an unstable tension with other ideals and standards of a good life. It can easily tip over into selfishness and a shallow form of individualism. It can lead us to overlook the fact that values are sustained socially, and that each of us must forge our own way of life in an ongoing dialogue with others: with those close to us, and with the ideals and standards of our culture. Nevertheless, though it is an ideal that becomes self-defeating if it is taken too far, it is unrepudiable by us moderns. Authenticity is so deeply woven into our cultures and our values that few, if any, of us can simply turn our backs upon it. It is true that some of us choose to embrace, or to remain in, ways of life that are in some ways antithetical to the ideal of authenticity – we join monasteries, or adhere to religions that regulate every aspect of our lives, even to the point of deciding who we shall marry and what careers (if any) we shall have. But even when we embrace ways of life that require us to cede control of our significant choices to others, we often justify our decision in ways that invoke authenticity: we find this way of life personally fulfilling; it is, after all, our way of being ourselves.

It is easy to see why the use of direct manipulations of the mind might be thought antithetical to the ideal of authenticity. To be authentic is to find one's way of life and one's values *within*; it is to make one's entire life an expression of who one truly is. But antidepressants, psychosurgery and the other technologies of direct manipulation introduce an alien element into the equation: after treatment with these technologies, I am no longer the person I was. Either I have changed, as a result of this intrusion from outside me, or (less radically) who I really am has been covered over by the foreign element. This cheerfulness, this sunny disposition, this is not really *me*; it is the antidepressants. As Carl Elliott, the bioethicist who has insisted most forcefully and persuasively on the problem of inauthenticity puts it:

> It would be worrying if Prozac altered my personality, even if it gave me a better personality, simply because it isn't *my* personality. This kind of personality change seems to defy an ethics of authenticity.
>
> *(Elliott 1998: 182)*

To this extent, psychotherapy is preferable to direct manipulation. Psychotherapy explores *my* self, my inner depths. It seeks coherence and equilibrium between my inner states, and between my inner states and the world. But direct manipulation simply imposes itself over my self.

One might illuminatingly compare the effects of direct manipulation in treating a mental illness to the effects of more familiar direct manipulations of the mind: drugs consumed for recreational purposes. When someone behaves aggressively, or breaks a promise, while drunk, they may plead for forgiveness, saying something to the effect of: "it was the drink talking. That's not who I really am." We may not be ready to forgive them, but we are likely to modify our indignation at their behavior at least somewhat, taking into account the extent to which the alcohol clouded their mind. In exactly the same manner as we may conclude that the drunk person was not entirely themselves, we may think that the person cured of depression by direct manipulation is not themselves. We may think the price, of a small degree of inauthenticity, is well worth paying for alleviation of the symptoms of a disease that is extremely serious, indeed life-threatening, but that is entirely compatible with acknowledging that the cost is nevertheless real.

SELF-KNOWLEDGE AND PERSONAL GROWTH

Psychotherapy, at least as traditionally practiced, aims at exploring the mind of the patient, in order to lead them to acknowledge and confront truths, often painful truths, about themselves. Psychoanalysis, for instance, aims at knowledge, and not just any knowledge, but knowledge concerning ourselves, which is – arguably, at least – the most important kind of knowledge any of us can ever achieve. To be sure, traditional methods of changing minds *need* not aim at knowledge. They may seek to change minds by deliberately distorting reality, by lying, for instance. And they may be indifferent as to whether they result in knowledge: some kinds of therapy teach ways in which to pursue our goals, or to pursue happiness, which are quite mechanical or which are indifferent to the truth (consider the use of self-affirmations: I am beautiful; I am confident; I am successful. Therapists who advocate their use do not generally caution that we should only use self-affirmations that are true; indeed, they often recommend that we choose our self-affirmations precisely because they are *not* true. By repeating them to ourselves, we are supposed to increase the chances that reality will slowly come to resemble the claim. They are more expressions of goals to be achieved than claims about our actual states). However, psychotherapy can, and perhaps usually does, aim at truth, and can therefore be a powerful means whereby we pursue self-knowledge.

However, at least apparently, psychopharmacology and other direct manipulations do not and cannot aim at truth. They are mechanical manipulations of the brain, and of the mind through the brain, characterized by the fact that they bypass our rational capacities. When someone becomes less depressed as the result of taking antidepressants, their mood does not lighten because they have been given *reasons* to be happier (as we might seek to alleviate the depression of a friend by listing all the goods things in life). Instead, the amount of a neurotransmitter, serotonin, in their brain has effectively been increased by inhibiting the reabsorption of the chemical.[3] Having more serotonin available is no reason to be cheerful! The depressed patient does not know more than they did before; they do not understand themselves, their self-narrative, and the causes of their depression any better than they did before. Once again, advocates of the presumption in favor of the traditional methods of changing minds can concede that the benefits of direct manipulations often outweigh the costs; in this case, the opportunity costs arising from forgoing a means to self-knowledge. Rather than arguing that direct manipulation is impermissible, they need only claim that traditional means are to be preferred, other things being equal. It is, they might argue, because only traditional means have the power to aim at truth and therefore increase our self-knowledge that there ought to be a presumption in their favor.

If the benefits of direct manipulations are supposed to lie primarily in their efficiency, their sheer speed at alleviating symptoms, a closely related objection holds that this very efficiency robs them of the power to assist in personal growth that is inherent in more traditional ways of coming to terms with suffering. Pain and suffering are a normal part of human life. Though they are, at best, unpleasant, they also offer us opportunities. Pain is adaptive: we feel pain because it is a reliable signal of something to which we need to attend, and of lessons we must learn. Those rare individuals who are congenitally unable to feel pain are at much greater risk of serious injury or death because they lack these generally reliable signals of somatic problems. For this reason, too much analgesic, or too effective an analgesic, is risky, leaving those who take it similarly exposed. But mightn't direct manipulations such as antidepressants constitute just such an analgesic for emotional pain? Emotional pain, like somatic pain, can be a signal that something is wrong: that our choices have not been wise, and that we ought not to repeat them, that our relationships need work, that the way we are acting toward others is inappropriate. Blocking these signals prevents us from learning from our failures, and therefore removes one of our most important opportunities for personal growth. Direct manipulation, if used to medicalize normal suffering, turns opportunities for growth into symptoms to be eliminated (Manninen 2006).

MECHANIZATION OF THE SELF

A further reason to favor traditional means of changing minds over direct manipulations is closely connected to the forgoing. Bypassing our rational capacities in order to change our minds might carry a cost that is potentially far greater than merely passing up the opportunity to gain self-knowledge: it risks the very existence of our *self*, as it has traditionally been understood. The self is, or has as an essential component, the capacity to respond to reasons. We are not machines, but living creatures, with rich inner lives constituted by our emotional and cognitive responses to our environment and to the people within it. When we treat ourselves *as if* we were machines, by modifying our brains, our emotions and our cognitive processes using direct means, we risk everything that makes us more than mere machines. If we treat ourselves as if we did not live in a space of reasons, we risk making it true, and that is to risk, literally, everything.

One way to understand the claim being made here is by analogy with the kind of disrespect we show others when we treat their emotional and cognitive responses as mere *symptoms*. Think, for instance, of one all-too-real response to feminists, especially in the early days of the movement. Critics rejected feminist arguments, but not on the grounds that they were false. Rather than engage with them *as arguments*, they were wont to reject them as *hysterical*; as expressions of psychological maladjustment. If I reject your arguments because I think they are false, and especially if I give reasons why I reject them, I manifest respect for you as a rational being. But if I reject your arguments without even engaging with them, because I see them as expressions of your psychology and not as rational responses to the world as you perceive it, I treat you with profound disrespect. I treat you as an object to be managed, not as a person to engage with. More generally, when we treat mental states, of ourselves or of others, as objects to be manipulated, we treat *ourselves* as things (Freedman 1998).

What's wrong with treating ourselves as things? Well, it may be that *being* a self requires being *treated*, and treating ourself, as a self. Human identity is relatively fragile. It can be disrupted or degraded by inappropriate treatment. We are self-interpreting animals, Freedman argues (following Charles Taylor), and the terms of our interpretations profoundly affect the kinds of creature we are. How we understand ourselves, the kinds of stories we tell ourselves about ourselves, actually affect the kinds of beings we are. So we must be careful to avoid the kinds of mechanistic explanations of our actions and thoughts that are appropriate to mere machines. We can appropriately explain why a computer responded in a certain way by referring to its internal states in mechanical terms, but treating each other as selves involves treating our responses as reflecting assessments of situations, not as mere mechanical processes. The computer responded like *that* because there is a bug in its program (or a malfunction in its coprocessor, or a power failure), but the person responded as they did because they thought he was rude (or whatever the case might be).[4]

The problem with Prozac, then (where "Prozac" refers to any chemical means of treating mental problems) is that it treats people in the manner appropriate to machines. Rather than treat someone's problems as expressing their reasoned (which is not to say rational) assessment of a situation, we treat them as expressing a malfunction. Freedman gives the example of Lucy, one of Peter Kramer's patients (Kramer 1993). Lucy is far too quick to see rejection in the behavior of others. For instance, when her boyfriend turns away to change the TV channel, Lucy feels ignored and hurt. Lucy's over-sensitivity to rejection is the result of her painful upbringing; her mother was murdered when she was ten, and her father was emotionally un-available. Her over-sensitivity is the product of a background which left her with a distinctive, and dysfunctional, manner of seeing the world. She *expects* to be rejected; she doesn't feel worthy of acceptance. Now, Freedman argues, if we treat Lucy's anxiety with Prozac, we might succeed in altering her manner of responding. Perhaps she will no longer be over-sensitive to rejection. But by giving her medication for her problem, rather than working through it with her, by talking and reasoning, laying bare the childhood trauma that leads her to respond as she does, we treat her as a thing and not as a person.

Of course, Lucy's response is affective, and there is a long-standing tradition that treats emotions as arational, or even irra-tional. But the dominant view in recent philosophy of the emotions, the view Freedman invokes and endorses, holds that emotions are at least partly cognitive (Neu 2000; Nussbaum 2001). Emotions are not merely visceral responses to situations; they reflect our assessment of these situations, and they are, in principle, open to justification. When all goes well, they reflect our beliefs, giving them a salience for us that they might not otherwise have had. My indignation, when I read accounts of the torture of inmates at Abu Ghraib reflects and reinforces my belief in the wrongness of the ill-treatment. My affective response is not a mere add-on, but helps guide my delib-eration (not only moral deliberation, but also prudential deliberation, as Damasio (1994) has shown). Freedman is surely on strong ground when she argues that it can be dehumanizing to treat an emotion as a merely mechanical response, rather than as a state with a cognitive content.

Moreover, Freedman argues, if we treat emotional responses or beliefs using merely mechanical procedures like psychopharmacology, a much worse threat is in the offing. The use of such means leads us to treat ourselves "in mechanistic terms", terms that are incompatible with our existence as free and responsible agents. But our view of ourselves and of one another as free and responsible agents, agents who choose between alternatives on the basis of reasons and who are subsequently accountable for their choices, is an essential component of our conception of humanity. We threaten our very existence as free, responsible and rational agents by treating ourselves mechanically. What will it profit us to gain mental tranquillity and lose our very selves?

TREATING SYMPTOMS AND NOT CAUSES

Another common objection to the use of direct means to manipulate the mind is that it merely covers over the symptoms of a problem, without getting to its root causes. Antidepressants in the Prozac family are SSRIs; they work by slowing down the rate at which serotonin, a neurotransmitter, is reabsorbed in the brain, thereby increasing the availability of the neurotransmitter for carrying messages across neural synapses. The theory behind the use of SSRIs is that depression is caused by a deficit of serotonin; therefore, we can treat it by increasing available levels. But treating serotonin levels directly may be missing the real roots of the problem.

Serotonin levels rise and fall in response to life events. For instance, among social animals, including human beings, serotonin varies as a function of status (Edwards and Kravitz 1997). Dominant animals have high serotonin levels, but if they experience a fall in the social hierarchy, their serotonin levels fall as well. They also exhibit depression-like symptoms: loss of appetite and of interest in everyday activities, withdrawal from the group, characteristic rocking movements and self-absorption. It is frequently suggested that these responses are adaptive (Watson and Andrews 2002): withdrawing allows one time to recuperate from the sudden decline in status, and from any wounds that may have been incurred in fights over hierarchy. Decreased serotonin is also associated with rumination and with hypervigilance, which are likely also adaptive responses: rumination ensures that all one's intellectual resources are concentrated on the problem of how to ensure that the decline in status is reversed or at least halted, and hypervigilance ensures that one is able successfully to navigate the dangerous environment of the low-status animal. In short, a fall in serotonin levels, and subsequent sadness, is not a disease. It is a rational response to external events.

Today serotonin levels are more likely to fall in response to various kinds of life events: losing one's job, or getting divorced. Nevertheless, it remains plausible to think of the response as adaptive and even as rational. It is normal to feel depressed in response to such events. Indeed, one might go further: failure to feel depressed in response to these life events would *itself* be pathological. These events *are* depressing, and if one simply brushes them aside and carries on cheerfully, one fails to appreciate their proper significance. The person who shrugs off the failure of a marriage, for instance, fails to appreciate the importance that intimate relationships have in a properly human life, which is a reliable indication that they fail to *live* a properly human life. The proper response to intimate relationship breakdown, the only response that takes the measure of its true significance, is deep sadness; a sadness which, moreover, persists for some extended period of time (think, for example, of how we look askance at someone who remarries very soon after divorce or the death of a spouse). Similarly, the appropriate response to the loss of a job might well be depression, as the unemployed person contemplates the struggle to pay the mortgage or the rent, to feed their family or to forge a new place for themselves within the social world.

None of this is to say that depression may not sometimes be a pathological response to life events. Depression is pathological when it is deeper and far more prolonged than life events warrant.

Depression *becomes* pathological: it is appropriate to react with lowered mood to the loss of one's job, but if someone is unable to shake off their depression – if, instead, it deepens and begins to interfere with their ability to find another one – then it may be pathological. Moreover, there is a huge qualitative difference between the ordinary melancholy we all experience when our plans go awry, and the malignant sadness (as Wolpert (2001) calls it) of clinical depression. Clinical depression is crippling and involves very significant suffering. It is, literally, life-threatening. We ought not to deny any of these points. Recall, we are not attempting to show that depression ought not to be treated, or even that it ought not to be treated with direct manipulations of the brain. Instead, we aim only to explain the common intuition that it is better, all things considered, to treat mental dysfunction with traditional means. It is perfectly coherent to think that if clinical depression can only, or most effectively, be treated by direct manipulation, then we ought so to treat it, but also to hold that direct manipulation ought to be avoided if possible. It is also perfectly coherent to think that *if* in a particular case it is only possible to treat symptoms, and not causes, it is far better to do so than not to treat at all, but that it is better still to treat causes, as well as, or instead of, symptoms.

The charge of treating symptoms only, while leaving the causes untouched, has been levelled at a variety of direct manipulations of the mind; most notably, the use of antidepressants to treat depression or anxiety and the use of Ritalin and similar drugs to treat ADHD. The behaviors characteristic of ADHD (on the assumption that there is any such thing as ADHD; some critics are sceptical) are, it is sometimes claimed, not the result of a dysfunction on the part of the individual child, but are instead the product of problems in the environment: overcrowded classrooms, unrealistic parental expectations, or a "culture of masculinity" that expects boys to conform to a stereotype centred on autonomy and independence (Pollack 1998). Medicating children may allow them to *cope* with this toxic environment, but will leave them unable to develop in their own way, and unable to achieve the full range of goods constitutive of a flourishing life.

Carl Elliott (1998) has developed this theme in a way that links it closely with the problem of authenticity. Authenticity can be contrasted with alienation; a state in which we feel estranged from our social world and cut off from sources of meaning. In seeking authenticity, we normally seek a place in the world that is fulfilling for us, and which satisfies our deepest needs as human beings. But (and here I go beyond what Elliott himself says), authenticity-as-fulfilment understood in this way has social preconditions. Only in social environments which are conducive to meaningful lives can authenticity-as-fulfilment be achieved. In less favourable environments, authenticity will be a less happy – literally and figuratively – affair. In some environments, authenticity consists not in fulfilment, but in the clear-headed acknowledgement that we confront serious and perhaps insoluble problems.

Authenticity must not be confused with happiness. The authentic individual is not necessarily happy, and the happy individual is not necessarily authentic. Elliott asks us to consider the example of the stereotypical conformist, an accountant living in the American suburbs. Suppose that such a person presents to a physician suffering from depression. Should the physician treat him with anti-depressants (or, indeed, with any other direct manipulations)? The case for treatment is simple: the man is suffering, and the physician has it within their power to relieve that suffering. But it is far from clear that in treating the patient's suffering, the physician actually makes them better off. Elliott contrasts two possible (inauthentic) suburban accountants (the qualification is necessary, since it is at least possible that someone could be an *authentic* suburban accountant). Both live a life of dull conformity to social norms which they have accepted unthinkingly, neither lives according to a conception of the good life they have reflectively endorsed. Both suffer a growing, gnawing, malaise, as their opportunities for a life endorsed from the inside slip away. But suppose that one of them now seeks professional treatment for their depression, and is prescribed Prozac. They respond well to the treatment, and their mood lifts. They are more energetic at work, and happier at home. But are they really better off than their counterpart across the road, whose despondency is untreated?

The point here is subtly different to the objection that in covering over our pain, Prozac obstructs a path to useful self-knowledge – knowledge that can enable us to achieve a better life and more satisfying relationships. The claim Elliott makes is that *independently of its instrumental value*, a clear-eyed appreciation of inauthenticity or other malaises is valuable. Even if there is no practical means available to the suburban accountant to achieve authenticity, even if seeing the truth comes at the cost of permanent and irredeemable psychic pain for him, he is better off for suffering that pain than his medicated counterpart.

There is more, far more, to a properly human life than mere happiness, as a little reflection on some possible ways in which humans can achieve happiness demonstrates. Most people fear the prospect of dementia, sometimes as much as or even more than death. They dread the prospect of having their mind, their memory and their very selfhood slipping away. But if happiness were all that mattered, this fear would be irrational. Dementia is not incompatible with happiness; though some demented individuals experience a great deal of frustration and unhappiness, some seem quite content. Our fear of dementia therefore seems to be due to our recognition that well-being consists in more than just feelings of contentment. Similarly, few of us believe that the life of the drug addict would be a good life, even if we could ensure a steady supply of high-quality drugs and suffered no adverse health effects (both of which are reasonable assumptions, for addicts who are wealthy). We think that a good life is a life not just of happy *experience*, but of contact with reality (Nozick 1974). Happiness, if it comes, is certainly to be welcomed, and perhaps it ought to be sought. But it is not to be sought at the expense of contact with reality. The happiness we seek is the happiness which comes through the achievement of intrinsically worthwhile goods, whether moral or religious goods, or the goods of family and home. If we must choose, we better honor our sense of ourselves as human beings if we choose reality over happiness.

But Elliott's contented accountant has made precisely the opposite choice. He has chosen happiness over a clear-eyed grasp of reality. To that extent, he may be *worse* off, and not better, than his unhappy counterpart. He does not live an authentic or a fulfilling life; he has merely lost the ability to respond appropriately to his empty life. He may *feel* better, but he does not *live* better.

Finally, and on a closely related note, it has sometimes been claimed that treating symptoms and not causes might foster political quietism (DeGrazia 2005). If mental illness is sometimes or often a response to a toxic environment, as many people claim, then we ought to respond to it by concerted political activity that aims at changing that environment. We are currently in the grip of a veritable pandemic of depression (the World Health Organization predicts that by 2020, depression will be the second most significant contributor to the global burden of disease). What explains this upsurge in depression? One plausible explanation is that the social conditions in which we live – the alienation and anonymity of big cities, the insecurity caused by globalization and shifts in employment, the threat of new diseases, political tensions, and so on – are incompatible with a flourishing life. Just as psychic pain gives us, as individuals, an opportunity to learn about ourselves and the ways in which our lives might be going off-track, so common emotional problems give us an opportunity, as a society, to learn about our political and social malaises. We ought to learn from our depression; we ought to use it as a guide to what is wrong with our world. Rather than medicating ourselves to cope with our toxic environment, we ought to change it.

We now have before us a range of the objections to direct manipulation of the mind. It is, I suggest, one or more of these objections that almost invariably underlies the intuition that such manipulation is questionable or problematic (at least when the intuition is not merely a response to the unfamiliarity of the new technologies); that it is preferable to avoid using direct manipulations when alternatives exist. Are these objections sound? The next chapter will be devoted to the consideration of these objections, as well as to the examination of the treatment/enhancement distinction that has played such a significant role in debates over the use of new technologies that increase the power of the mind. As we shall see, considering the treatment/enhancement distinction points us in the direction of two more objections against the use of neuro-technologies: that such technologies are a form of *cheating*, and that they threaten to exacerbate existing *inequalities*.

End notes

1. In transcranial magnetic stimulation, powerful magnetic fields are used to induce electrical changes in the brain. In deep brain stimulation, an electrode is surgically implanted in the brain; the electrode is attached to an external source of current that can then be controlled by the patient. Deep brain stimulation has had encouraging results in the treatment of movement disorders arising from Parkinson's disease.

2. One of the most important contemporary philosophers of authenticity, Charles Taylor, has traced the slow growth of the ideal of finding one's measure within, in his magisterial work *Sources of the Self* (Taylor 1989). On the extent to which village life enmeshed the individual in a network of mutual surveillance and constant enforcement of strict and all-encompassing moral norms, see Darnton (1985).

3. At least that's the case if the antidepressant is an SSRI: a selective serotonin reuptake inhibitor. SSRIs are by far the most commonly prescribed antidepressants, but others are still used. Though different antidepressants work in different ways, this does not affect the point here, which is that none of them work by giving the subject *reasons* to be happy.

4. Of course, there are circumstances in which it *is* appropriate to adopt what Peter Strawson (1962) has famously called "the objective attitude" to another person, at least temporarily: when the person is not responsive to reasons. But adopting the objective attitude is a last resort, a response to a dramatic (if sometimes short-lived) breakdown in humanity. It should not be entered into lightly, with regard to ourselves or to others.

The presumption against direct
manipulation

In the last chapter, we set out the objections that seem to underlie the
presumption in favor of traditional means of changing minds (hereafter, "the presumption"). In this chapter we shall consider these
objections in detail. Before we begin treating them, however, we need
to consider another, more general, question, one that cuts across all the
other objections and across a range of possible neurological interventions. Many people – laypeople, philosophers, bioethicists and neuroscientists – have importantly different responses to actual and
potential neuroscientific (as well as medical) interventions, depending
upon what they are being used *for*. Interventions to *treat* diseases and
impairments are regarded as significantly more permissible (perhaps
even obligatory) than interventions aimed at *enhancing* normal capacities. Treating disease is generally regarded as an intrinsically
worthwhile activity, and we are therefore under a (possibly defeasible)
obligation to engage in it, but enhancing already normal capacities is a
luxury, which is at best permissible, and not obligatory, and at worst
impermissible. Different thinkers make different uses of the treat-
ment/enhancement distinction. For some, it marks the difference
between the kinds of medical interventions which it is incumbent
upon the state to provide, and the kinds of interventions which can
permissibly be bought and sold, but need not be provided as a matter of
justice; for others, it marks the difference between interventions
which are permissible, and those which ought to be banned. Despite
these disagreements, there is a broad consensus that the treatment/
enhancement distinction marks a difference that is morally significant.

The traditional home of the treatment/enhancement distinction is medical ethics. However, it seems just as pertinent to the field of neuroethics. Suppose that the presumption against direct manipulation can be sustained. In that case, these manipulations are to be avoided, whenever possible; they can be used only when they give us the sole, or the sole practicable, means of treating conditions that impose significant suffering on patients (and those close to them). In that case, it follows quite directly that the use of direct manipulations to enhance already normal capacities will always be impermissible. Moreover, if the treatment/enhancement distinction can be sustained, it provides us with additional reasons to doubt the permissibility of enhancements, over and above that provided by the presumption: enhancements constitute a kind of *cheating*, and would exacerbate existing *inequalities*.

ENHANCEMENTS AS CHEATING

Suppose Billy and Beth are both scheduled to sit an important examination. Both are talented students; both are hardworking and conscientious. Both are looking for that extra edge in the exam, since they know that performing well on it will open doors to better employment opportunities. Both therefore avail themselves of the full range of means traditionally employed to achieve success. They both sit practice examinations, look at past papers and talk to people who have already been through the process, seeking advice and helpful hints. But Beth goes further: she takes Ritalin, which is widely used by college students to enhance concentration and to boost performance on problem-solving tasks (Farah 2002; Farah and Wolpe 2004). Her performance is correspondingly better than she would have achieved without the drug. Her final score is a couple of precious percentage marks higher than Billy's, and she has pick of the rewards that come from success at the exam. Billy is normally a gracious loser, but not this time. When he learns that Beth's performance was drug-enhanced, he feels cheated.

Drugs and other biological interventions that enhance sporting performance have received a great deal of attention from ethicists (Mottram 2003; Savulescu *et al.* 2004). But the problems that arise from the use of enhancements of the mind can be expected soon to dwarf those arising from their use on the sports field. With our aging populations, there is a huge potential market for drugs which slow or even reverse the loss of memory and cognitive function typical of dementia. Of course, few people would object to such *treatments* of a tragic disease. But these same drugs may prove useful in *enhancing* the memories of normal adults (Farah 2002; Glannon 2006a). Research into drugs that enhance learning in different ways is also well advanced. The adult brain learns at a slower rate than the child's, and part of the reason seems to be that the child's is more plastic. Some researchers are therefore investigating ways of enhancing learning by increasing neural plasticity. One promising line of work explores the role of gamma-aminobutyric acid (GABA) in normal learning. GABA is a neurotransmitter that plays an inhibitory role in the human brain; in normal skill-acquisition, GABA levels fall, allowing the brain to rewire itself, and thus lay down the pathways that will underlie the skill. Ziemann and his colleagues (2001) have published preliminary results, from studies of human subjects, suggesting that deliberately manipulating GABA levels may increase plasticity, and therefore enhance skill acquisition. Ziemann *et al.* suggest that this might provide us with a therapy to aid the recovery of patients who have suffered some kind of neurological insult. But – if the technique proves safe and effective – it may find a bigger market among normal people looking for that extra edge, or a short cut to new skills and knowledge (Gazzaniga 2005).

Antidepressants are already sometimes used to enhance the lives of individuals who do not meet criteria for any psychiatric disorder. Of course, most people who take such medications look to them for a boost in mood, but, whether as an intended effect or incidentally, antidepressants may also aid them in achieving goals in their work, study and relationships. Small-scale studies of the effects of SSRIs on normal subjects indicate that they make people more cooperative and less critical of others (Knutson *et al.* 1998) – traits which are likely to be attractive to employers. Other studies have confirmed that healthy subjects given antidepressants show greater social affiliative behavior, associated, perhaps paradoxically, with a decrease in submissiveness (Tse and Bond 2002; 2003). In many ways, antidepressants seem tailor-made for achieving the personality profile stereotypically associated with success. And there is evidence (most of it anecdotal) that people taking antidepressants are more successful (Kramer 1993).

But it is easy to see why many people would begrudge them success achieved by pharmaceutical means. Just as it is widely regarded to be cheating to use steroids to achieve athletic success, so we might regard the use of psychopharmaceuticals to enhance memory or concentration as a kind of fraud. Here's one way of justifying this intuition: it is a deeply held principle of modern Western societies that opportunities ought to be distributed according to merit. Thus, jobs ought to be open to talent, not reserved for the members of some hereditary caste, or for the members of a particular race or gender. Rewards should be *deserved*. But Beth does not deserve her greater success. She worked hard, true, and hard work is deserving of praise. She is also talented. But Billy is just as talented, and worked just as hard. He therefore deserves as much success as does Beth. Beth achieved greater success, and perhaps she did it within the rules. But she contravened the *spirit* of the rules. She cheated.

Note that this objection to the use of direct interventions is limited only to their use as enhancements. Were Beth suffering from a disease that prevented her from using her talents, few people would begrudge her the use of psychopharmaceuticals, or whatever the treatment might be. Rather than constituting cheating, her use of psychopharmaceuticals would simply correct for her disadvantage, in the same manner as, say, eyeglasses correct for short-sightedness. It is because Beth uses the drugs to raise herself above her already normal, or better than normal, level that Billy feels that she has cheated. The same point applies to our next objection, the objection from inequality.

INEQUALITY

Enhancements of the mind like those we have just reviewed are already available and may become commonplace. But it is extremely unlikely that they will be available to everyone who wants them anytime soon. The cost of pharmaceuticals puts them beyond the reach of the literally billions of people who live in extreme poverty, mainly in developing countries. Indeed, those drugs which must be taken continuously if mental function is to remain enhanced (such as Ritalin and SSRIs) are out of the financial reach even of much of the population of the developed world, at least in the absence of government subsidy. Other possible neurological enhancement technologies, such as the portable transcranial magnetic stimulation device envisaged by Allan Snyder (Osborne 2003), as a way to bring out the savant-like abilities he and his colleagues believe to be latent in us all (Snyder *et al.* 2003), would probably prove even more expensive. So the new enhancements will be available, in practice, only to the wealthier members of our society.

But these people are *already* better off than average, and their advantages extend to their minds. They may not be more intelligent than their fellow citizens, but they are better placed to develop their intelligence to the full. They send their children to the best schools, where they receive the best education; private tutoring is available to them if it is needed. More importantly, perhaps, they are brought up in an environment in which thought is respected and in which intellectual achievement is seen as a genuine possibility, a possibility for them in particular. It is not a strange world, from which they are alienated or to which they do not think they can ever belong. Their parents are professionals – lawyers, physicians, academics – and the world of professional achievement beckons to them. Moreover, they have better health care and better nutrition, both of which are conducive to higher intelligence. Birth weight, which reflects the nutritional and health status of the mother, is correlated with IQ, even when we restrict our attention to the normal range of weights, thereby excluding children born into extreme poverty (Matte *et al.* 2001).

Higher socio-economic status is already associated with higher intelligence (Hunt 1995). But if neurological enhancements become widely available, we can expect the gap to grow ever greater, both between countries, and between the wealthy and less wealthy citizens within countries. Since intelligence, in turn, is a key to prosperity and therefore further wealth, neurological enhancements are likely to speed up the rate at which a circle, which is already in motion, turns: enhancement leads to greater intelligence and success, which leads to wealth which enables further enhancement. Meanwhile, the less well-off languish in their unenhanced state. Now, there are several reasons to worry about the exacerbated inequalities that these enhancements might produce. First, they might (further) diminish feelings of social solidarity. The rich may not feel that they are in the same boat as the poor, so different are they from one another, and this might translate into a reduced willingness to contribute to the general welfare. They might demand a lowering of tax rates, failing which they might move their assets offshore. They might refuse to contribute to campaigns which aim to alleviate famine and the effects of natural disasters around the world. They may regard the poor as natural slaves (in Aristotle's phrase), who are born to serve their needs. Second, many people regard inequality, at least *undeserved* inequality, as intrinsically undesirable. The wealthy have been lucky: lucky in their genes, lucky in the environment into which they were born and lucky, in our scenario, that they are able to translate their existing advantages into neurological enhancements. Since we do not deserve our luck, we do not deserve the extra advantages it brings; correspondingly, the poor do not deserve their lower status and their lower standard of living.

PROBING THE DISTINCTION

Though most writers on the topic are convinced that a defensible treatment/enhancement distinction can be drawn, there is little agreement as to how best to draw it. There are two main approaches: the distinction can be defended by way of the contrast between disease and non-disease states, or by reference to the notion of species-typical functioning (Jeungst 1998). I shall argue that both these approaches have insurmountable difficulties, and that the treatment/enhancement distinction ought to be abandoned. It cannot, I shall suggest, do the work that writers on the topic hope for it: it cannot provide us with an *independent* standard to which we can appeal to settle moral arguments. Instead, it is already (at best) a thoroughly moralized standard. We ought, therefore, to recognize that it is a moralized standard, and assess it on moral grounds.

Treatment, as the word suggests, might be defined as medical intervention aimed at curing, reversing or halting the progression of diseases and disabilities. On this view, an intervention would count as an enhancement only if it is *not* aimed at treating disease. Unfortunately, the distinction between disease and other undesirable conditions is itself rather unclear. We might hope to define "disease" in terms of alterations of somatic function as a result of non-endogenous elements, where an endogenous element is anything specified in our genome. But – quite apart from the problem, to which we shall return, of making sense of the notion of something being specified in our genome – this won't do. *Normal* functioning is itself dependent upon a range of external elements, from the bacteria which help our digestion and which help maintain the health of our skin and eyes, to the nutrients we need to absorb from the environment in order to remain alive. Now, suppose that Beth is more intelligent than Billy because her "gut flora" enables her to absorb nutrients from food more efficiently, and this has given her a developmental advantage over him. Does Billy have a disease? If he does, it is caused by the *lack* of an external (external, that is, to his genome) element. Perhaps Billy's intelligence is within the normal range, though lower than it might have been. In that case, is medical intervention an enhancement, not a treatment? If we say that it becomes treatment as soon as Billy's IQ falls below the normal range, then, it seems, it is not the disease conception of the distinction to which we are appealing, but the species-typical account.

Part of the problem for the disease-based approach to the treatment/enhancement distinction is that the concepts of disease and disability are far more malleable than proponents are willing to recognize. A "disability" might be regarded as any impairment of functioning which departs far enough from the social norm. What counts as a disability is therefore relative to the norm: dyslexia is a disability only in literate societies (Buchanan *et al.* 2000), and being tone deaf is a disability only in societies which speak a tonal language. Of course, it might be replied that we are only interested in the extent to which an impairment counts as a disability here and now, and that therefore the fact that an impairment would or would not be a disability elsewhere (that it might even be an advantage) is irrelevant. But to appeal to departure from the norm, here and now, is to give up the disease-based defence of the treatment/enhancement distinction in favor of the species-typical conception. Alternatively, we can appeal to our intuitions about disease to defend the distinction. But the treatment/enhancement distinction is supposed to give us a means of evaluating whether a proposed intervention aimed at correcting for an impairment is permissible (or obligatory, or ought to be state-funded, depending upon the account) or not. If we appeal to the notion of disease to defend the distinction, and then appeal to intuition to defend the conception of disease we prefer, we implicitly appeal to intuition to defend the distinction – and in that case we have abandoned the claim that the distinction offers us an independent test of our intuitions. In that case, it is likely that it is in fact our *moral* judgments about the permissibility of intervention that are driving our intuitions about the distinction, rather than the other way round. Indeed, I suspect that that's precisely the case.

There is another, deeper, problem with drawing the distinction between treatment and enhancement on the basis of the disease model. But the problem – that in fact no sense can be made of one term of the contrast, and therefore of the contrast itself – obviously generalizes beyond the disease approach. I shall postpone discussion of it until we have the second major approach to the distinction firmly before us. I turn now to the second popular approach to distinguishing between treatment and enhancement.

The species-typical functioning approach is primarily associated with the work of Norman Daniels (1985; Buchanan *et al.* 2000). Daniels argues that *treatment* is medical intervention aimed at restoring the patient to normal functioning. In this approach, as in the first, disease is invoked, but it does not play a foundational role. Instead, what counts as disease or disability is defined by reference to normal or species-typical functioning. *Treatment* is medical intervention aimed at *disease or disability*, where *disease or disability* is adverse departure from normal functioning. An attractive element of this account of the distinction is that it gives us a natural explanation of why enhancement is less important, from a moral point of view, than treatment. Treatment aims to restore individuals to normal functioning, not because the normal is somehow intrinsically good in itself, but because normal functioning is necessary for equal opportunity. In Daniels' account of the aims of a just health system, health care is designed to restore and maintain individual's access to their share of "the normal range of opportunities (or plans of life) reasonable people would choose in a given society" (Buchanan *et al.* 2000: 122). Since equal opportunity is (extremely plausibly) itself a valuable good, worth protecting, restoring the ability of individuals to pursue it is itself worthwhile.

The normal functioning view aims to restore individuals to their baseline capacity, the capacity that is *naturally* theirs. Diseases are departures from this state; so are impairments due to past unjust social practices and discrimination. But simply being less intelligent than average is not, on this account, a disease or impairment that we are morally obliged to treat. My lack of intelligence, or of good looks, or athletic ability, is simply the result of my bad luck in the natural lottery, and such bad luck does not impose any obligations on others. We ought to restore people to the natural baseline that is theirs, in virtue, presumably, of their genetic endowment. Raising them above that baseline is not treatment, but enhancement.

Obviously, this view depends upon our being able to identify a natural (or "natural," as Buchanan *et al.* 2000 would have it) baseline from which disease or disability is a departure. The problem with this approach is simply that we can't do this. The very idea is biological nonsense. To show this, it is necessary to make a short excursion into the way in which genes function in building phenotypes – the observable characteristics of organisms.

All commentators, including Buchanan *et al.* (2000) reject the idea of genetic determinism. That is, we all now recognize that our genome does not simply encode our traits. The relationship between possession of a gene and the development of a phenotypic trait is a complex and mediated one. To be sure, there are some genes and gene-complexes that lead to predictable, usually adverse, consequences across the range of accessible environments. But most genes, and pretty much all genes for traits that are within the normal range, do not work like that. Instead, their phenotypic effects are the result of the way they interact with the environment and with each other.

Despite the fact that everyone rejects determinism and accepts interactionism, many people continue to speak of the genome as a "blueprint," which "encodes" traits; and about the natural baseline of capacities which is ours in virtue of our genome. None of these ideas make any sense, in the light of interactionism.

The effect of any particular gene on the phenotype (leaving aside those that cause the relatively few congenital impairments, such as cystic fibrosis and Down's syndrome, which produce adverse effects in all accessible environments – though even they merely complicate the picture, they do not falsify it) is the product of the way it interacts with the environment external to it, where that environment includes other genes. Not only do genes not have any determinate impact outside that environment, we cannot even assign to them a *tendency* outside a particular environment. The gene associated with high intelligence in environment X may be a gene that is associated with low intelligence in environment Y – and the two environments may not be all that different. In more technical terms, the *norm of reaction* for a given genotype is never *additive*. A norm of reaction is the graph representing the variation of a given phenotypic trait as a function of environmental variation. For instance, a norm of reaction might plot the predicted adult height of a plant (with its genotype held fixed) as a function of one environmental variable such as sunlight, or nitrogen in the soil. The norm of reaction is additive when the relationship between the environmental variable and the trait is linear: an increase in the variable causing a proportional increase or decrease in the variable and a decrease having the opposite effect. It is non-additive if the relationship is not so straightforward: if, for instance, increasing the amount of sunlight increases the height of the plant up to a certain point, beyond which further increases actually *decrease* height. All norms of reaction studied so far have been non-additive, and the overwhelming likelihood is that this will hold true for all possible norms of reaction (including the norms of reaction for those congenital traits mentioned above) (Levy 2004).

Thus, there is no natural (or even "natural") baseline against which we can measure departures. Because phenotypic traits vary as a function of the way the environment is structured, because they do not have *any* determinate effect, not even a tendency, outside a particular environment, talk of what a person's capacities would have been in the absence of a disease is either entirely empty, or it presupposes a determinate environment. If we are presupposing an environment, though, then it is permissible to ask why *that* environment. Suppose that Jorge and Joaquin both apply for a job, and are given a battery of tests to measure their intelligence and problem-solving abilities. Joaquin outperforms Jorge, and is offered the job. In Daniels' account, Jorge has no legitimate complaint, if the difference between their achievement is not due to a history of unjust discrimination. Let's assume that's the case; let's assume that neither belongs to a group that is discriminated against, either now or in the recent past. Nevertheless, suppose (realistically) that Joaquin's advantages – his better education and health care – are partly responsible for his higher achievement. What reason do we have to say that Jorge's level of achievement reflects a natural baseline, given that in a range of accessible environments he would have achieved more (and in a further range he would have achieved less)? Why take *this* environment as natural?

One possible move at this point would be to abandon the claim that the environment in question is natural, and therefore the correlative claim that the baseline is natural. We could instead look for a normatively defined baseline: we might say that the capacities that an individual deserves are those that they would possess in a *just* environment. Indeed, something like this kind of view may account for whatever surface plausibility Daniels' definition of the baseline possesses. In a Nozickian (1974) account of justice in distribution, any distribution of assets, no matter how unequal, is just so long as the history of acquisition of assets is not unjust, where injustice in acquisition is defined essentially in terms of theft, fraud and so on. This view has the counterintuitive implication that gross inequality, indeed absolute poverty, is not unjust so long as it is inherited poverty (and the poverty cannot be traced back to fraud, theft or other crimes). Daniels' definition of the baseline, according to which only certain classes of environmental influences count as illegitimate, commits him to an analogous, though less extreme, view of justice in distribution of traits. So long as there was no injustice, as Daniels defines injustice, in the history of acquisition of these traits, we are to take their distribution as just, *even though there are possible environments in which the distribution of traits would have been radically different.* In other words, Daniels is committed to regarding the actual environment as just, or at least just enough. This is a normative assessment: environments are regarded as just or unjust not on the basis of their "naturalness," but on the basis of the distribution of traits.

Now, this is a coherent view. Note, however, that like the disease-based account of the treatment/enhancement distinction, this view does not give us what defenders of the distinction want from it: an *independent* (because natural and non-normative) standard to which we can appeal in making moral judgments. Instead, it is itself a normative view through and through. If that is a weakness, however, from the point of view of those who are looking for an independent standard, it is also a strength from another point of view. Once we have the normative commitments of the view on the table, we can begin to assess them on normative grounds. We can begin the debate over whether gross inequality in capacities is itself unjust, when neither those who are better off nor those who are worse off have done anything to deserve their relative abilities, or whether such inequalities are only unjust when they are the product of a grossly unjust history. As I have argued elsewhere against Nozick (Levy 2002a), given that no one deserves the conditions into which they are born, no one deserves their relative advantages, and for that reason we have a (*ceteris paribus*) obligation to correct for gross inequality. In any case, once we see that the treatment/enhancement distinction rests upon a normative base, we ought to abandon it, as a focus for discussion and as a reference point in debate, and instead direct our attention to the plausibility of the normative commitments upon which it rests.

In other words, in assessing the suggested baseline against which to judge whether an intervention is an enhancement or a treatment, we need to ask ourselves whether the causes of the capacities in question are themselves just, as well as whether the resulting distribution of capacities is ethically permissible. Since our topic is cognitive enhancement, it is worth spending a little time reviewing the ways in which social and political choices influence the distribution of cognitive capacities. We have already glimpsed some of the ways in which our environmental transformations alter cognition by offloading it onto external props, in the section on the extended mind. Here I shall simply mention some of the more prosaic environmental factors which are relevant to intelligence.

Measured intelligence has risen consistently over the past century, across the world. The increase has varied, with some groups showing only *relatively* modest gains of around three points per decade, while others increased at twice the rate. But the effect (known as the Flynn effect, after the political scientist who first documented it (Flynn 1994)) is nearly ubiquitous. Now, it is still somewhat mysterious what underlies these gains, but we can exclude genetic changes at once. There may be selection pressures for increased intelligence, but the effect is far greater than such pressures could explain (given the slow reproduction rate of our species). Three factors have plausibly been proposed as explaining the rise: better nutrition, better education and alterations in the environment (Neisser 1997). We know, from studies of animal models, that simply enriching the environment in which the young are raised has a significant impact upon problem-solving abilities. Rats raised in an enriched environment perform significantly better at maze navigation tasks than rats raised in an impoverished environment (impoverished, that is, in terms of stimuli like toys and nooks to explore); rats from strains bred to be "maze dull" outperform rats bred to be "maze bright" if the former are raised in an enriched environment while the latter are not (Kaplan 2000).

Holding that the current distribution of resources in the world, or within one country, represents a natural baseline against which to measure departures is arbitrary and morally unjustifiable. We can be sure that if the distribution of resources were altered, some individuals would do better, and in some cases far better, than they do now (and some worse). We do not know if there is an optimal distribution of resources or an optimal environment for increasing people's cognitive abilities, but we do have every reason to think that we are nowhere near to achieving such a distribution (on the contrary; there is evidence that in some places IQ has fallen marginally, and that environmental changes are to blame (Teasedale and Owen 2005)). It is therefore morally inappropriate to take any current distribution as a baseline, as well as scientifically unjustifiable.

The inability to set a baseline against which to measure normal functioning will obviously prove fatal to an account like Daniels', but its effects spread beyond this particular approach to the treatment/enhancement distinction. In fact, without a baseline to appeal to, *all* conceptions of enhancement, at least all which look to the distinction for an independent test of permissibility, are in trouble. Medical interventions that are commonly regarded as treatments, as well as those that are regarded as enhancements, increase the capacity or well-being of patients. In that, minimal, sense, they are all enhancements (when they are successful). For a very wide range of interventions, it is true to say that the subject would be better off as a result than they would be in their absence. This counterfactual claim can't pick out enhancements, because it is true of too wide a range of interventions. My intelligence might be enhanced by, say, transcranial magnetic stimulation, in the sense that I might become capable of savant-like feats of which I am currently incapable. But my intelligence can also be enhanced by learning: if I devote myself to a program of arithmetical tricks, I can no doubt improve my ability, perhaps remarkably (if I am prepared to spend enough time and energy on the project).

We could, of course, always decide to *set* a baseline by reference to non-moral criteria. We might, for instance, choose one standard deviation below the average (or the mean, or the median) as the baseline: anyone with a capacity or characteristic falling below this threshold would have the right to have it raised. But if we were to do so, we would be engaged in a deliberate act of choice, and should see ourselves as such. The grounds for the choice would not be solely natural; we would not have identified an Archimedean point which really separates obligatory treatment from supererogatory or impermissible enhancement. The grounds for our choice would instead be moral and political. These are, I suggest, precisely the right grounds upon which we should be making these choices; indeed, as I have argued, they are probably the grounds upon which, implicitly, we *currently* divide interventions into "treatments" and "enhancements." It may be that instead of setting a baseline, it would be better to ask ourselves whether, in the absence of intervention (and holding the rest of the environment fixed) the impairment in question is significant enough to warrant the intervention. Once we see ourselves as making a moral choice, the debate over the right grounds for this choice can begin in earnest; at present the attempt to identify an illusory baseline merely obscures the genuine grounds for intervention.

Abandoning the treatment/enhancement distinction in favour of an importance of intervention test will also allow us to capture the undoubted fact that many interventions which intuitively fall on the enhancement side of the divide are far more urgent than others which are traditionally regarded as treatment. Enriching the environment of children (in the manner of "Headstart" programs) who can otherwise be expected to perform at a lower level than their wealthier peers is surely more important than treating certain allergies, when the latter do not have a significant impact on the quality of life of sufferers (which is not to say that we ought not to treat these allergies; as well as asking how significant is the impairment, we also need to know how extensive are our resources, in order to assess whether we ought to treat them). In any case, and no matter how these moral debates are settled, we must abandon the treatment/enhancement distinction as an independent basis for moral judgment.

ASSESSING THE CRITICISMS

How ought we to respond to the criticisms of direct manipulations of the mind which apparently motivate the presumption against such manipulations? In the rest of the chapter, I shall consider the objections one-by-one. It might be helpful, however, to signal the conclusion of this overview here. I think that we ought to concede that at least some of the points made by the critics are weighty, and that we ought therefore to hesitate before we use direct manipulations. We ought, that is, to assess *each* possible use to see whether it might not be preferable to avoid it, for one or other of the reasons offered. But, I shall argue, the larger claim that these reasons are widely seen as supporting – that traditional means are always preferable to direct manipulations, and that there is always a cost associated with the use of the latter – is false. Though there are reasons to be cautious in the use of direct manipulations, I shall claim, there is no reason to think that each and every use of such means is somehow suspect. Very often direct manipulations are perfectly permissible, and sometimes even preferable to traditional means of changing minds; we can therefore use them, on ourselves or on others, in good conscience. In other words, we ought to drop the presumption in favour of traditional means, and instead engage in the hard work of assessing each proposed use of direct manipulations on its own merits.

Authenticity

Authenticity, as we defined it in the previous chapter, is the search for a way of life that is distinctively one's own. The authentic individual looks within, to find his or her own "measure" (Taylor 1991). It is this conception of authenticity that motivates worries like those expressed by Elliott (1998); that the use of direct manipulations risks loss of contact between the individual and his or her authentic self. However, Elliott overlooks the fact that authenticity need not only be inward-looking. We can achieve authenticity by looking within, but we can also achieve it by *self-creation*. We do not have to remain content with the kinds of people we are; we can seek to change ourselves, and we can do this within the horizon of the ideal of authenticity.

The conception of authenticity emphasized by Taylor and Elliott looks to the preexisting self to set standards. In this conception, we live authentically to the extent to which our lives are expressions of who we, most deeply, really are. But there are other notions of authenticity, both in the philosophical literature and influencing everyday life well beyond the bounds of academic philosophy. The notion of authenticity associated, above all, with Jean-Paul Sartre is importantly different, even opposed, to the notion presupposed by Taylor and Elliott. Authenticity for Sartre (1956) *cannot* consist in expression of a pre-given self, for there *is* no pre-given self. Sartre's argument for this claim doesn't bear up under examination; nevertheless the claim itself is true. What *could* constitute my essence, to which I am bound to conform? Some people continue to claim that personality is encoded in the genome, but as we have just seen, in reviewing the way that genes actually interact with the environment to produce phenotypes, that's simply false. A gene that contributes to the development of a personality trait – say, a tendency to introspection – might have contributed instead to a quite different trait like extroversion in a different context. An example: recently Terrie Moffitt and colleagues have investigated the relationship between genes and violence. They found that men who possessed a particular allele of one gene *and* who were maltreated as children were significantly more likely to exhibit violent behavior than men who possessed either the gene alone, or who had been maltreated but lacked the gene (Caspi *et al.* 2002). It is clear that the allele is not a "gene for" violence, at least in the sense that having it does not predispose the person toward violence. It is a gene for violence *given* a particular environmental context.

It might be replied that the fact that personality traits are not encoded in the genome is irrelevant. Authenticity might be understood to mean, not harmony with a *pre-given* self – a self that is innate in us when we are born – but with the self *as it is*, however it comes to be. Those mistreated adults who also possessed the relevant allele were not *innately* disposed to violence, but they *were* disposed to violence. The personality they came to possess was, authentically, theirs, and authenticity demands that they conform to it somehow (not by expressing their violent disposition, one hopes, but by expressing other aspects of their essential self, or by sublimating their violence and channelling it into socially benign activities). So defenders of authenticity as harmony with a given self need not commit themselves to biologically implausible views.

However, we cannot contain the interactionist point in the suggested manner; we can't limit it to childhood development without being entirely arbitrary. Why should our personality at, say, eighteen be sacrosanct? In fact, people do continue to change throughout their lives, sometimes subtly, sometimes quite drama- tically. And very often we do not think there is anything wrong with such changes. Consider the cases of Ruby and Elly. Both seek treat- ment for longstanding, though minor, depression (I stipulate that the depression is minor in order to avoid winning the argument cheaply: even critics of direct manipulation usually agree that we should use it if it is the only way to avoid significant suffering). Ruby's doctor prescribes an SSRI, and after several weeks of taking it Ruby feels her mood lift. She is more outgoing and confident than ever before, and both her professional and social life improve. Friends and family remark on the change in her. Elly's doctor, meanwhile, suggests treating her depression without chemicals. In fact, she suggests that Elly take up an exercise regime. Elly begins jogging and going to the gym, and in a few weeks her mood begins to improve. Six months later, she is doing as well as Ruby; once again the change in her is remarkable (on the effects of exercise on depression see Blumenthal *et al.* 1999; Salmon 2001).

The first thing to notice is that very few people will be inclined to accuse Elly of inauthenticity. Sometimes it is appropriate to worry that a friend is acting out of character. We might be anxious for her welfare because we think she's far outside her comfort zone. We might think that either she hasn't really changed at all – she just pretending, perhaps well enough to fool herself – or that the change is so shallow that it's unlikely to be sustained. We fear that the time is near when the mask will fall; she will be revealed for who she really is, and that when that happens she will suffer shame, humiliation, or worse. But these fears are predicated on the belief or suspicion that the change is neither deep nor permanent. If she *has* changed, then we can't accuse her of inauthenticity. Since there is no inner essence to which she is compelled, indeed *able*, to conform, there is no reason at all to accuse someone who changes of inauthenticity (so long as they satisfy the Sartrean conditions on authenticity: roughly, they refuse to make any excuses for their choices, but instead take responsibility for them). Elly's change might be entirely authentic; similarly, we are not generally inclined to accuse those who go through religious conversions or similar life-changing epiphanies – the man who leaves his desk job and his staid existence to perform famine relief in the third world; the woman who leaves her husband and the suburbs to live in a lesbian relationship in a commune, or what have you – of inauthenticity, no matter how great the apparent change in their lifestyle and personality.

But if we should withhold the charge of inauthenticity so far as Elly is concerned, then why should we treat Ruby any differently? Of course, we might worry that Ruby's transformation is less secure than Elly's. But there is no reason to assume that that's the case. Indeed, it may be that it is *more* secure: taking a pill once daily is surely easier (side effects permitting) than adhering to an exercise regime. We may think that the difference in the *means* of transformation equates to a moral difference: altering one's neurochemistry is interfering with the self in a way that qualifies as inauthentic, whereas exercise is not. But that won't stand up to examination either. In fact, exercise is successful at relieving depression, at least in part, because it functions (in much the same way as antidepressants) to increase the amount of serotonin available for transmitting signals across neural synapses.

Elliott, as we saw, argued that if Prozac gives us a new personality, we become inauthentic: the new personality is not truly *ours* (1998: 182). But that's simply false: it *is* ours. It's different to our old personality, to be sure, but so what? Why should we be bound to that old personality? What grounds do we have for telling Ruby that though she *feels* cheerful and successful, she's not really? Cheerful and successful is as cheerful and successful feels and does. Elliott's charge apparently rests on the romantic, and biologically implausible, idea that we have an innate personality (DeGrazia 2000). Once we realize that selves are continually recreated and transformed, throughout life, we shall lose the urge to accuse someone of inauthenticity on the grounds of character change alone.

As a matter of fact, at least some people who take antidepressants *experience* the transformation as authentic. Peter Kramer (1993) reports many instances where patients identify with the self they experience while on antidepressants. Thus, when he took them off the medication they would sometimes return voicing an odd complaint: "I'm not myself." Kramer notes how strange the claim sounds. "But who had she been all those years if not herself?" (1993: 19). Nevertheless, the patients' claim is better grounded than Elliott's. The true self is the self that *actually* exists; so long as the alteration is sustained and sustainable, and goes deep enough – so long, that is, as we can genuinely attribute the new personality to them – then there is no reason not to regard it as theirs *authentically*.[1]

Self-knowledge and personal growth

Giving someone serotonin is not offering them a reason to be cheerful, nor is to helping them to understand what made them depressed in the first place, but giving them a course of psychotherapy might enable them to come to understand themselves better. Compare two agents cured of their depression, one by psychotherapy and one by antidepressants. The first will possess significant knowledge that the second will not: knowledge about himself (about his history and about the structure of his psyche), and about his relationship to the world (about the kinds of life events which caused or contributed to causing his depression, and about their true significance and the extent to which depression is a rational response to them). The person cured by direct manipulation knows none of that: they know only that they feel better as a result of taking a drug. Since self-knowledge is surely a valuable good, we have reason to prefer traditional means of changing minds to non-traditional.

Unlike the charge of inauthenticity, I think this charge has some bite. We really do sometimes have reason to prefer traditional means of changing minds to non-traditional, on the grounds that the former are more conducive to self-knowledge than the latter. However, this fact does nothing to justify a *general* presumption in favour of traditional means, for two reasons. First, it will frequently be the case that we have no reason to prefer traditional means to non-traditional on the grounds of self-knowledge; second, and more significantly, we shall sometimes have reasons for precisely the *opposite* preference, on these same grounds.

People who seek treatment for depression and mental illness may lack self-knowledge, in the sense that they may not understand what, in their personal history, caused their problems. But that's far from always being true. Sometimes, they understand the sources of their problems already; the PTSD sufferer is an obvious example. Consider the patient that Kramer calls Lucy. Freedman (1998), arguing against the use of direct manipulations, believes that Lucy's problems stem from "false beliefs, [that] are grounded in something like a *mistake in reasoning*" (1998: 143). Lucy falsely interprets her boyfriend's changing the channel on the TV as a rejection of her; therapy, Freedman claims, should be aimed at helping her to see her error. But Freedman's interpretation of the case is wrong, as Kramer's description of Lucy makes clear. Lucy is intelligent and globally rational; she recalls her personal history clearly and she knows that her over-sensitivity to rejection is a product of this history. She does not, as Freedman claims, need help to see that her response is irrational; she already *knows* it is irrational. That's what brings her to treatment in the first place.

So Lucy does not enter therapy in order to acquire true beliefs about the source of her problems. She understands herself and her reactions perfectly well. She wants help preventing a response of hers that she, rightly, regards as irrational and unjustified. She does not need nor seek self-knowledge.

Suppose, however, that a course of psychotherapy would be just as effective in helping Lucy, and suppose, plausibly, that psychotherapy would contribute to her self-knowledge (even if not of knowledge regarding the origin, in her personal history, of her pattern of response). Perhaps she will acquire a *richness* of understanding that she doesn't currently possess; suppose, further, that she is unlikely to gain this understanding from antidepressants. In that case, there is indeed, in her case, a reason to favor psychotherapy over antidepressants (other things being equal). Self-knowledge *is* a great good. However, there are reasons to think that things are rarely likely to be equal. Though self-knowledge is a good, it is one good among others. Life is short, and we have time and opportunity only to pursue some of the many valuable goods on offer. If someone has a choice between, say, pursuing self-knowledge and investing the time and energy in their scientific work instead, this seems to be a choice they are entitled to make. There is no reason why someone cannot rationally and ethically choose to pursue a valuable good other than self-knowledge.[2] And it will frequently be the case that this is the kind of choice confronting people contemplating different kinds of treatment. Psychotherapy is time-consuming (as well as expensive). Freudian psychotherapy is notoriously lengthy, extending over many years. It therefore has high opportunity costs. Indeed, on the overwhelmingly plausible assumption that there are routes to self-knowledge other than psychotherapy, it may be that choosing the expensive and time-consuming option of psychotherapy, rather than direct interventions that are quicker and cheaper, involves a sacrifice of opportunities for self-knowledge.[3]

Second, it is neither true that psychotherapy, even if it is successful, is always a means to self-knowledge, nor that psychopharmacology is never a means to self-knowledge. Ironically, on some measures the depressed seem to have a more accurate self-perception than the non-depressed (Alloy and Abramson 1979;

Alloy 1995). To that extent, treatment of depression is, from the point of view of truth alone, a mixed blessing: it leads the subject to self-knowledge on some scores, and to greater illusion on others. Moreover, psychotherapy does not always focus on the true sources of a problem. Instead, it uses whatever seems to work: this might mean getting to the root of the problem, or might mean employing non-truth-conducive strategies for controlling it. Some (successful) methods employed by cognitive-behavioural therapists, for instance, are relatively mechanical in form: for instance, treating phobias by teaching subjects to associate the conditioned stimuli with relaxing scenarios. Psychotherapy is not a synonym for truth-seeking.

Moreover, as Kramer notes, psychopharmacology can itself be conducive to self-knowledge. Indeed, it seems to have helped Lucy herself to achieve a greater degree of understanding of her own behavior. Lucy experienced significant side effects, and was not on antidepressants for very long. But – Kramer claims – her brief period of medication gave her a new perspective on her behavior; as a result "[s]he became more open to examining her responses to rejection" (Kramer 1993: 103). Patients may be better able to examine their own emotions and reactions when they are no longer paralyzed by depression; direct means can be means to truth, as well as to healing. It is worth noting that there is growing evidence that patients respond best to a combination of psychotherapy and psycho-pharmacology (Keitner and Cardemil 2004); it may be that psycho-pharmacology enables psychotherapy, precisely because it makes the pursuit of truth easier.

In any case, though it is certainly possible to pursue self-understanding when we pursue mental health, why should we always prefer means to the latter that also provide the former? People do not usually think that if we can choose between two treatments for an entirely somatic illness – kidney disease, say – we should always choose the one that offers the incidental benefit of self-understanding. Suppose kidney disease could be given a talking cure, in which we explored the origins and cause of the disease. We would still choose the kind of treatment for the disease by reference to criteria like cost, effectiveness and convenience. Why should mental illness be any different?

There are sometimes reasons to prefer psychopharmaceuticals to psychotherapy on the grounds of self-knowledge; probably more often, there will be little to choose between them on these grounds. That is not to say, however, that we ought not to be alert to people using direct manipulations inappropriately. Psychic suffering does indeed sometimes offer us an opportunity for self-knowledge (and indeed for other kinds of knowledge as well: our emotional distress may be a response to problems in our environment, and not just in the ways we respond to it). Normal psychic pain ought not to be medicated away; it is only when we have good grounds to judge that our emotional distress far outruns its cause that we ought to be seeking to cure it. Our troubles can also be opportunities; opportunities for knowledge and for growth. As Manninen (2006) reminds us, we ought to be especially careful in making these judgments for others, particularly for children. It is likely that coming to terms with their share of emotional pain is a necessary condition of maturity; we do them no favors in medicating away their pains too quickly.

But the fact that normal pain offers us an opportunity for learning and for growth does not entail that we can never morally and rationally choose to medicate it away. Knowledge is only one good among others, and we can rationally trade it off for one or more of these other goods; it may even be that we can ethically and rationally make this choice on behalf of our children. Moreover, we ought not to see the claim that treating psychic pain is sometimes inappropriate as applying only to direct manipulations. Some kinds of psychotherapy, too, may be used prematurely to alleviate normal distress. In any case, though there are cases in which we should hesitate to use direct manipulations, on ourselves or on others, because we are better off working through our distress than in curing it quickly, this fact does nothing to justify the presumption. In many cases direct manipulations are appropriate; sometimes they are clearly preferable to traditional means of changing minds precisely because they *facilitate*, rather than preventing, self-knowledge and personal growth.

Mechanization of the self

Some of the points made above with regard to both authenticity and to self-knowledge generalize to the question of the mechanization of the self. That is, some of the traditional means of changing minds mechanize the self to just as great an extent as the new neuroetherapies do. Some psychotherapies, we have seen, seek to manipulate the self rather than to approach it via argument (think, for instance, of the technique of desensitizing patients to the object of their phobias); some traditional means of treating depression and mental illness are every bit as mechanistic as antidepressants. Recall Ruby and Elly once more: neither sought to alleviate their depression by reviewing reasons to be cheerful; rather both sought to alter their neurochemistry, one by antidepressants, and the other by exercise. Why should suspicion fall upon one means of changing minds and not the other?

It may be that the suspicion which falls upon direct manipulations has its source in the illegitimate transfer of intuitions regarding some kinds of manipulations, in cases where they are genuinely problematic, to others in which they are not. It is surely (defeasibly) wrong to manipulate the minds of other people without their knowledge. Putting antidepressants in someone's coffee is disrespectful of their autonomy, even in many cases in which they would clearly benefit from the antidepressants. It is also (defeasibly) wrong to override someone's wishes. Both of these are instances of paternalism, and paternalism always requires special justification. We are justified in acting paternalistically (roughly) only when the agent's autonomy is genuinely and significantly compromised, such that they are not able to act in their own best interests, and they have also not planned for this loss of autonomy, for instance by making an advance directive while competent. Paternalism is also often justified when someone poses a significant risk of harm to others. But there is a legitimate presumption against paternalism: we need to be quite sure that someone's autonomy is significantly compromised or that they are a genuine risk to others before we intervene. Hence our justified resistance to manipulations which lend themselves to paternalistic treatment.

The history of psychiatry contains a number of shameful chapters in which direct manipulations – electro-convulsive therapy (ECT), lobotomy and drugs – have been used for social control rather than for cures, and in which people were treated as things. But it doesn't follow, from the fact that direct manipulations have a shameful history in psychiatry, that such means cannot be used in an ethically appropriate manner or that traditional treatments are always superior. The same direct manipulations that can be used coercively or paternalistically can be used rationally, by agents themselves, to expand and defend their autonomy and not to undermine it. Sometimes agents experience significant distress as a result of an enduring condition that does not have rational content, or in which the symptoms outrun any rational content. Some examples:

> Depression can be (to employ terms that are no longer fashionable) endogenous, rather than exogenous; that is, rather than being caused by genuinely distressing life-events, it can be without rational explanation (or be much deeper and more persistent than triggering events justify).
>
> Obsessive-Compulsive Disorder (OCD) is always without rational content, and is typically recognized as such by the sufferer. It might be rational to check that the stove is off once, or even twice, but, unless something has happened to make rechecking appropriate, it is not rational to go back a fourth or a fifth time. OCD sufferers, who are generally globally rational and may even be highly intelligent, appreciate this fact as clearly as anyone. Yet they feel an almost overpowering urge to check and recheck: to check lights and stoves and doors; to engage in rituals

that stave off feelings of anxiety, sometimes even to inflict harm on themselves. OCD seems to share a great deal of phenomenology and symptomology with other disorders on the impulsive-compulsive spectrum: Tourette's syndrome, kleptomania and some paraphilias and impulse control disorders are similarly characterized by an impulse to perform an action, which may be ego-dystonic, followed by an increasing sense of tension which can only be relieved by repeating the action.

(Skodol and Oldham 1996)

Many delusions have causes that do not rationalize them. Sufferers from the monothematic delusions profess a false belief, which they cling to in face of the evidence and which they will not acknowledge is false. In other ways, however, they may remain globally rational. A sufferer from Capgras's delusion, for example, believes that people close to them – family or close friends – have been replaced by replicas: alien invaders, spirits, robots, or whatever else their cultural beliefs might suggest as potential candidates. Yet they remain rational in other areas of their lives. Indeed, delusional patients are sometimes able to appreciate the absurdity of their delusion, acknowledging that if they heard their story from someone else, they would find it hard to believe.

(Alexander, Stuss and Benson 1979)

These illnesses differ from one another in one respect that is central to our discussion: the degree to which sufferers have *insight* into their condition. Depressed patients typically lack insight into their depression; they take their feelings of worthlessness and hopelessness to be justified by their capacities and their situation. Sufferers from monothematic delusion have a little, but only a little, more insight: they may recognize that their delusion is bizarre, and that they would disbelieve anyone who professed it. Sufferers from OCD may have comprehensive insight into their condition: they may recognize that their rituals are senseless, and may even understand their causes as well as anyone.

Degree of insight matters because it often correlates, roughly, with the degree of paternalism represented by a potential intervention. If a patient has insight into his or her condition, they may request treatment and cooperate with the measures recommended. If they lack insight, they may resist treatment; in these cases treatment is appropriate only if it satisfies the conditions that justify paternalism (for instance: the patient is not autonomous and the intervention has a reasonable chance of restoring their autonomy, or the patient is a danger to themselves or others). Now, as a matter of fact, psychotherapy has been shown to be effective in treating some sufferers from all the above conditions. Cognitive-behavioral therapy (CBT) is the treatment of choice for OCD; alone in milder cases and combined with medication in more severe. It is also often very effective for depression. CBT is less useful for delusions, but even here some successes have been recorded in treating medication-resistant delusions (e.g. Valmaggia *et al.* 2005). But is there a presumption in favor of such treatments for these conditions, other things being equal?

Many of the things we said about self-knowledge are applicable to the question at hand. When a response to the world has a rational content that is commensurate with triggering events, it is prima facie disrespectful to manipulate the mind to moderate the response, even if doing so is in the interests of the patient. Emotional responses are cognitive responses, when they are operating properly, which allow us to orient ourselves to the significance of an event, and which appropriately guide our exploration of it (Jones 2004). They prompt us to ask the right questions, and to respond in the right kinds of ways. The man whose wife dies *should* feel devastated; if he doesn't (and the relationship was not itself pathological) then we have good reason to think less of him, or of his mental capacities. He doesn't understand what the death of an intimate partner *means*, what is its proper place in human life and in his life in particular, if he does not respond with something approaching despair, at least for some period of time. Someone who medicated or hypnotized him so that he felt indifferent to the loss – or merely upset by it – would prevent him from appreciating its significance. They would harm him, by preventing him from properly understanding the unfolding narrative of his life.

But in cases in which the content of the emotional response is excessively disproportionate to the stimulus, manipulation may not be disrespectful. Suppose that the feeling of despair is not a response to life events, or that it is a response that is far out of proportion to the objective import of the stressor that brought on the episode. Though it is true, as Freedman says, that emotional responses are in principle justifiable, it does not follow that each emotional response is *justified*, or even that it is seen by the agent whose response it is as a rational response to eliciting events. Return to Lucy's case. Lucy is a rational agent, as rational as you or me. She simply has some emotional responses that are irrational (so do I; so, I'm willing to bet, do you). If this is correct, Freedman's description of her is misleading. Freedman claims that Lucy thinks her feelings of rejection, every time her boyfriend changes the channel, are justified. But this is extremely unlikely; if Lucy is as rational as I claim, then she cannot think that changing the channel *is* rejection. Indeed, if this is what she thought, she would have been unlikely to have made her way to Kramer's clinic. It is far more likely that Lucy knows that her response is irrational, but she can't help having it. She might well use just this kind of language: "I know it doesn't mean anything, but I can't help seeing it as a rejection." She does not, as Freedman claims, need help to see that her response is irrational; she already *knows* it is irrational. That's what brings her to treatment in the first place.

In that case, it seems quite appropriate – with, and only with, Lucy's informed consent, of course – to treat her depression using "merely mechanical" means. We bypass her rational faculties, but we do so to treat an illness that itself, by her own reckoning, bypasses reason. We should always treat people's affective responses with the respect they deserve, and in this case they deserve little respect. Lucy sufferers from an illness, rather than from, say, an idiosyncratic way of viewing the world. Though we are obligated to respect people's rational reactions, we are not obligated to respect their irrational responses – not when *they* acknowledge the irrationality.

The endogenous/exogenous distinction is somewhat crude. There are probably few "pure" case of endogenous depression, entirely uncaused by life events or external circumstances (indeed, as the considerations in favour of the extended mind illustrate, we cannot draw any hard-and-fast internal/external distinction). Nevertheless, so long as we are aware of its limitations, we can justifiably invoke it. I suggest the following principle: *to the extent that depression is endogenous*, there is no presumption against treating it in ways that bypass the rational faculties of the agent. Almost all real cases of depression are mixed; they are responses, in part, to real life events. To the extent that they are, there is a presumption in favor of taking the response seriously. This might translate into using talk therapy *as well as* pharmacological treatment, or in some other way acknowledging the (partial) rationality of the depression. Even so, if pharmacological intervention is the only practical method of treating it, or if psychotherapy involves costs – in money, energy or time – that the patient is unwilling to pay, then we ought not to withhold the most effective and efficient treatment from them.

Suppose (plausibly, given the details of the case) that Lucy's depression is a mixture of endogenous and exogenous factors. How should we treat it? Is there an obligation to supplement psycho-pharmacology with psychotherapy? As we have already noted, Freud believed that it was not enough to know the source of one's neuroses; you had to be able to properly appreciate the merely abstract knowledge, by working through it. If Lucy enters psychotherapy, she might be able to work through her problems, and alter the interpretive frame through which she sees others' actions. No doubt, treating her in this manner respects her as a human being; perhaps it is *more* respectful than the alternative of giving her antidepressants (alone). Even if that's the case, however, even if psychotherapy is more respectful than direct manipulation, it doesn't follow that direct manipulation would be disrespectful of her as a rational being.

She is able, rationally, to *ask* for antidepressants. She wants to bring her avowed and rational assessment of her boyfriend's actions into line with her emotional responses. Precisely *because* emotions are partly cognitive, because they are in principle open to rational justification, Lucy can see that her response is irrational, and take steps to alter it. If she chooses biochemical means, rather than psychotherapy, she does not thereby step outside the space of reasons. She is reinforcing herself as a rational being, not abdicating rationality. The *aim* of psychiatric treatment, no matter the means, is to restore the patient to full rationality, whether that means allowing her to come to see her former beliefs and responses as irrational or, as in Lucy's case, forestalling a response whose irrationality she already clearly sees. Given that this is the case, then even if the means bypass her rational capacities, her status as a rational agent is respected.

I claimed above that direct manipulation is appropriate when the response to an event is *excessively* disproportionate to its objective import. The qualification is necessary to deal with some hard cases, in which agents' responses seem, from some angles, to be inappropriate, yet in which we are rightly loathe to intervene. Consider Bernard Williams, (1981) example of the man who, through absolutely no fault of his own, runs down and kills a child. His vehicle was in good condition and well maintained, he was concentrating on the road, he responded appropriately to the emergency, but there was nothing he could do to prevent tragedy when the child darted out in front of him. In that case, we are likely to attempt to comfort him, telling him that it wasn't his fault and that he shouldn't feel so bad. But, as Williams points out, if he takes our advice to heart too quickly, we shall be dismayed. If he says, "I guess you're right," and cheers up and goes to the cinema, he gives evidence of a lack of appreciation of the seriousness of what he has done. His fault or not, he has caused the death of a human being, and he ought to feel very bad about that. But there is still a sense in which the reaction we expect of him is *also* inappropriate, inasmuch as the emotions we expect him to feel – not merely regret, but also guilt – are not good guides to *his* role in the unfolding of events. Should he feel only regret, we shall blame his lack of moral seriousness, yet if he feels guilt we shall reassure him. Cases like this are puzzling, but they constitute no *special* problem for us. It would certainly be wrong to manipulate him into feeling better about his actions; by the same token, it would be wrong to talk him into premature cheer.

It is often appropriate for us to treat ourselves as mere machines. We do it all the time: when we go for a run to make ourselves feel better, when we count to ten before we speak in anger, even when we go into the sunshine to dispel melancholy. We do not act inappropriately when we do so. In a sense, we act entirely appropriately since we *are* machines, or at least built out of thousands of mechanisms. Just as we can recognize this fact without threatening our status as rational agents, so we can manipulate ourselves without mechanizing ourselves. Of course, to regard ourselves as *just* mechanisms would indeed threaten our rationality; similarly, to manipulate ourselves *too much* would threaten our agency. But manipulations engaged in with open eyes, and with the end of restoring rational agency, can be entirely appropriate.

There is no support for the presumption here. There are, however, difficult problems, concerning when it is appropriate to use means that bypass agents' rational faculties. Cases like Lucy, where a globally rational agent autonomously requests treatment are easy; so are cases in which an agent is globally irrational, and in which direct manipulation would restore reason (there is no point addressing ourselves to an agent's rational faculties when these faculties are absent). The difficult cases are those in which an agent has islands of preserved rationality, of a greater or lesser extent. In that case, should we see a request from her as expressing an autonomous desire to be restored to fuller reason? Should we see a refusal of treatment as rational? These are difficult questions, which ought to make us hesitate before we apply direct manipulations too casually. But they do not justify a general suspicion of these interventions.

Treating symptoms, not causes

We can dispense with this objection quickly. It is surely true that direct manipulations can be used to treat symptoms and not causes. So, for that matter, can psychotherapy. Indeed, psychotherapy for psychosis often is deliberately designed to accomplish just this. Rather than, say, aiming to eliminate the voices the patient hears, it aims to get them to reconceptualize them: to regard them simply as symptoms of their illness and not as commands from authority figures (Dickerson 2000). Sometimes, as this example shows, treating the symptoms of an illness is perfectly appropriate, inasmuch as doing so can be sufficient to restore the patient to something approaching full rational autonomy.

Nevertheless, we should admit that direct manipulations can be used to treat symptoms inappropriately. It may, for instance, be inappropriate to use a manipulation in order to allow a person merely to cope with a toxic environment, at least when the option of improving that environment is available (once again, other things – like cost – being equal). However, there are two further points that must be recognized. The first is obvious: that direct manipulations can be abused does nothing to establish that they are not often appropriately used; they may appropriately target symptoms, and not causes, or they may be used to target causes directly (bear in mind the distinction between endogenous and exogenous depression: when depression is not an appropriate response to external events, treating it via manipulating brain chemistry may just *be* treating its cause).

The second point is only slightly less obvious, but it is often missed. It is this: having direct manipulations available alters what counts as a toxic environment, and therefore moves the goalposts so far as the appropriateness of treatment is concerned. Consider Erik Parens' objection to the use of direct manipulations (Parens 1998). Parens argues that such manipulations may incline us to target suffering individual bodies and minds, rather than "the complex social conditions that produce that suffering" (1998:13). For instance, if overcrowded classrooms produce inferior academic performance, we may find it easier and cheaper to use Ritalin to compensate for the deficiencies of schools, rather than fix them. Now, in many actual cases Parens may be quite right. If he is, however, it cannot be because Ritalin allows us to achieve, at a lower cost, *precisely the same* results (in terms of academic performance and well-adjusted students) as better classrooms and more individualized teaching. If it does, then Ritalin is clearly *superior*: if it has the same benefits, and lower costs, then we should use it (and use the savings elsewhere, where the money is needed). No, if spending on classrooms is to be preferred to spending on drugs, this must be because the benefits of each alternative are *not* the same. This might be for many reasons: because Ritalin has side effects that are undesirable; because it is expensive and not all parents will be able to afford it; because though it allows for adequate academic performance, it has costs in terms of students' psycho-social development, and so on. In other words, Parens is quite wrong to think that the problem with using direct manipulations is simply a question of *means*. It is results that matter, not means. We cannot infer from the fact that an environment *would be* toxic in the absence of Ritalin that it really *is* toxic when Ritalin is used. Toxic is as toxic does; if we are not poisoned by a substance because we regularly ingest the antidote, then it is not poisonous for us (so long as we can be sure that we shall continue to have the antidote available). An overcrowded classroom before Ritalin is available may have the optimal number of students once it is in use (once again, unless the drug has costs that change the equation).

We cannot, therefore, condemn direct manipulations on the grounds that they will *necessarily* cause the systematic worsening of our environment. Nevertheless, they might have a tendency to do so, especially when they are pushed by powerful industries and by governments seeking to save money. They may be used to allow people to cope with toxic environments, as a cost-cutting measure. But we ought not to reject such manipulations in principle because they *could* be used to bad ends; it is only when they actually, or are likely to, worsen people's lives that we ought to be critical of them.

Cheating and inequality

In the discussion of the enhancement/treatment distinction we introduced two further threats: that the use of neurological enhancements could constitute cheating, and that they might lead to, or worsen, inequalities. Having outlined those threats, we then examined considerations which threw the entire distinction between treatments and enhancements into doubt, at least as an independent standard for assessing moral permissibility. Nevertheless, it remains important to examine these two threats, for they continue to seem powerful objections to direct manipulations. Even if the distinction between treatment and enhancement does not stand up to scrutiny, it is clear that some uses of interventions are unnecessary; we may continue to feel that such unnecessary interventions ought to be especially suspect, and that the cheating and inequality objections provide part of the reason why this is so.

The worry that enhancements constitute cheating and the worry that they will cause or exacerbate inequalities are closely linked. If someone gets away with cheating – at an examination, in a sporting event, or whatever it may be – their performance is usually better, and their rewards are correspondingly greater. So cheating leads to unequal outcomes. The fear of inequality may just be the fear that people are able to convert wealth into other, unearned, advantages, and these advantages into further wealth; these conversions might well be regarded as forms of cheating – cheating on the social contract, as it were.

However, it is hard to sustain the charge that the use of enhancements is *necessarily* cheating. An athlete cheats if they use a performance-enhancing drug that is proscribed by the rules. They cheat because the other competitors have a legitimate expectation that *no one* will use the drug. It can't be the *use* of the drug, all by itself, that constitutes cheating. If the rules allowed the drug, then it wouldn't be cheating. To be sure, it may be that access to the drug would be very unequal: it may be very expensive, and therefore available only to athletes from wealthy countries like the United States and Germany, and not to athletes from Kenya or Ethiopia. Perhaps that's a reason to object to the use of the drug, but consider how many performance-enhancing interventions we currently allow, in the knowledge that access to them is unequally distributed. Training facilities in the developed world differ greatly from those in the developing world; Western athletes have access to nutritionists, sports scientists, psychologists and equipment that is the best in the world. They are given supplements and advice, designed to extract from them the best possible performances. There can be no doubt that all this extra help enables them to run faster, to jump higher, to have more endurance than they would otherwise have had. Why isn't this cheating? Because this kind of extra help is permitted by the rules, whereas the use of anabolic steroids is not.[4]

The situation is relevantly similar with regard to cheating on intellectual tasks. The use of calculators and notes is cheating under some exam conditions, but not others; if the rules permit them ("open book exams") then it is not cheating. And of course there are already a wide range of performance-enhancing technologies that are available, at a cost that ensures that only a privileged minority will be able to make use of them. As we have already noted, diet and general health are closely linked to intellectual performance; moreover, only the relatively wealthy can afford to hire tutors or to send their offspring to foreign countries in order to be immersed in their language and culture. The French sociologist Pierre Bourdieu (1986) coined the term "cultural capital" to refer to the accumulated knowledge, explicit and implicit, which enables individuals effortlessly to navigate complex social environments, including the environment of the educational system. Writing a good academic essay requires mastery not only of the concepts being taught, but also of the ability to adopt the right tone: to shape one's sentences appropriately, and to use the relevant vocabulary in the relevant manner. In many ways, this is a skill that is more difficult to master than the concepts that are explicitly taught; like all such social knowledge, it is hard to acquire cultural capital by deliberate effort, but easy to acquire it by extended exposure, especially if the exposure comes early in life. For this reason, the children of professionals, of parents who expose them to intellectual discourse and make a variety of books and cultural experiences available to them young, are at an important advantage. Without (apparently) cheating, they turn their early cultural capital into academic success, and thence to economic capital. They pass on all of these benefits to their children: the capacity to buy the best nutrition, the best health professionals, the best teaching in the best schools *and* the cultural capital to take full advantage of all these benefits.

Indeed, neuroscience itself is beginning to demonstrate the truth of these claims. Neuroscientific research on the impact of environmental deprivation on the mind demonstrates that our mind/ brains can be deformed not only by genes, disease, drugs and alcohol, "but also by the socio-economic circumstances of our childhood in equivalently physical mechanistic ways" (Farah 2006 et al.: 285). Blair et al. (2005) also stress the ways in which environmental stressors impact negatively on the brains of children, especially on hippocampal development. As they graphically put it, "environmental stressors may lead, effectively, to brain damage" (2005: 35). Long before psychopharmaceuticals and neuroscientific technologies became available, environmental differences led to inequalities in cognition, by impacting directing on the brain.

Might neurological enhancements exacerbate these inequalities? They might. Should we worry? I think we should, but the worry has an interesting implication. We should realize that there is nothing *special* about neurological enhancements, so far as the concerns with cheating and inequality are concerned, and that we should therefore turn the worry back upon our *existing* social and political practices. Given that cognitive function, and the underlying neurology, is already shaped by environmental factors, given that wealth is already converted into cognitive advantage and poverty into neurological deficit, we ought to be as much, or more, concerned about existing inequalities as those that might come.

We noted previously how widespread is the fear that great inequalities could result from a market in neurological enhancements. We can express the rationale for the underlying worry in the following principle:

> Any enhancement available only to the wealthy, which would allow them to achieve a greatly enhanced level of functioning and open up opportunities to them which are not available to the less well-off, ought not to be permitted.

But as we have just seen, such enhancements are already available to, and widely used by, the wealthy; they consist in the superior schooling, nutrition, medical care and other advantages that wealth can buy. Consider the current life expectancy of a child born today in Sierra Leone versus that of a child born in the United States: thirty-eight years for the former, and seventy-seven for the latter. This difference is strongly correlated with income. Sierra Leone has a per capita Gross National Product (GNP) of just $160, whereas the United States has a GNP per capita of $30 600. Infant mortality figures paint a similar grim picture.[5] Within countries, disparities in life expectancy also follow income lines. It is uncontroversial to suggest that these disparities, which are reflected across a range of important indicators, are in very important part the result of differences in income. If we are worried that wealth can be converted into very significant enhancements which are not available to others, then we ought to be worried by these gross disparities.

The inequality worry is a genuine one: we really have reason to fear that making enhancements of the mind available will benefit the wealthy to a disproportionate extent, both within and across nations.

Already existing gaps can be expected to grow. However, though this is a serious problem there is nothing new about it. The gap between wealthy nations and less wealthy has been growing for centuries, much more rapidly recently than ever before:

> The income gap between the fifth of the world's people living in the richest countries and the fifth in the poorest was 74 to 1 in 1997, up from 60 to 1 in 1990 and 30 to 1 in 1960. [Earlier] the income gap between the top and bottom countries increased from 3 to 1 in 1820 to 7 to 1 in 1870 to 11 to 1 in 1913.
>
> *(Pogge 2002: 100)*

We should worry about inequality, especially when it is growing rapidly, wherever we find it and however it is caused. That is a reason to worry about neurological enhancement, but about much else besides, and probably far more urgently.

Let me mention one further objection often heard with regard to direct interventions before concluding: they *individualize* suffering (Kaplan 2000). When direct manipulations are the treatment of first choice, mental illness or less than optimal functioning comes to be regarded as a problem with individuals: they have something wrong with *them*. But, as we have seen in discussing norms of reactions, assigning the proportion of responsibility for a trait, physical or mental, due to the individual and that due to the environment is really meaningless: phenotypic traits are the joint product of genome (and other internal developmental resources) and environment, and it is in principle impossible to disentangle the contribution each makes. Seeing mental illness as the individual's problem is therefore, strictly speaking, false (in all but the most unusual cases). Worse, it can be politically regressive. First, it discourages us from seeking social and political solutions to problems. It may be that we could reduce the amount of suffering in a fairer and more effective manner by changing social structures, rather than by medicating individuals (or by using psychotherapy). To mention some obvious instances: people are less likely to be depressed if they have work available, if that work pays them enough to ensure their self-respect and if that work is satisfying. Providing that kind of work might be a more effective treatment of depression than millions of prescriptions of SSRIs (which is not to suggest that no one would be depressed in the best society; some people are depressed, through no fault of their own or of anyone else, because – for instance – of the way their genome interacts with an environment which is well suited to most people).

Second, individualizing suffering tends to lead to individuals having to bear the costs of treatment (Kaplan 2000). If someone is depressed, and depression is a medical condition which is the individual's problem (if not, quite, their fault) then fixing it is something for which they ought to take responsibility. It might simply be bad luck that they have this problem, and we owe them compassion and support. Nevertheless, it is *their* problem, for which they must take responsibility. In fact, it is only their problem in the trivial sense that (typically) they suffer most from it. So far as causation is concerned, it is no more theirs than anyone else's. Their misfortune is to find themselves unable to flourish in a set of conditions for which they are not responsible (usually, at any rate), and their misfortune could just as well have been ours.

We can now see why the charge of promoting political quietism has bite. Many mental illnesses are produced or exacerbated by social conditions, and often (though not always) those are social conditions which are independently undesirable. For instance, though the malignant sadness of clinical depression may outrun its causes, in the sense that it is deeper and more persistent than the event that triggers it warrants, it is still nevertheless generally triggered by events to which sadness is an appropriate response, and often these events are the product of social circumstances: loss of job, loss of sources of social support, and so on. If we treat the depression by focusing on the individual, we miss an opportunity to improve our society, to the benefit not only of the depressive individual, but, potentially, of all of us.

There is, however, an important caveat that must be mentioned here. These problems – the inequality worry, the individualized treatment worry, and the political quietism worry – are not raised exclusively by direct interventions. Whenever treating mental illnesses or lowered functioning is approached first and foremost in terms of treatment of the individual, and not of improvements of social conditions that contribute to the problem, the individualization of suffering and consequent political quietism is a likely result. Individualized treatment is not limited to direct manipulation; it is equally a feature of psychotherapy. So if we should worry about direct interventions on these grounds, we should also worry just as much about some kinds of traditional means of changing minds. Moreover, the inequality objection also applies equally to many traditional means. If psychotherapy enables those who undergo it to function better, then that, too, is another way in which existing inequalities might be exacerbated (especially given that psychotherapy is *more* expensive than many direct manipulations). This is really an obvious point, if we stop and think about it: teaching is one of the oldest methods of changing minds we have, and one of the most respected, but its quality varies from time to time and place to place, and one of the most effective ways of ensuring that we get the best is by paying for it.

CONCLUSION

There are, indeed, reasons to worry about direct interventions into the mind. Use of antidepressants, or more drastic manipulations, can indeed lead us away from self-knowledge and they can indeed inappropriately mechanize the self. They can also be used to treat symptoms while leaving causes untouched, they can contribute to inequality and promote political quietism. But there is nothing intrinsic in the new neuroscientific technologies that raises these worries. Traditional, non-invasive, techniques of changing minds can have the same problems. They can be just as mechanical, can bypass reflective capacities just as surely and have proved potent means of perpetuating inequality.

To be sure, traditional means of manipulating minds have an important advantage that direct manipulations do not: they include the one means which does address itself to the whole person and their rational capacities: the presentation of evidence and argument. There is nothing in the new technologies that has this feature; though direct manipulations can be used to *enhance* rational capacities, they succeed at this using means that bypass them during treatment. On the other hand, traditional means include many techniques that are not addressed to the rational agent. These traditional means of bypassing rational capacities have no advantage over the newer direct manipulations. The treatment of many mental illnesses, and even problems in living, often requires a combination of techniques that address themselves directly to the agent as a rational person and techniques that bypass their rational capacities; given that we require such bypassing techniques, there is no reason to prefer traditional over newer manipulations. Direct manipulations, when they are used appropriately, often have as their goal the restoration of the person as a rational, autonomous agent. Many psychotherapists today combine talk with medication, because they find that the medication makes the patient better able to cope with the distressing feelings evoked by the therapy, or better able to adjust their behavior in the ways recommended. These are admirable goals, and they are not the less worthy for being pursued, in part, through direct manipulations.

One of the themes of this book is that the distinction between the inner – the brain, the genome, the authentic self, and so on – and the outer, the publicly accessible environment, cannot bear the weight all too often placed on it. Interventions in the mind can proceed from the inside, via direct manipulation, or from the outside, by environmental alterations, and the difference between these ways of proceeding is not, by itself, significant: it does not predict outcomes and has no moral import. Effects on the mind are the product, in very important part (though, if the extended mind hypothesis is true, far from exclusively) of effects on the brain, and we change the brain as inexorably and as importantly by acting directly on it or by addressing the person as a rational agent (neuronal connections in your brain have altered as the result of reading these words). If antidepressants increase the amount of serotonin in the synaptic cleft, so does improving the quality of an agent's life, or improving their diet. There are many ways of pursuing mental health and of creating the self; they can all be misused (even addressing the person as a rational agent can be misused: we can simply lie, presenting evidence that has been fabricated), and none is intrinsically good or bad. We need to assess them one by one, in the context in which they are used and examining the details of their application, before we accept or reject them.

End notes

1. Erik Parens (2005) would no doubt regard this line of argument as shallow and one-sided. For Parens, we ought to acknowledge that we are attracted to both sides of this debate: the Sartrean that celebrates self-creation and the side represented by Elliott (and which ultimately descends from Kierkegaard) that preaches the wisdom of accepting what is handed down to us. I don't doubt that Parens is right, inasmuch as we all feel the force of the Kierkegaardian appeal to gratitude. But this side of the debate ought not to be given any weight, no matter its intuitive appeal, since the notion of a self that is given to us, and for which we ought to express gratitude, is not coherent. Some of our intuitions (as indeed the cognitive sciences show) are expressions of heuristics, biases or sheer irrationalities; to this extent they ought to be disregarded in moral argument.
2. Manninen (2006) argues, contra Kant, that there is a perfect duty to acquire self-knowledge. It is surely far more plausible to hold that if there is any such duty, it is imperfect: that is, we can rationally and ethically choose to forgo fulfilling it if so doing is necessary for achieving another valuable good.
3. It should be noted that some other forms of psychotherapy are much less time-consuming. Cognitive-behavior therapy, for instance, which teaches patients strategies to break the link between situations and habitual responses, as well as to alter thinking patterns that are counterproductive,

has been shown to be effective after just a few sessions (Hazlett-Stevens and Craske 2004). Interestingly, therapies which are not time-consuming are also generally less truth-conducive: rather than aiming at bringing the patient to understand the causes of their problems, they aim to give them strategies for coping with them, strategies that may be quite mechanical in nature (e.g. counting to ten before acting).

4. Admittedly, there are differences between taking anabolic steroids and vitamin supplements, other than the fact that the first is prohibited and the second is not, which might be thought to be relevant to the question of why one is cheating and the other is not. Most obviously, steroids have deleterious health effects; that might be part of the reason that they are widely regarded as illegitimate. There is, many people believe, a constitutive or at least a close link between sporting performance and health, such that a means of achieving sporting excellence that undermines health is contrary to the internal ends of sports. However, not all banned performance-enhancing technologies are deleterious to the health of athletes, and not all permitted means are healthy. Blood doping, in which an athlete is given his or her own red blood cells to boost oxygen-carrying capacity, is quite safe if it is carried out under medical supervision. On the other hand, professional sport (especially contact sports) involve so much wear and tear on the body that even without drugs there are significant health risks.

5. Source, *The New Internationalist*, April 2000.

4 Reading minds/controlling minds

Much of the interest and anxiety provoked by new and developing neuroscientific technologies is centered around two issues: the extent to which these technologies might allow their users to read the thoughts of people, and (as if that prospect was not disturbing enough) the extent to which these technologies might actually be used to control people. Some commentators believe that one or both of these issues are pressing, in the sense that the relevant technologies will soon be available; some even believe that these technologies already exist. In this chapter, we will ask how worried we should be. Are these technologies imminent? And if they are, are they as threatening as they appear?

MIND READING AND MIND CONTROLLING
There has been a great deal of interest in the possibility of "brain reading" as a lie detection technology. The problems with existing lie detectors are well known: they produce high rates both of false positives and of false negatives, and they can be "beaten" by people who deliberately heighten their responses to control questions, which are used to establish a baseline for comparison. In its overview of current lie-detection techniques, the US National Research Council concluded that there is "little basis for the expectation that a polygraph test could have extremely high accuracy" (National Research Council 2003: 212). The reasons for this conclusion are many: because the responses measured are not uniquely involved in deception, because they include responses that can be deliberately controlled and because the technology is difficult to implement in

the real-world. The authors conclude that further research and investment can be expected to produce only modest gains in accuracy. For these kinds of reasons, conventional polygraph results are inadmissible as evidence in most jurisdictions.

It is recognition of the severe limitations of current lie detection technologies that is responsible, in important part, for the current interest in lie detectors that directly "read" the mind. Polygraph machines are sensitive to changes in somatic states such as skin conductance (changes in the resistance of the skin to electricity, which is a good indicator of increased sweating), heart rate and blood pressure. Now, the problem with these measures is that, at best, they are only correlated with deliberate deception. They are indications of increased nervousness, and can be manipulated. Moreover, even with a naïve subject who does not know how to manipulate these responses, the correlation between the responses and deliberate deception is far from perfect; hence the false positives (where these responses peak but the subject is not lying), and the false negatives (where the subject is lying, but their somatic responses do not reflect this fact). Proponents of neurologically based lie detection argue, apparently plausibly, that such technologies would not be subject to these limitations. It might be possible to fool a system that measures only stand-ins for lies, but it is not possible to fool a system capable of honing in on the lies themselves. Of course, lies are not directly detectable, but the technology might be capable of doing the next best thing. Thoughts are realized neurologically; in the jargon of cognitive science, they have neural correlates. The correlation between the lie and its neural correlate is, by definition, perfect. Hence, if the lie detection technology can hone in on the neural correlates of lies, it will not give false positives or false negatives, and it will not be able to be fooled. Brains do not lie.

The problem with this line of thought is obvious. Though it is certainly true that every thought has a neural correlate – to say that is just to say that thoughts are realized in brains, so the claim should be uncontroversial to anyone who does not believe in substance dualism – it does not follow that for every *type* of thought there is a *distinct* neural correlate. Indeed, the latter claim is rather implausible, given that there are endless ways in which thoughts might be categorized ("concerning animals with fewer than four legs," "concerning either my maiden aunt or a ming vase," "concerning an odd number of elephants" – the categories are limited only by our ingenuity). But the idea that we can detect lies by honing in on their neural correlates requires that to the thought-type "deliberate deception" there corresponds one, or at any rate a tractable number, of distinct neural correlates. Unless and until we develop the technology to translate neural correlates into thoughts (a prospect we shall consider later in this chapter), we can only hope to detect lies if we discover that there is something distinctive about deliberate deception; something we can look for in brain scans.

So reliable neurological detection depends upon there being something neurologically distinctive about deliberate deception. Is there? There are various proposals for such distinctive correlates, either of the entire class of deliberate deception, or of various smaller segments of that class. Perhaps the best-known technique of neurological lie detection, "brain fingerprinting," targets one possible distinctive correlate. Brain fingerprinting does not aim to detect any and all deliberate deception; instead, it is aimed at detecting *guilty knowledge*. The technology uses memory and encoding related multifaceted electroencephalographic response (MERMER), which combines electroencephalography (EEG) data from several sites on the scalp. Electrodes are attached to the subject's scalp at several sites, and brain activity is measured while the subject is asked questions or shown pictures. If the subject recognizes a picture or is familiar with the content of the question, they are supposed to exhibit a characteristic response, the P300 wave (so called because it occurs 300 milliseconds after the stimulus). If they do not have the relevant knowledge, the amplitude of the P300 wave will be significantly smaller.

MERMER and brain fingerprinting are the brainchildren of Lawrence Farwell; Farwell has aggressively commercialized the technology, through his company Brain Fingerprinting Laboratories. Farwell claims that brain fingerprinting has several advantages over polygraphy. Because the P300 wave is involuntary, it does not depend upon the cooperation of the person being tested (with one exception: the subject must sit still during testing). This makes it especially suitable for testing people who might be planning a crime, for instance suspected terrorists. The tester might show them bomb-making equipment, and examine their EEG. Most importantly, Farwell claims that brain fingerprinting cannot be manipulated. Whereas clever criminals can beat conventional lie-detection tests, they cannot control the involuntary P300 response. In one test of the technology, subjects were instructed to attempt to conceal the knowledge being probed; nevertheless the guilty knowledge was detected. There were no false positives, false negatives or indeterminate cases (Farwell and Smith 2001).

Farwell and colleagues claim these kinds of results are a spectacular vindication of brain fingerprinting. However, there are a number of problems with the technology. First, the method of analysis used by Farwell is proprietary and undisclosed; for that reason there cannot be independent testing of its validity. What few tests there are for brain fingerprinting come exclusively from Farwell's laboratory. Independent testing is, of course, the gold standard of good science; in its absence, we are entitled to a high degree of scepticism (Wolpe et al. 2005). Moreover, even assuming that Farwell's tests have been scrupulously conducted, and his own investment in the technique has had no effect in biasing his results (consciously or unconsciously), his sample sizes are too small to yield a great deal of confidence.

Moreover, there are difficulties concerning the ecological validity of the technology; that is, the extent to which the findings can be generalized to the world outside the laboratory. It requires carefully controlled situations; in particular, it requires that the tester possess information that they know will be available only to the perpetrator of the crime. Sometimes such information will be known, but probably only in the minority of cases (Tancredi 2004). Suppose the subject exhibits a P300 to images of a terrorist training camp. Should we conclude that they have trained as a terrorist, or that they watch CNN? In fact, in the only field study to date on the technology, it performed at around chance accuracy (Miyake *et al.* 1993).

Finally, it appears that Farwell may well be wrong in thinking that P300 detection methods cannot be beaten. The P300 wave is a response that is produced when the stimulus is meaningful to the subject; it can therefore be manufactured by any method that makes irrelevant probes (used to set the baseline for comparison of wave amplitude) meaningful to them. Apparently, this is not very difficult. Rosenfeld and colleagues (Rosenfeld *et al.* 2004) instructed subjects to perform a variety of covert acts in response to irrelevant stimuli: wiggling toes, pressing the fingers of the left hand onto their legs and imagining the experimenter slapping them in the face. These countermeasures were sufficient to defeat Farwell's six-probe paradigm. Reaction-time data remained a significant predictor of guilt on a one-probe variety of the test, but this is of little comfort to proponents of MERMER-based guilty knowledge tests; the six-probe test is necessary to avoid too great a rate of false positives as a consequence of subjects' finding the probe meaningful for coincidental reasons.

It is apparent that the P300 test has not, so far, lived up to the hype. However, it may well improve, as the hardware gets more sophisticated, the algorithms that interpret the data are refined and the experimenters find better ways to probe guilty knowledge. Moreover, the P300 test is only one of several deceit-detection technologies currently under investigation, some of which are also aimed at detecting lies by reading brains. Langleben and colleagues (Langleben *et al.* 2002) used fMRI to scan the brains of subjects engaged in intentional deceit; they discovered that areas of the anterior cingulate cortex and the superior frontal gyrus were more active during deception than when subjects responded truthfully. Once again, there are questions concerning the ecological validity of the technique: how well will it generalize from the controlled laboratory with willing subjects to the outside world where conditions are uncontrolled and subjects are uncooperative? Even in the laboratory, the accuracy of the test is not all that high: it showed a between-group difference between deceivers and the truthful, but the effect is not great enough to identify individual deceivers with a high degree of confidence. In addition, technical limitations of fMRI – its relative lack of spatial and temporal resolution – will probably need to be overcome before the test has an acceptable degree of reliability. Once again, however, the technology and the testing methods can be expected to improve.

What does the foreseeable future hold? I think it is safe to claim that the kind of mind reading technology which is most feared, which can scan the brains of subjects and reveal intimate details about their thoughts, without their knowing that they are under the mental microscope, is (at least) a long way off. The most promising methods of mind reading require that we build up a set of data on an individual subject: we need to establish a baseline for responses we know to be truthful, against which to compare the probes of interest (see Illes *et al.* 2006 for review). Conditions must be carefully controlled and the subject (relatively) cooperative. Moreover, neither EEG equipment nor, especially, fMRI equipment, is anywhere near portable or concealable. We can expect to see mind-reading technology that is of some help in detecting deception in the laboratory, and that can therefore be used in the kinds of situations in which polygraphy is employed today, long before we see covert surveillance of thoughts – if indeed that ever turns out to be possible.

What about laboratory tests for mental states and dispositions other than lies? Once again, work is proceeding along several fronts. Many studies have shown brain alterations associated with chronic schizophrenia; the possibility therefore exists that the disease could be diagnosed on the basis of brains scans (Farah and Wolpe 2004).

Some researchers claim to have discovered identifiable neural correlates of normal personality traits. The work of Canli and colleagues (2001; 2002) is the best known and most interesting in this vein. They found that extraversion was correlated with particular kinds of responses to images with positive emotional qualities, whereas neuroticism was associated with differences in responses to images with negative emotional content. Phelps and colleagues (2000) used fMRI to study the responses of white subjects to photographs of black faces. They found a correlation between the degree of activation of the amygdala and negative evaluation of blacks. We shall return to this study shortly.

What are the prospects for a genuine mind-reading machine – one that is capable of interpreting brain states more generally? Outside of personality traits, neuroscientists have had some success in detecting the neural correlates of the orientation of lines to which a subject is attending (Kamitani and Tong 2005); when subjects viewed a visually ambiguous figure, the researchers were able, on the basis of fMRI data, to determine how the subject was resolving the ambiguity. Once again, the data was interpretable only after an initial "training" run was used to establish a baseline. Quiroga et al. (2005) claim to have been able to isolate neural correlates of a much wider range of representations. In their small study, they apparently showed that representations of a single person, building, or a single class of objects – e.g., cartoons from The Simpsons – are encoded in such a way that, no matter how they are presented, they activate specific neurons. Thus, one of their subjects had a neuron that responded preferentially to pictures of Jennifer Aniston, no matter what angle the picture was taken from, and relatively little to pictures of other people, famous or non-famous. Another subject had a neuron that responded preferentially to pictures of (what he took to be) the Sydney Opera House, as well as to the words "Sydney Opera," but not to other buildings or people.

This study used recordings of single neurons, rather than fMRI or EEG techniques. It might seem to provide the basis for a much more powerful mind-reading technique, since the range of thoughts that it could detect is far wider than other techniques. However, there are good reasons to suggest that it will not result in a mind-reading machine anytime soon. First, the technology is invasive, requiring electrodes to be implanted deep in the brain (Quiroga and colleagues were only able to carry out the experiment because they had a pool of intractable epileptics, who required surgery, to draw on. Electrodes are implanted in the brains of such subjects to locate the foci of seizures, to allow the surgeon to locate the precise area for intervention). Second, once again the technique required training and cooperation. Even if we could get single neuron recordings from subjects, we could not interpret them unless we already had a set of data showing correlations between the firing of the relevant neurons and particular mental states. Third, the authors themselves caution that the fact that they were able, in the short time they had available, to discover pictures to which the individual neurons responded suggests that the neurons probably respond to other images as well. If the Jennifer Aniston neuron responded *only* to pictures of Jen, it would be nothing short of a miracle that the researchers had been able to hit upon its precise stimulus. But if the neurons respond to many different images – and perhaps to sensations and abstract thoughts as well – then even the possession of single-cell recordings plus a set of correlation data will not be sufficient to tell us what the subject is thinking. We may have to conclude that he is thinking about Jennifer Aniston, or parliamentary democracy, or Friday Night Football, or a pain in his toe, or something else for which we don't have any data yet.

The development of a general mind-reading technology, able to read the thoughts of people even in the absence of preliminary training and the establishment of a baseline, is possible only if there is a great deal of commonality in the neural correlates of mental states across persons. That is, it will only be possible to construct a device to read the thoughts of anyone – whether for the purposes of detecting potential terrorists or selling them cola – if it is possible to construct some kind of translation manual, which details the correlations between particular brain states and particular thoughts. If my thought that "elephants are gray" has neural correlates which are very different from your thought that "elephants are gray", then constructing the translation manual will be difficult or impossible (impossible if there are few commonalities across the population; difficult if the differences are tractable – for instance, if there are identifiable groups, between which the neural correlates of thoughts differ markedly, but within which there is a great deal of commonality – just as there is a great deal of commonality within, but not between, the vocabularies of different languages).

Moreover, even the construction of a mind-reading machine reliably able to read the thoughts of a single person, upon whom the machine has been trained, depends upon our thoughts having stable neural correlates across time. Perhaps my thought that "elephants are gray" today has a very similar neural realization to the same thought, in *my* head at least, tomorrow, but perhaps next week, or next month, or next year, it will be quite different.

There is already evidence for some kinds of commonalities within and across subjects. The method used by Kamitani and Tong (2005) to detect the orientation of lines to which a subject is attending uses data from extensive testing of the visual systems of monkeys; from this data, we know that orientation is represented in the early stages of visual processing in ways that are consistent across primates. However, the degree of consistency is not sufficient to underpin the development of a mind-reading machine: an initial set of data is necessary to make the neural activity meaningful. Thanks to the data on the primate visual system, we know where to look for orientation-tuned neurons, but gathering data on individual subjects remains indispensable for applying the technique.

It's not difficult, however, to think of ways in which this data could be gathered unobtrusively; that is, without the subjects' being aware that it is taking place. We could flash lines in such a way that subjects had their attention attracted to them, and use this information to hone in on the relevant neurons. Perhaps we could, but so what? This is, after all, a relatively uninteresting mental state: it is difficult to imagine a realistic scenario in which knowing the orientation of lines to which subjects are attending is important enough to justify the massive investment necessary to justify designing and building a machine able to provide such information. Moreover, even if such a machine were in existence, we would have little reason to worry about it. There are good reasons to worry about a loss of privacy, but few to worry about the loss of this kind of privacy in particular. Apart from a very few, very peculiar, situations, none of us will be worried if others are capable of determining the orientation of lines we are attending to.

But mightn't the results be capable of generalization; that is, mightn't we expect to be able gradually to expand the range of mental states we are capable of detecting? The answer depends, once again, upon the degree of commonality in the neural correlates of thoughts across subjects and within subjects across time. The visual system, especially the early visual system, is *relatively* (the emphasis is very necessary here) simple, and the relationship between its contents and what it represents relatively easy to decode. It may turn out, for all we know at the moment, that more complex and abstract thoughts have neural correlates that are far less stable across time and across subjects. In recent work, Haynes and colleagues were able to identify whether a subject had chosen to add or to subtract two numbers with seventy percent reliability (Haynes *et al*. in press). Arithmetical operations are at a greater level of abstraction than visual perception, but this is still a long way off from complex conceptual thought. Indeed, such operations, and all the other kinds of mental states that we have hitherto been able to detect via fMRI, may be subserved by brain *modules*, innate brain structures dedicated to specific tasks. If an important cognitive task regularly confronted our distant ancestors in the environment of evolutionary adaptation, then a module may have developed to perform it efficiently. Since brain modules are (typically) discrete entities, and perform a regular function in a predictable way, we can expect that it will prove relatively easy to decode their processes, in such a way as to be able to predict their output. But our more abstract beliefs are unlikely to be processed by modules. Instead, they are far more likely to be handled by domain-general mechanisms. In general, the higher the level of abstraction of a thought, and the more it pertains to matters which were likely to be variable in (or entirely absent from) the environment of evolutionary adaptation, the lower the probability that belief acquisition and retention will be handled by modular mechanisms: since these conditions will usually be satisfied by the kinds of beliefs we are likely to be concerned to keep private, we have little reason to think that past successes at detecting neural correlates predict disturbing kinds of future successes in these areas.

These considerations suggest that detecting neural correlates of more abstract thoughts will prove far more difficult than detecting the neural correlates of the kinds of thoughts processed by modules. Moreover, it may be that domain-general thoughts have neural correlates that are far more varied across subjects, and perhaps even across time within the brain of a single subject. It might, that is, turn out that the neurons involved in *my* thought that "elephants are gray" are located in quite different regions of the brain to those involved in the very same thought in *your* mind; it might even turn out that across time the location of the neurons involved in that thought in *me* shifts. The degree of neuroplasticity – the ability of the brain to reorganize itself – is much lower in adults than in children, but we now know that new neural cells are produced throughout the lifespan. Cell death is compensated for, at least to some extent, and new learning forms new neural connections. It would be surprising, then, if the neural correlates of particular thoughts were entirely unaltered over the lifespan. There is evidence, indeed, that *precisely* the same mental state never occurs twice, at least for some classes of mental state. The act of recalling a past event seems subtly to alter the memory, so that when the event is recalled a second time, it is the remade memory that is recalled. Older memories are also altered by the context of recall, and by newer memories since laid down (Schacter 1996). It may be that a very large number of our mental states, especially our complex thoughts which represent the world as being a certain way, are reshaped by our causal history: since our brains develop as a result of the interaction of endogenous resources with the environment, *my* precise history of learning and perception will shape the morphology of my brain (Rose 2005). Which neurons activate when I represent Jennifer Aniston will depend on when I learned about her; in what context, both internal and external. This context will certainly differ from person to person.

Useful, or threatening, mind-reading machines are not going to be built soon: not, at least, mind-reading machines capable of detecting the details of complex thoughts. Machines that detect, say, emotional arousal are another matter: given that the structures for emotional processing are relatively discrete, and relatively invariant across individuals, such machines are an in-principle possibility. Whether these machines would be more useful for lie detection than existing polygraph technology is, however, a moot point: they probably could be beaten in the same kinds of ways. After all, people do have some indirect control over their thoughts: we can learn to control our emotional arousal, at least temporarily, and in at least some situations (meditators are proficient at this skill).

The most immediate ethical problem arising from these new techniques of measuring the neural correlates of mental states stems from the dangers of premature adoption (Wolpe *et al.* 2005). The aura of prestige and objectivity which surrounds science generally is perhaps even stronger in relation to the science of the mind at its cutting edge. When neuroscience is applied to produce what are apparently pictures of thoughts, especially when the technologies are surrounded by hype (some of it, though not the bulk, originating from reputable scientists) these pictures are apt to be given a weight they may not deserve. Reporting on Farwell's P300 technique, the Discovery Channel described it as providing "an infallible witness". ABC news reported that the technology read the mind of subjects too quickly for them to have time to lie. Unsurprisingly, Farwell has reproduced these breathless reports on his corporate website. Right now, with public insecurity heightened by fears of terrorism, governments are desperate to be seen to be doing something to minimize risks. Across the world, respect for human rights and justice is taking a backseat to measures designed to secure victory in a war against an invisible enemy. In this climate, worries about the risks of new technologies are unlikely to be given the weight they deserve. Despite repeated warnings about the unreliability of conventional lie-detection technology, several US governmental agencies, including the FBI and the CIA, routinely screen their own employees with polygraph machines (Aldrich Ames, who sold American secrets to the KGB while working for the CIA, passed several polygraph tests designed to detect espionage). Unsurprisingly, governments are beginning to implement brain fingerprinting technology. India moved to introduce the technology in 2004 (*The Hindu*, September 4, 2004). At present polygraph results are inadmissible in most jurisdictions. There is, as yet, very little case law on brain fingerprinting. It is to be hoped that it, too, is ruled inadmissible; at present levels of reliability it cannot be trusted to help decide important questions of truth and justice.

MIND CONTROL

If it is worrying to contemplate the prospect that neuroscientific technologies might one day be used to read our minds, how much more worrying is it to think that they might be used to control us? Mind control could take one of two forms: it might cause the body of a person to move against their will, or, more worryingly still, it might work directly on their will (as it were): causing them to behave in the way desired by the controller, while leaving them with the illusion that they are in charge. Covert means might be used not only to get people to *do* what others want, but to get them to think, desire and believe what others want. If methods of controlling minds neurotechnologically can be devised, our autonomy, our rightly prized ability to shape our lives according to values that *we* endorse, would be under threat.

Are covert means of controlling minds or behavior achievable, at least in principle? There is already evidence to suggest that they are: if we cannot bring people to believe precisely what we want or to do precisely what we want, by neurotechnological means, at least we can influence what they think and what they do. The most obvious way of controlling minds is through the use of psychopharmaceuticals, which influence mood and therefore have effects on belief and behavior: the person with an elevated mood can be expected to put a more positive spin on evidence than the person in a darker mood; moreover depression is strongly linked to inactivity and withdrawal, while alleviating it can be expected to produce more extroversion. These effects, while far from subtle, are global rather than precise, so can't be used to control behavior and thoughts to order. Nevertheless, this kind of manipulation could be used to limit our autonomy to some degree.

Might more precise techniques be developed? Most writers regard the suggestion as science fiction (e.g., Greely 2004), but there is some evidence to suggest that they are wrong. Consider the effects of transcranial magnetic stimulation (TMS) on voluntary action. TMS involves the precise targeting of rapid pulses of powerful magnetic fields on the brain. It has yielded promising results in the treatment of depression. Brasil-Neto and colleagues (1992) studied the effect of TMS on movement choice. Subjects were asked to move either their left or their right hand at a signal: the choice of movements was theirs alone. Simultaneously, their motor cortex was magnetically stimulated. Subjects showed a marked preference for the hand contralateral (i.e., on the opposite side) to the stimulation. Yet they experienced the choice as free and uninfluenced by any external factor.

We can therefore already influence people's voluntary choices. Can we alter their beliefs? One way to alter people's beliefs is by inserting false memories, or deleting real ones. I leave this fascinating topic for the next chapter.

MIND READING, MIND CONTROLLING AND THE PARITY PRINCIPLE

I mentioned above that we would need to return to Phelps and colleagues' (2000) fMRI study of the neural correlates of racism. Phelps *et al.*, recall, found an association between negative evaluation of blacks and amygdala activity (the amygdala is involved in processing of emotions, and especially of fearful stimuli). Now, the interesting thing, for our purposes, is that in order to show a correlation between racism (or more precisely negative evaluation of black faces) and amygdala activity, the researchers had first to find a way to measure the degree of racism of participants. One way of going about this is simply to ask them. But few people are willing to identify themselves as racist these days. Notoriously, racist attitudes are frequently denied, not only to others, but even to oneself. Relatively few racists believe they are racists.

Fortunately for the sake of the experimental design, there are existing, well-validated, methods of measuring racial prejudice. Phelps *et al.* (2000) used two methods of measuring prejudice, the implicit association test and an eyeblink startle test. The implicit association test tests for bias, defined as a preference for one group over another, where the preference may not be conscious. The test works by asking subjects to sort positively and negatively valenced items (such as words) into one of two categories, which are also racially coded. The racial coding of the terms is altered in subsequent rounds. For instance, subjects might be asked first to sort words into the categories of "good or white" and "bad or black;" then to sort them into the categories "good or black" and "bad or white." Subjects sit in front of a computer monitor upon which words and faces are displayed. Suppose they are engaged in the first task, sorting words into "good or white" or "bad or black." In that case they are instructed to press a button on the left whenever a black face or a negatively valenced word – "pain," "hurt," "agony" – appears on the screen, and to press a button the right whenever a white face or a positively valenced word – "beautiful," "pleasure," "joy" – appears.

They then perform the second task, sorting words into "white and bad" or "black and good", again signalling category by pressing a button (of course, the order in which the two tasks are undertaken is varied randomly across subjects and across trials, in order to ensure that the results do not reflect simple order effects). The implicit association test is designed to measure racial bias by measuring relative reaction times: if it takes a subject longer to associate positive terms with black faces than with white faces, the person shows a preference for whites; the extent of this prejudice can be measured by the disparity between reaction times as well as the number of coding mistakes made (you can do an implicit association test yourself: several websites have versions of it, testing not only implicit associations for race, but also for gender, religion and sexuality).

Most whites show some tendency to associate positive terms with white faces more quickly than with black faces, and conversely with regard to negative terms. This is probably a more or less inevitable result of growing up in a culture in which negative stereotypes of blacks are common. Indeed, black Americans do not escape the effects of these stereotypes, though – unsurprisingly – they are more resistant to them than are whites. Black Americans show no in-group favoritism on average, whereas white Americans do; instead they show much more varied responses, with some of them showing an implicit bias in favor of white faces (see Dasgupta 2004 for a review). Similarly, most subjects show a preference for heterosexuals over homosexuals, and males over females; once again, gay men and women are sometimes subject to the same preferences as heterosexuals, and females show a preference for males. It is not so much the existence of the preference that is of interest, when we are concerned with individuals; it is the magnitude of the preference. Someone counts as prejudiced (by this measure) only when they exhibit a significantly larger than average preference for one group over another (the existence of an overall preference for one group over another is of interest in itself, of course: it tells us something very important about our societies).

The second test Phelps *et al.* used to establish the existence of a prejudice among their subjects was a test of the startle response. The startle response – the reflex that causes us to jump in response to a sudden loud noise – is expressed in many ways, including a reflexive (and therefore involuntary) eyeblink. The startle response is augmented by negative or fear-provoking stimuli (Lang *et al.* 1990). This fact provides us with another means of measuring prejudice – or at least the extent to which (say) black faces are negative or fear-provoking for a subject. By measuring the extent to which the eyeblink startle response is augmented while black and white faces are shown to the subject, we can measure the extent to which such faces are negatively valenced or fear-provoking for them.

Phelps *et al.* (2000) were only able to establish a correlation between amygdala activity and in-group preference, then, because they were able to measure in-group preference first, and they measured this preference using non-invasive techniques. In order to establish a baseline for comparison with their fMRI measure of racism, they used the tools of cognitive psychology: they used measures that are environmental rather than internal, exterior rather than interior. People who worry about the – so-called – mind-reading abilities promised or threatened by the new neurosciences often express the concern that these invasive techniques might threaten our "brain privacy" (Farah 2005). These concerns have provoked calls for the preservation of a right to "cognitive liberty" (Sententia 2004). Cognitive liberty, the argument runs, must be directly protected because it faces new and unprecedented threats. Whereas previously freedom of thought could be effectively protected by guaranteeing freedom of expression, in this new climate, where our mind/brains can be "read," we need new protections, protections which extend into the privacy of our skulls. But these responses need to be carefully rethought, in light of the fact that "mind-reading" is best done, today and for the foreseeable future, from outside the mind.

Generally, the best way to discover what someone is thinking is to ask them. They are able to describe the contours of their thoughts with a detail and a subtlety, using that marvellous tool, language, that far surpasses any other method we have available (or are likely to, probably ever). But when we ask someone what they are thinking they have the option of refusing to answer, lying or telling only part of the truth. These are, of course, options we exercise everyday, in ways that are innocuous or even beneficial. Someone asks us how they look, and rather than cause unnecessary pain or embarrassment we say "great;" someone asks us a question we regard as inappropriate and we gently change the subject. The worry about neuroscientific technologies is that they threaten to take this power away from us: it won't matter whether we want to reply or not, because the technologies will scan our brains and extract the information in any case. But this worry, if it is genuine, should not be focused on neuroscientific technologies: the techniques of psychology are at least as effective in revealing information about us without our consent.[1]

Of course the psychological techniques require elaborate set-ups: cooperative subjects (though they need not know what the techniques are measuring), large amounts of expensive equipment and trained operators. Might the neuroscientific techniques be more effective as covert measures of our minds than anything psychology can produce? There's no reason to think so. EEGs, fMRIs and other neuroscientific techniques are more expensive, harder to conceal and require even more cooperative subjects than measures of startle responses, not less. No doubt these techniques can get cheaper, smaller and easier to use, but the same can be said for the techniques of psychology, should anyone be interested in developing them. If the one could be used, in principle, for covert scanning of the contents of the mind, so could the other. It's relatively easy to see how measures of the startle response could be covertly conducted. We can display relevant stimuli (e.g., pictures of black and white faces) in a way that people can't fail to notice them, and then produce loud noises: gathering this data shouldn't be any more difficult than measuring amygdala activity.

Indeed, some of the new lie-detection technologies currently under investigation measure external responses, not internal. Some researchers seek to build on Paul Ekman's research on facial expressions as indicators of deception. Ekman argues that involuntary "micro-expressions" give us away when we lie. Micro-expressions are facial expressions which occur so briefly that they are undetectable by untrained observers; they are also difficult to produce voluntarily and difficult to suppress voluntarily (Ekman 2003). They are therefore reliable signs of deception – not perfect, but at least as good as anything that more interventionist technologies have to offer. By scanning the faces of subjects with video cameras, and interpreting the results with software designed to detect the relevant micro-expressions, some researchers hope to develop reliable lie-detection methods (Gazzaniga 2005).

Ironically, if they succeed they will do so by building upon one of humanity's most ancient capacities. The ability to detect deception has probably been selected for in the evolutionary history of humanity: for a social animal like human beings, being able to trust wisely is an important ability. Despite this fact, we are not all that good at it, probably because at the same time as evolution has selected for the ability to detect deceivers, it has selected for the ability to deceive (and possibly even self-deceive) (Trivers 1985). Whatever the explanation, most of us don't do all that well in detecting deception (DePaulo 1994), generally performing close to chance. However, some people *are* good at detecting deception: some of the members of groups with a professional interest in detecting deception, and who practice the skill regularly, perform very well at the task. Interrogators from the CIA and from police forces, and clinical psychologists with a special interest in detecting deception perform well above chance at the task, without any special equipment (Ekman *et al.* 1999). If we are worried about the ability of others to discover what is on our minds, it is not only neuroscientific technologies, and not even the techniques of cognitive and social psychology, that we must worry about; it is also the ordinary skills of mind reading that human beings possess, and which can be honed to a high degree of accuracy.

What about controlling the mind? Can our thoughts be constrained, limited and directed by others without the use of neuroscientific technologies? This kind of thought control has been the goal of repressive governments and cultural and religious authorities for millennia; more recently advertisers have got in on the act. I think it is reasonably obvious that these people have had some success; sometimes quite spectacular success. Consider the success of some societies in bringing members of oppressed or severely disadvantaged groups to accept their situation as just. In one study of attitudes to health, widows and widowers in India were asked to rate their health. Widows rated their health significantly better than widowers; in fact their health was significantly worse on average (Nussbaum 2000). It is plausible to suspect that widowers in India, which is still an extremely sexist society, have higher expectations and a greater sense of entitlement, as a consequence of attitudes prevalent in their culture. This sense of entitlement translates into dissatisfaction with their health when it is less than optimal, but women, with a much lower sense of self-worth, accept much greater impairments before they complain. Ideas prevalent in a culture are usually absorbed by the majority of its members, even when these ideas conflict with their real interests; the finding that black Americans often show a bias against black faces in the implicit association test demonstrates the same phenomenon.

One difference between this process of absorption and the kind of mind control that some people fear from neuroscientific technologies is that there is no one – certainly no single person – at the controls. Indeed, the people in a position most strongly to influence the ideology of a culture, the religious, political and cultural leaders, are often themselves in the grip of these very same ideas. It is, very probably, unusual for a leader to seek entirely cynically to manipulate the masses; instead they usually seek to inculcate ideas and to reinforce them at least in part because they take them to be true.

Moreover, even if they do seek to manipulate others for entirely cynical ends, this method of changing people's minds is a blunt instrument. It certainly doesn't work perfectly, and it is better at some things than at others. It can lead us to have biases that we don't endorse, but it works less well at changing our conscious beliefs and some people are quite good at resisting it.

Nevertheless, this kind of external control can be used, quite cynically, to get us to perform actions that are not in our interests. Advertisers have been very successful in making certain kinds of useless consumption compulsory: they have ensured that most of us cannot avoid giving quite expensive Christmas gifts, for instance, even when these gifts are not really wanted or appreciated. Britons alone spend around two billion pounds annually on *unwanted* Christmas presents (Smillie 2004). These are gifts that most of us don't want to purchase, often entirely useless (not to mention tasteless) novelty items, and which the recipients don't want to receive. They are exchanged because Christmas gift-giving, *commercialized* gift-giving, has become an almost inescapable fact of contemporary life. Advertisers have brought us to do what they wish, for their benefit, and that of their clients, and not for ours. Is neuroscientific mind control any more threatening?

Rest assured, moreover, that advertisers are keeping abreast of developments in all the sciences of the mind. Though there would be a horrified response if they were working at internal means of mind-control – TMS, for instance – no one seems to mind so long as they seek more effective methods of external control. Work in social psychology on the phenomenon of loss of control, the so-called ego-depletion hypothesis, is currently under investigation by marketers. We will examine ego-depletion in some detail in a later chapter; very briefly the idea is that self-control is a limited resource, which is depletable in the short-term and which only gradually returns to its initial level. If you want to make someone buy a product that they desire, but which they prefer, all things considered, not to purchase, you ought to ensure that their self-control resources are depleted when they confront the option of purchasing it. This can be done by requiring potential purchasers to engage in self-control tasks, which deplete their resources, before they are presented with the option of purchasing. One way this might be done is simply by exposing them to many opportunities to consume: they can successfully resist the early temptations, but repeated exposure will lead inevitably to consumption, if the subject doesn't remove themselves from the scene of temptation. It goes without saying that shopping malls present us with constant temptations in precisely this manner.

To my knowledge, no one has tested the hypothesis that repeated shopping opportunities are ego-depleting all by themselves. However psychologists have tested whether ego-depletion affects the propensity to consume, as well as whether it affects subjects' evaluation of consumer items (Vohs and Faber, 2003). Ego-depleted subjects are more willing to buy, and will pay higher prices, at least in the laboratory. Marketers seeking ways to control our behavior are far more likely to use this kind of technique than to resort to the use of more invasive techniques. They can structure the environment to produce the behavior they want, and they can do so more effectively in this manner than they can using the tools of neuroscience. Most people are not as worried about this kind of manipulation as they are about neuroscientific technologies. But the differences are not important. Both manipulate behavior, and they do so for purposes that are not those of the people who are manipulated. Both can result in changes in beliefs, and in the actions which express those beliefs. The way in which these alterations come about doesn't seem to matter, from a moral, or a political, point of view. If there are good reasons to be concerned about the first kind of manipulation, there are equally good reasons to care about the second as well.

CONCLUSION

In this chapter, we have seen that there are no *special* reasons to worry about neuroscientific mind reading or mind control; the kinds of powers that neuroscience promises in the near future pale in comparison to the mind reading and control techniques already in existence, in power and in precision. Autonomy is an important good, and we ought not to surrender it lightly: for this reason, we ought to be concerned about mind control and mind privacy (since autonomy matters, largely, to allow us the space to develop and pursue our own conception of the good, not only without direct interference from others, but also without the moral pressure that might come from observation). But we ought not to be concerned especially about internal means of manipulating or reading the mind: not unless and until far more powerful techniques come into existence than currently seem practical.

Thus, the issues of brain privacy and mind control demonstrate the ethical parity principle in action: we see that the very same reasons we have to fear neuroscientific mind reading and mind control apply, with at least equal force, to existing techniques, and perhaps even more to new discoveries coming not from neuroscience but from cognitive and social psychology. Of course, we need only the weak version of the parity principle to make the point. But it is worth remarking that the very success of weak ethical parity might constitute indirect evidence for the strong principle, by helping to support the extended mind hypothesis itself. If the extended mind hypothesis is true, then we have as much reason to be concerned about external manipulations as internal, since both can equally target the mind *itself*. And indeed, it seems that we ought. Given that we think with cognitive resources which extend beyond our skulls, into the environment, given that we rely for our cognition on resources that extend across space and across time, it is far from surprising that neuroscience is not *uniquely* perilous.

End note

1. Canli (2006) dissents. He provides what he takes to be "empirical evidence that data derived from brain scans can be better predictors of behavioral measures than other types of measures" (2006: 174). However, his

evidence shows no such thing. What he demonstrated is that fMRI data better accords with measures of behavior than personality questionnaires do. Two points should be made about this data. First, it is unsurprising that fMRI measures, which measure moment-by-moment states, better measure these states than questionnaires that seek to measure stable personality traits. Second, Canli established the accuracy of his fMRI measurements by calibrating them against a baseline that was itself behavioural: reaction times in an emotional word test, and self-reported subjective emotional ratings. Nothing in his experiments showed that these – behavioral – measurements are unreliable. Indeed, Canli's experiment *cannot* show this, in principle, since the experimental design depends upon taking these measures as a baseline.

5   The neuroethics of memory

One scenario which simultaneously fascinates and horrifies many people is the prospect that our memories could be altered by others. The number of films depicting this kind of scenario bears witness to its fascination; think of *Total Recall*, *Eternal Sunshine of the Spotless Mind* or *Dark City*. The prospect of losing our memories, or having them replaced with false recollections, exerts such power over us because we all recognize, more or less clearly, that our memories are, in some sense, *us*: our very identities (in one sense of that multiply ambiguous term) are constituted by our past experiences insofar as we can recall them and insofar as they shape our present behavior, thoughts and desires.

The so-called memory criterion of personal identity was originally proposed by John Locke, the great seventeenth-century English philosopher. Locke argued that a person at time *t* was the same person as an individual at some earlier time if at *t* they are able to remember experiences of that earlier individual. Locke's criterion came under attack almost immediately, and with good reason: philosophers like Thomas Reid pointed out that the memory criterion was circular. Memory *presupposes* personal identity, and therefore cannot constitute it. I can only remember things that actually happened to me; that's part of the very definition of memory (if I seem to remember being abducted by aliens, but I was never in fact abducted by aliens, I don't actually *remember* being abducted by aliens; "remember" is a success word and is only appropriately applied when the event actually happened, and the recollection is appropriately caused by the event). Nevertheless, Locke was clearly onto some important aspect of identity. He was wrong in thinking that memory provides a criterion of persistence of identity across time, but it does constitute our identity in a different sense.

Marya Schechtman usefully distinguishes between two senses of personal identity. The traditional debate in philosophy, the one to which Locke took his memory criterion to be a contribution, seeks answers to what Schechtman calls the *reidentification* question: the question of whether an individual at *t* is the same person as an individual at another time. There are circumstances in which the reidentification question actually matters (for instance, we might be concerned with questions about when individuals come into and go out of existence, because the answers seem to bear on issues like the moral permissibility of abortion and the moral significance of sustaining the life of individuals in persistent vegetative states). But in everyday life we are usually far more concerned with Schectman's second question, the *characterization* question: the question of which mental states and attitudes, as well as the actions caused by such states, belong to a person. When we talk about someone's identity, it is generally this sense of identity we have in mind. Think of the phenomenon of the "identity crisis": someone undergoing an identity crisis does not wonder whether they are now the same person (in the reidentification sense) as another past individual; they wonder whether their values and projects are the kinds of things they can authentically identify with.

In this sense of the word, our identities *are* very importantly constituted by our memories. At least, they are constituted by our beliefs, plans, policies and values, and these things exist across time. What *really* matters to me is not just a matter of what I think matters to me now; it is revealed in my behavior over the long-term. This is not to say that I can't change my mind – conversions on the road to Damascus really happen, after all. But a genuine conversion must itself be ratified by a long-term change in behavior; a short term conversion is merely an aberration. Our identities, in this sense, are diachronic entities: I am the sum of my plans and policies; I work towards a goal and I understand myself in terms of my background – where I'm coming from, as we say, is where I come from (my religion, my community, my language group and ethnicity, my family). Memory links my past to my future self, and makes me the person I am.

Hence, I suggest, our horrified fascination with the idea of losing our memories. Would *I* survive if my memories evaporated? In what sense would I still be the same person if my memories were replaced by false ones? Hence the fascination not only with false memories, but also with amnesia: not just films like *Eternal Sunshine of the Spotless Mind*, in which the protagonists deliberately erase some of their own memories, but also films like *Memento* and *50 First Dates*, in which characters struggle to cope with catastrophic memory loss. We also see the same horrified fascination in our responses to dementia, which we see, rightly or wrongly, as the gradual unravelling of the person themselves.

Neuroscientific knowledge and the technologies it might spawn are relevant to our memory-constituted identities in several ways. Most directly, it might give us the means of altering our memory systems, in more or less dramatic ways. Dramatic (potential) alterations include the deliberate deletion of memories, or the insertion of false memories; less dramatic alterations include the enhancement of our memories, perhaps beyond their current capacities, or the treatment or prevention of memory loss. More immediately, we may already have the ability to modulate the emotional significance of memories in certain ways; a power that promises great benefits, but which also, used inappropriately, might carry great risks. Understanding the significance of this power is one of the most pressing issues in all of neuroethics, simply because the techniques needed to put it into practice may already exist. We shall explore this question fully later in this chapter; for now, let us turn to the question of the insertion or deletion of memories.

TOTAL RECALL

Is it possible to insert false memories into the mind of a person? Developing the power to alter or insert memories requires a far better understanding of the precise manner in which memories are encoded than we currently possess. There are two obstacles to our being able to insert memories, one technical and one conceptual. Overcoming the technical obstacle requires unravelling the mechanisms by which memories are stored and retrieved, and then using this knowledge to develop a technique whereby memories can be mimicked. We have made great progress at the first half of this task: we understand how memories are first stored in the medial temporal system, in the form of enhanced connections between neurons, with a particular pattern of connections constituting a particular memory (though we are far from being able to "read" the memory just by examining the connections between the neurons). We know that memories that persist are transferred out of the medial temporal system and distributed across networks in cortical regions (Schacter 1996). Because short-term memories and consolidated memories are stored in different regions of the brain, the ability to recall events long past can be preserved even when the ability to lay down new memories is lost. There are cases of patients who, through disease or brain injury, live in an eternal present, entirely unable to recall events for more than a few seconds, and who therefore do not know where they are or what they are doing. These unfortunates typically retain memories of their childhoods; in general, the older the memory, the more resistant it is (a phenomenon known as Ribot's law).

Inserting memories requires not only that we understand memory storage, how a pattern of neural connections constitutes a memory, but also memory retrieval: how the pattern is reactivated. Here, too, we are making great strides, though perhaps it is fair to say that we know less about retrieval than about storage. There is evidence that retrieval is, in part, reconstruction: that what is recalled is an amalgam of the original event as it occurred, and the retrieval cues which prompt recall (Schacter 1996). The memories we recall are influenced by the goals we have at the moment of recollection, our intervening experiences and our reinterpretations. Hence, each time that (ostensibly) the same event is recalled, it will in fact be subtly (and perhaps not so subtly) different: first, because the retrieval cue will be different in each case (since the context of retrieval is necessarily different each time), and therefore the combination of stored memory and retrieval cue will be unique; and second because the stored memory itself, the so-called engram, will have changed by the very fact of having been recalled. As Schacter (1996: 71) puts it, "we do not shine a spotlight on a stored picture" when we recollect; instead, we reconstruct the past event using stored cues.[1]

Retrieval seems to work through the matching up of a cue to an engram; if there is a sufficient degree of match, the memory is recalled. The process is mediated by a kind of index, which keeps track of the engrams scattered through cortical regions. Inserting a memory would therefore require not merely altering the connections between neurons in such a manner as to mimic a real engram; it also requires that the indexing system be deciphered and mimicked. The technical challenge is immense, and may in fact prove insurmountable. We may never understand memories in sufficient detail to know what neural connections would be needed to create a false memory, and even if we one day acquire this knowledge, understanding what is involved is one thing, being able to recreate it ourselves is quite another. Insertion of false memories, using direct intervention into the brain, is at best a long way off.

Suppose that we one day overcome the many obstacles that currently stand between us and the ability to insert false memories. It is probable that even then there would be quite severe limitations on the content of the false memories that could be inserted, limitations that stem from the *holism* of mental content. By the holism of the mental, I mean the way in which mental content is usually involved in manifold meaningful links to related content. Daniel Dennett (1978) has explored the ways in which this holism limits the content that could be inscribed directly in the brain, had we the technology. Suppose that we wanted to implant the false memory that Patty visited Disneyland with her younger brother when she was five, when in fact Patty has no younger brother, and suppose we know what neural connections must be made in order to create this memory and how this memory must be indexed to be available for recall; we go ahead and make the changes required. Now suppose we ask Patty about the trip: "Do you recall any holidays with your brother when you were a child?" What will Patty say? She'll probably be confused, saying something like "I seem to recall a trip to Disneyland with my brother, but I don't have a brother." For a proposition that must occupy a relatively central position in someone's web of beliefs, it's not enough (apparently) just to wire it in: one must also wire in a whole set of related beliefs. For Patty to recall a trip to Disneyland with her brother, she must recall that she has a brother, and recalling *that* will require a large set of related propositions and memories. Recalling the existence of a brother implies recalling innumerable everyday experiences involving him (sitting down at the breakfast table together, playing together, and so on) or recalling an explanation for why the brother was absent from everyday life, and where he is now. Beliefs do not generally come as isolates in the mental economy of subjects. Instead, they come in clusters, and the more central to our identity (in the characterization sense of the word) the larger the cluster. Central experiences and relationships do not come all by themselves; instead, they spread their shadow over almost all of our mental lives.

Patty will expect herself, and will be expected by others, to be able to recall all kinds of information about her brother. The isolated thought, that she went to Disneyland with him when she was five, in the absence of a whole network of related memories will probably seem more like a hallucination than a veridical memory or belief. Memories of experiences that are central to our lives imply many other propositions, beliefs and memories. Suppose, then, we attempt to wire in not just the single memory, that Patty went to Disneyland with her younger brother when she was five, but enough of the network of beliefs that that memory implies to make it stable enough to be accepted by Patty as veridical. We shall probably discover that this network needs to be very extensive. Each of the propositions implied by the proposition that Patty went to Disneyland with her younger brother when she was five itself implies further propositions: propositions about her brother's friends, propositions about their parents (did they favour her over her brother, or vice versa? Did they worry about him? Was he naughty child?) and these propositions imply yet further propositions. Moreover, some of them might conflict with memories and beliefs that Patty already possesses: memories of loneliness, perhaps, or of envy of those with siblings, memories of being asked whether she had brothers and replying negatively, and so on. Will we delete these memories? If we don't we risk the failure of our attempt to wire in the memory: when Patty realizes that her new memory conflicts with others, she may revise one or the other, dismissing it as a dream; the less well-embedded memory (the one with the fewest rational connections to other memories) will probably be the one to go. But if we do delete these memories, we shall also have to delete the network of propositions that *these* memories imply, and so on for these implied memories in turn.

Inserting a memory or a belief almost certainly does not require that we insert every other proposition that it might imply, and erase every proposition with which it conflicts. Our mental economy is not so coherent as all that. If we were pressed on our beliefs long enough, we could all detect some conflicts within our own web: beliefs about friends that are contradictory (that Janine is selfish; that Janine has on several occasions gone out of her way to help others at some cost to herself, or whatever it might be). But the conflicts and incoherencies had better not be too obvious: if they are, either our web of beliefs is in danger of unravelling, or our status as (reasonably) rational agents will be under threat. One possibility is that Patty will end up looking for all the world like a delusional subject. Sufferers from the classic delusions – Capgras' delusion, in which the person believes that someone close to them has been replaced by an impostor, Cotard's delusion, in which they believe they are dead, somotaparaphrenia, in which they deny that a limb is theirs, and so on – often exhibit the same paradoxical belief structure as might someone who recalls that they went to Disneyland with their younger brother, and that they have no younger brother. It's often observed that delusions are in many ways incoherent. Someone who believes that they are dead retains the usual understanding of death. They know that dead people don't tell others that they are dead. But they are apparently untroubled by the discrepancy. Similarly, sufferers from Capgras' delusion often fail to exhibit the kinds of emotional responses we would expect to the belief that someone close to them has been replaced by an impostor: they don't call the police, nor do they worry where their real husband or wife has gone and how they're getting on. They are very stubborn in affirming their delusional belief, but also sometimes seem to believe the direct opposite. There have been numerous attempts at explaining, or explaining away, the paradoxical patterns of belief of the deluded (Currie 2000; Bayne and Pacherie 2005; Hamilton forthcoming). This debate need not detain us here. All we need do is to note that inserting memories might undermine the coherence of the subject's beliefs, and thereby the rationality of the subject, in the same kind of way as do delusions.

It should be noted, however, that the limitations on inserting false memories that stem from the holism of the mental will affect some false memories and beliefs more than others. The greater the degree of conflict between the false memory and existing memories and beliefs, the more difficult it will be to insert the memory (and end up with a rational subject). Some memories will cohere quite well with the subject's existing beliefs; the holism of the mental will present no obstacle to their insertion. Anything which could well have happened but didn't (that you had ice-cream cake and a balloon on your fifth birthday; that you got a parking ticket two years ago – obviously the content of such plausible false memories will vary from subject to subject, and from culture to culture) could be inserted without this particular problem cropping up. The holism of the mental is therefore only a limitation on our ability to insert false memories, not an insurmountable obstacle. It is, however, an extremely important limitation, for the following reason: in general, the more important the false memory to be inserted – where important beliefs are either those central to the agent's identity, in the characterization sense, or those which might be expected to have had a significant impact on then – the more connections there must be between it and subsequent memories and beliefs, and therefore the greater the difficulties posed by the holism of the mental. It will prove relatively difficult to convince someone that they were kidnapped by aliens five years ago (since they should have subsequent memories that depend on that event: memories of telling the police, their friends, their doctor; memories of nightmares and fears, and so on).

False memories can be important without being deeply embedded into an agent's mental economy: some kinds of relatively commonplace events can be significant. Therefore, the holism of the mental does not make the implantation of important false memories impossible. On the contrary, it is *already* possible to implant significant false memories. The most promising (if that's the right word) results in memory insertion today do not involve cutting-edge neuroscientific techniques. They involve much lower-tech techniques of suggestion and prompting. Elizabeth Loftus has shown that these techniques can be quite effective at inducing false memories in normal subjects. We are highly suggestible creatures, and suggestible in surprising ways. Loftus discovered, for instance, that recall of traffic accidents was sensitive to the questions asked of subjects: if they were asked how fast the cars were going when they *smashed* into each other, they recalled higher speeds than if they were asked how fast they were going when they *hit* one another; moreover, they were more likely falsely to recall seeing broken glass if asked the former question (Loftus 2003). Hundreds of studies have now been published showing that subjects exposed to false information about events they have personally witnessed will frequently incorporate that information into their later recollections (Loftus 2003). Misleading questions seem to fill gaps in subjects' recall: the proportion of "don't recall" responses drops after subjects are primed with misleading information, and the false information takes the place of such responses.

Loftus has even been able to create memories out of whole cloth. In one famous study, she had family members of subjects describe to her events from the subjects' childhoods. She then retold these stories to the subjects; unbeknownst to them, however, she added one false recollection (of having been lost in a shopping mall at age five, including specific details about how upset they were and how they were eventually rescued by an elderly person). About twenty-five percent of subjects falsely recalled the event; many claimed to recall additional details (Loftus and Pickrell 1995). Later work, by Loftus and others, now suggests that the proportion of people who will confabulate false memories in this kind of paradigm is actually slightly higher: around thirty-one percent. Moreover, the false memories need not be banal: people may confabulate unusual and traumatic false memories (Loftus 2003). To ensure that the memories are truly false, and not actual events recalled only by the subject, impossible events are sometimes suggested. For instance, subjects were brought to recall meeting Bugs Bunny at Disneyland (Bugs is a Warner Brothers character, and would never be found at Disneyland). Sometimes the false memories are very rich and highly elaborated; often the subject expresses great confidence in their veracity.

These memory distortions also occur, unfortunately, outside the laboratory. Gazzaniga (2005) provides a recent and striking example. In 2002, Washington D.C. and neighboring Virigina and Maryland were terrorized by a sniper, who for three weeks targeted random individuals, killing ten. During these panicked three weeks, several witnesses reported seeing the sniper driving a white truck. In fact, the sniper drove a blue car. What happened? First, a witness who had seen a white truck near the scene of one of the shootings falsely recalled seeing the sniper in the truck. The media picked up on the false recollection, and broadcast descriptions of the truck.

The expectation that a white truck was involved then primed witnesses' memories, leading them to falsely recollect seeing such a truck (2005: 125).

In fact, our memories are far less reliable then we typically think. We incorporate false information and suggestions, advertently or inadvertently given to us by others, into our memories; we create composite memories out of similar scenes; we transpose details and even central incidents from one memory to another, and our expectations lead us to recall details that never occurred. Skilful manipulators can use these facts about us deliberately to distort memories; more frequently clumsy interrogators inadvertently lead others to falsely recall events that did not take place. There is plentiful evidence that police interrogation of eyewitnesses sometimes leads to false recollections. Part of the evidence is circumstantial, and comes from studies of convictions later overturned on the basis of DNA evidence. In one study of forty such cases, fully ninety percent of the convictions were based at least in part on eyewitness testimony (Gazzaniga 2005: 131). In some cases, of course, the witness may have lied, but often they seem just to have got it wrong.

The unreliability of eyewitness testimony, at least as it is currently elicited, is extremely significant, given that an estimated 75 000 cases annually are decided on the basis of such testimony in the United States alone. What mechanisms lead people falsely to recall seeing a suspect at the scene of a crime? An important part of the explanation lies in the manner in which the *source* of a recollection can be forgotten. A witness to a crime may be shown mugshots before they are asked to pick out the suspect from a line up. They may then confidently identify a suspect, recognizing that they have seen him before. But they may have seen his picture in the mug shots, rather than seeing him at the scene of the crime. Suspects have even come to mistake their imaginings about a crime scene for recollections of it, and have consequently confessed to a crime they did not commit (Schacter 1996). Even memories of traumatic events, which seem seared into our brains, can come to be distorted over time (though such traumatic memories tend to be resilient in their central features). Since memories are so easily contaminated, they should only be relied upon, in a legal setting, if they are elicited sensitively; unfortunately, police are largely ignorant of the need to avoid such contamination and may sometimes inadvertently lead witnesses to confuse what they saw with what the interrogators describe or suggest.

Advertent or inadvertent memory distortion also occurs in other contexts. Consider the phenomenon of repressed memory and its recovery. The repression of memory may indeed be a real phenomenon: there is evidence that people sometimes do become amnesic for traumatic events (Schacter 1996). But there is much less evidence that they can recover these memories, and the evidence that exists is equivocal and open to dispute. On the other hand, the evidence that memories, however sincerely held and detailed, can be entirely false, is overwhelming. Importantly, we have no way to distinguish real memories from false: neither the person whose "memory" it is nor observers, no matter how highly trained, can confidently distinguish true memories from false. Confidence, vividness, detail – none of these factors distinguish true memories from false.[2] It may be possible to recover veridical memories of past traumas, but unless there is strong *independent* evidence of the veracity of the recovered "memory," we should regard such memories with suspicion.

The fact that recovered "memories" are more likely than not false (perhaps *far* more likely) matters greatly: there have been many court cases, criminal and civil, which are mainly or even entirely based around such recollections. Many people have gone to jail, convicted largely, often exclusively, on the basis of recovered memories. Many of these convictions are certainly wrongful, in the sense that the person did not in fact commit the crimes of which he or she is accused; *all* of them are unsafe. Consider one well-known case, that of Paul Ingram. Ingram, a sheriff's deputy, was accused of molesting his daughters, on the basis of their recovered memories (after a member of the daughters' church, who claimed to have the gift of prophecy, told one of them that God had told her that the daughter had been abused). Ingram claimed not to recall any abuse, but at the urging of his pastor and a therapist, Ingram began to "remember." The girls' accusations rapidly became more bizarre: they claimed they had been raped and forced to bear children, who were then sacrificed in a Satanic ritual attended by other towns-people. Ingram duly recalled many of these supposed events. He pleaded guilty when the case came to trial, and was sentenced to twenty years imprisonment.

During the trial, Ingram was extensively tested by Richard Ofshe, a social psychologist. Ofshe wanted to know how suggestible Ingram was. As Loftus had shown, many of us are vulnerable to having false memories implanted in us, but could a memory of sexual abuse be created out of whole cloth? Ofshe fabricated a false memory for Ingram: he told him that Ingram's son had reported that he and Ingram's daughter had been forced to have sex in front of him. In fact, no one had made any such allegation. Ingram failed to recall the incident at first, but after praying and meditating, he developed a detailed memory of the event. In part on the basis of Ofshe's obser-vations, Ingram attempted to change his plea to not guilty, but he was too late: the court rejected his plea (Schacter 1996). He served fourteen years before being released in 2003.

The guilty parties, in many cases of recovered memories, are the therapists and counsellors who encourage their emergence. Sometimes recovered memories might appear spontaneously; more often, they are coaxed and cajoled by well-meaning but ignorant advisers. Some psychotherapists use techniques – encouraging patients to visualize events they cannot recall, or to pretend that they happened – which are known to be effective in producing false memories, or in otherwise bringing people to mistake imaginings for reality (Loftus 1993). Recovered memories may, occasionally, be veridical. But they seem far more likely to be false, and they are certainly never reliable enough to serve as the basis for a criminal conviction. When people believe themselves to recover memories of abuse, they suffer a great deal of pain: the memories are no less traumatic for being false, the sense of betrayal by loved ones no smaller. They suffer and their families, often their entire local community, suffers as well. Moreover, as Loftus (1993) points out, the cycle of recovered memory and exposure risks producing other victims: genuine victims of childhood sexual abuse (almost all of whom never forget the abuse) may be disbelieved, tarred with the same brush as those who recover "memories" of abuse.

Reflecting on the ways in which memory is already subject to distortion and manipulation ought thus to give us pause. Though the power that neuroscience might offer to distort memories raises serious moral and political qualms, no less serious are the problems that currently beset us. Induced memory distortions, deliberate or accidental, already impose high costs: innocent people convicted of crimes they did not commit, families torn apart by accusations of abuse, investigations going astray because witnesses incorporate false information into their recollections. We do not seem close to any new neuroscientific technology that might help us avoid these problems: the drugs currently in development that promise to enhance memory seem not to protect us against its suggestibility. But there are direct ethical implications of our growing *knowledge* about memory, the way it works and the ways in which it fails. We ought to be far less trusting of eyewitness testimony. The mere fact that someone sincerely claims to recognize the perpetrator of a crime should not be sufficient grounds for conviction, all by itself. Only when we can be sure that the memory is uncontaminated – that no one has suggested to the witness that this person is the criminal, that there has not been a failure of source memory, so that the person genuinely recognizes the individual, but is mistaken as to where they have previously seen them – should we rely upon such testimony. But avoiding such contamination is near impossible. This being the case, eyewitness testimony must be treated sceptically: only when it is corroborated (by other witnesses, or, preferably, independent evidence – DNA, fingerprints, cameras, and so on) should it lead to conviction.

MEMORY MANIPULATION

Suppose that significant memory manipulation, of the kind envisaged in films like *Eternal Sunshine* and *Total Recall*, becomes possible. What ethical questions would this raise? I have advocated the parity thesis throughout this book. But the parity thesis does not commit us to thinking that all the problems that new technologies might present have already been anticipated. Far from it: the parity thesis only commits us to saying that *the mere fact that* a technology is new and unprecedented, or that it involves direct interventions into the brain using new neuroscientific knowledge and techniques, does not give us reason to think that it raises new, or even – necessarily – especially great, problems. But if the direct manipulations of memory envisaged in science fiction films ever do become possible, there is good reason to think that the problems they pose would indeed be unprecedented.

Memory alteration and erasure could cause harm to the person him or herself, or to others. The harms to self which could potentially result would not be unprecedented in *form*, though they may be unprecedented in *degree*. What is the nature of these harms? Recall the reasons that memory matters so much for us. Memory is significantly constitutive of our identities, in what Schectman calls the characterization sense of identity. Our memories help us to make sense of our actions and our personalities, by situating them in the context of an unfolding narrative. Our most important actions get their significance from their place in this narrative: we engage in them in order to further projects which have their origin in the past, and which continue into the future. I type this sentence *in order to* finish this paragraph, and I aim to finish this paragraph *in order to* finish this book; and I want to finish this book *in order to* ... what? We can trace the significance of this work to me ultimately all the way to what Sartre (1956) called my fundamental project, which is my way of living my life. Perhaps I aim (at a level slightly less fundamental than the one Sartre had in mind) to boost my CV and get a better job, thereby to increase my income and my personal comfort, or perhaps I aim at recognition from my peers, or at increasing the amount of knowledge in the world. In any event, the meaning of my action is constituted in very important part by the threads that link my past to my future.

Now, as Schectman recognizes, our personal narratives are never wholly consistent or coherent. The suggestibility of memory, and the way it alters with recall, ensures that each of us is likely to misremember certain events. A certain amount of incoherence need not matter, nor a certain amount of falsity. It is a difficult matter to identify the point at which incoherence or falsity ceases to be innocuous. Part of the problem stems from the fact that more than one kind of good depends upon the kinds of narratives we construct for ourselves, and that these goods can conflict. Narratives are routes to self-knowledge, which is a good that is – arguably – intrinsic, that is, valuable in its own right, as well as a good that is instrumentally valuable inasmuch as it allows us to achieve other goods (since knowing one's own strengths and weaknesses allows one to plan future actions more effectively). But narratives can also be instrumentally valuable independently of their truth.

An example will make this clearer. The American philosopher Owen Flanagan (1996b) has related how one of his own childhood memories proved instrumentally valuable to him. Flanagan had, he tells us, very few friends as a young child. But he did have one close friend, Billy, with whom he spent many happy hours playing. Later he lost touch with Billy, but the memory of this important friendship gave him the confidence he needed to approach people and make new friends. Years later he discovered that his Billy memories were almost entirely false. Billy had been the son of one of his father's colleagues, and had visited the Flanagans just once. Owen had indeed played with Billy, but they had never been friends. The close and long-lasting friendship was a fabrication, built upon the flimsiest of foundations – yet the influence of the "memory" had been very real. It really had contributed significantly to Owen's later success at making friends.

Flanagan's memory was false, and therefore could not contribute to his self-knowledge. Yet it was instrumentally valuable, helping him to achieve goods that mattered to him. More usually, we can expect instrumental value and intrinsic value to coincide, for the following reason: generally, being able to achieve the goods that matter to us depends on having true beliefs, both about ourselves and about the world. If you want to avoid danger, it helps to be able to accurately distinguish tigers from trees, and to know how good you are at outrunning the former and climbing the latter. If Flanagan had no social skills and no capacity to develop them, his false memories would not have been instrumentally valuable to him; it is only because – by chance – his false memories were not an inaccurate guide to his capacities that they proved useful.

The more central a capacity to the agent's sense of themselves, and the more central to the projects they undertake, the more important it is for them to have an accurate sense of it. Flanagan went on to become a prominent philosopher of mind; it was therefore important to him to have a good sense whether he was more talented intellectually or on the sporting field. For most of us, the kind of work we do is central to our sense of identities, in the characterization sense. Friendship, family and relationships are also central to this sense of identity, and it will be correspondingly important for each of us to have true beliefs about them. It does not matter very much whether each of our memories regarding our interactions with those closest to us are accurate, so long as our general sense of the shape of the relationship – of its narrative course – is accurate (Schechtman 1996). Reminiscing with family and friends we occasionally discover events concerning which we have divergent memories. It doesn't matter much, so long as each of us is correct in our general sense of the importance we have for each other, the place we each occupy in others' lives and their affections.

However, with regard to many of our memories, truth or falsity does matter. This suggests one important reason why erasing certain memories can constitute a significant harm to oneself. Some of the memories we might be tempted to erase are relatively inconsequential: all those petty embarrassments and humiliations which haunt each of us. But some of our memories, including some of our most painful, are important guides to our abilities and limitations. They constitute self-knowledge, and this self-knowledge is – at least – instrumentally valuable to us. If our lives are to go well, we require the ability to learn from our experiences: from the ways in which we failed, as well as the ways in which we succeeded. Erase our memories, and we leave ourselves at the mercy of impulses of the moment. The person who erases their failures from their memory risks being a dramatic illustration of Santayana's dictum that "those who cannot remember the past are condemned to repeat it."

Though the harms to which we could subject ourselves as a result of memory erasure would, plausibly, be more dramatic than anything we can currently produce, they would not be entirely unprecedented. People can already learn to cultivate their memories of incidents, or take steps to repress them. Experiments have shown that subjects instructed to forget items, such as a list of words presented to them, have some success at the task: though their ability to recognize words as having appeared on the list is unaffected, their ability to retrieve them uncued is reduced (Whetstone and Cross 1998). If it is possible to have some effect on one's own recall over the space of a single short experiment, it is surely possible to produce a more dramatic effect over a longer time span. Nevertheless, this is unlikely to prove as drastic as the effects of the kinds of memory erasure envisaged in science fiction.

If the harms to self made possible by such technologies could be unprecedented, at least in degree, the harms to others they could bring would be quite novel. Showing that this might be so could prove important, because considerations of autonomy normally trump considerations of self-harm. That is, if my actions will harm no one but myself, then it would normally be wrong for others to coerce me into refraining from them. I have the right to harm myself. But I do not have the right to harm others without their consent. If, therefore, memory erasure might harm others, we might permissibly prevent its use.

How might memory erasure harm others? In several ways. Our narratives, which form the core of our identities, in the characterization sense, are not merely personal and private stories. Each of us is perpetually at risk of what psychologists call *confabulation*: inventing more or less plausible stories that bear little relationship to reality to explain what we do and why. Without a public check on what happens to us, the risk that we shall slip into unchecked fantasy is high. Once again, the way memory works is important to this process. *Source memory*, our memory for where we acquired a piece of information, is dissociable from *semantic memory*, our memory for facts (Schacter 1996): it is this fact that accounts, in part, for eyewitness misidentifications. The dissociation of source memory from semantic memory explains how people can perfectly innocently come to believe their own fantasies, and this, too, has had tragic real-world consequences. It is therefore very important, for our self-knowledge, that we associate with people who can corroborate important elements of our life story. Now, if I erase my memories of you, I risk harming myself. But I also risk harming you: I remove myself, permanently and irrevocably, as a reference point against which you can check your self-narrative.

Moreover, even if we succeed in retaining accurate memories of the major events in our lives, we would likely be damaged by our inability to share them with those who feature centrally in its unfolding narrative. In the past decade, philosophers have devoted a great deal of effort to understanding the concept of *recognition*, first introduced into philosophy by the great German philosopher Hegel. Hegel saw that it was very important for us social animals that our worth be recognized by other people. But, as he also saw, our sense of self-worth depends upon recognition from others that we ourselves think worthy of recognition in turn; moreover, the recognition must be freely given if it is to be valuable. The absence of this kind of recognition is, as more recent philosophers have emphasized, profoundly damaging to our identity (once again, in the characterization sense of identity with which we are here concerned).

Why should recognition be so important to our identity? As Charles Taylor (1995) points out, this is a consequence of the extent to which our identity is *dialogical*: we understand ourselves in terms which we fashion in dialogue with others. Whereas other animals have (at best) only a very rudimentary culture, which does not significantly shape them, we humans are essentially cultural animals, and culture is by definition something which exists only intersubjectively: as a result of the interaction of human beings. Our identity is profoundly cultural, and it is therefore up for negotiation and renegotiation in the stories we tell one another. Of course, as we mature we internalize this story-telling; we begin to construct our narratives for ourselves. But, even in cultures that place a high value on the autonomy of the individual, the extent to which we can ever entirely break out of the dialogical mode is limited. We engage in lifelong conversations with others – actual conversations, with those from whom we seek recognition, and internal conversations, with those who have passed from our lives.

Now, as profoundly damaging as a lack of recognition of someone's *worth* might be, how much worse is the failure even to acknowledge that they have played a significant role in one's life *at all?* We cannot demand recognition of others: if relationships fail, we cannot prevent our lovers from walking out. We do not have a right to their time and affection, nor even to their attention. Sometimes, we must move on. But we can reasonably expect that our former lovers will at least acknowledge that we once *had* a relationship. We sometimes advise friends to try to forget their mistakes, to put them entirely behind them. In the worst cases, we might mean it literally: one might do better to entirely forget an abusive relationship (so long as the memory will not help us to avoid a repetition). But in more run-of-the-mill cases, the advice is more metaphorical. Though we know it is hard to pull it off, we often think that in acknowledgement of the significance of the relationship ex-lovers ought to remain friends, or at least cordial to one another. Of course, often this is not psychologically possible – when the relationship is broken off acrimoniously, perhaps after bad behavior by one or the other partner. But even in these cases, the coldness with which the former lovers might treat one another when they meet is a form of recognition. It has been said that hate is not the opposite of love, since both are forms of responding to the individuality of the other. The profound indifference that is the product of true forgetting, however, might be far more damaging to our sense of worth than mere hate, or the mere refusal of recognition.

Why is this profound indifference so damaging to our sense of identity? When we have had a long and significant relationship with another person, our identity-constituting narrative now incorporates that relationship into its core. The relationship might be conceptualized as the culmination of an important plot-line, as it were, in the way in which relationships are often understood in many movies. If the other person then erases the memory of that relationship from their mind, there is an important sense in which it is as if it never was. There is little practical difference, for us, between actually having had the relationship and merely having fantasized it.

Now, it is one thing to say that erasing a memory would cause harm to other people, and quite another thing to say that it is – all things considered – impermissible to erase the memory. There are many things that are morally wrong, but which we are nevertheless – morally and legally – permitted to do. We may, for instance, lie to each other, without fear of legal sanction. We can begin to delineate the limits of what we are permitted to do by considering John Stuart Mill's *harm principle* (Mill 1985). The harm principle simply states that each of us has the right to act as we like, so long as our conduct does not result in harm to (non-consenting) others. According to Mill, no one can legitimately prevent others from doing anything which does not infringe the harm principle; we cannot prevent others from doing things just because we find them distasteful, or even because we believe (or *know*) that they will later regret doing them. We may advise and persuade, but we cannot coerce, except when harm to others is threatened.

Applying Mill's harm principle yields the result that memory erasure is permissible when it harms no one, or when it harms only persons who have consented to it. But, as we have just seen, memory erasure would sometimes harm other people as well. Does that imply that, in those cases at least, it is impermissible? Not necessarily. The harm principle captures our sense of what is permissible and what is forbidden only roughly. Think of the case of lying once more: lying to those close to you may well harm them, yet we do not coerce adults into telling the truth (except in a judicial context). If we examine the rationale for the harm principle, we can come up with a better test for distinguishing permissible and impermissible acts.

The harm principle is plausibly taken to be designed to protect the *autonomy* of individuals. The idea is this: each of us has the right to pursue his or her own conception of the good life, without coercive interference from others. Historically, this idea emerged for merely pragmatic reasons, in response to the wars of religion that racked Europe in the wake of the Reformation (Rawls 1993: xxvi). The alternative to finding a *modus vivendi* – a means of getting along with one another – was endless and ruinous war. But by the eighteenth century, the doctrine of tolerance for other ways of life was increasingly recognized as a *moral* principle. We have a *right* to pursue our own conception of the good life. Part of the justification for this idea came from political philosophers pondering the purpose of the state. Many philosophers argued that the state existed only to allow autonomous individuals to pursue their own projects; since the state is constituted by the free adhesion of individuals, its legitimacy depends upon allowing each to pursue their projects without interference. It is precisely this doctrine that is expressed in the American Declaration of Independence: each of us has the "inalienable right" to the "pursuit of happiness" (as each of us sees it); the end of government is to secure these rights, and therefore when a government "becomes destructive of these ends, it is the right of the people to alter or abolish it."

Autonomy, the freedom to pursue our own conception of the good life without interference, is such an important good, for us in the societies founded on the principles of liberal political thought, that a certain amount of harm to others is tolerated in its pursuit. If, in pursuing goals fundamental to my conception of the good life, I cause you harms that are relatively superficial – which do not affect your fundamental interests, do not prevent you from pursuing your conception of the good life and do not put you at an unfair disadvantage – then I do not wrong you. Some people, for instance, are offended by the sight of gay couples. But since pursuing a relationship is a fundamental part of living a good life, on most people's conception, we need a very strong reason to prevent anyone from having such a relationship. The fact that some people are offended, even physically revolted, is not sufficient reason. In general, we are allowed to cause relatively minor harms, if we have no other practical way of pursuing goals and projects central to our conception of the good life.

The permissibility of memory erasure depends, therefore, not only on *whether* it harms others, but also on the extent of that harm. If we have the right to a sphere of liberty, within which we are entitled to do as we choose, our minds must be included within that sphere. No one may prevent me from thinking what I like, desiring what I like or fantasising what I like; my thoughts are my affair, and no one else's. It is only when we choose to act upon our thoughts that they become, potentially, matters for the state to pronounce upon and for morality to control. Thus, I must be permitted to remember what I like. It is my mind, and my mind *is* me (more or less; it is at any rate an essential part of my identity, in the characterization sense). If my freedom is to be worth anything, it must include the liberty to change my mind, figuratively or literally. Indeed, Mill himself said as much: "Over himself, over his own body and mind, the individual is sovereign." (1985: 69).

Now, it should be obvious that the extended mind hypothesis greatly complicates the picture. Were the mind confined to the skull, then there would be a strong presumption in favor of the individual's freedom to shape his or her own mind. But since the mind extends into the world, altering one's own mind might entail altering the mind of others. Hence the presumption in favor of sovereignty over one's own mind is weakened. Though the extended mind hypothesis complicates the picture, however, it does not fundamentally alter it: the individual remains, for almost all practical purposes, sovereign over their own brain, if not their mind. There remains an important asymmetry between the brain and the extended mind. The brain of each individual *always* figures in the realization of their own mental states, but the brain of one individual figures in the realization of the mental states of others less often. The most common cases of this type probably involve extended memory stores, when people rely upon one another for recall of important events. Since these cases are relatively rare, and the mental states involved often rather unimportant, cases in which we harm others directly – by actually interfering with their significant mental states – by altering our brains will be relatively rare, and we shall continue to remain sovereign over our brains. However, there are some cases in which the mental entwinement of two individuals is so extensive that altering the brain of one will cause the other significant harm. As Wilson notes (2004: 210), this is part of the reason why the death of a loved one can be so disabling, and why certain kinds of betrayal are so devastating.[3] When we consider the permissibility of someone choosing to alter their brain-based memories, such harms will figure in the costs. Generally, even then people ought to remain free to alter their own minds, though we might permissibly prevent them from so doing if their reasons are trivial.

For these reasons, it seems that despite the fact that memory erasure might harm non-consenting others, it will usually be permissible. Does it follow from this fact that moral assessment of it is pointless? No: we assess things from the moral point of view for many reasons, not just to see whether they should be banned. There are, after all, actions intermediate between forbidding and ignoring: we can advise, exhort, praise and disapprove, others and ourselves. We can educate and inculcate the best values. It doesn't follow from the fact that we decide to permit something that we must approve of it, nor that disapproval may not be very effective in discouraging others (and ourselves) from utilizing it. Moreover, ethics is concerned not only with what is permitted and what is forbidden, but also with ideals and virtues; questions of what kind of persons we should strive to be.

Additionally, given that the technology of memory erasure does not yet exist, morally assessing it can help guide our actions, as individuals and as citizens. Though states may not be justified in banning memory erasure, they are not thereby required to encourage its development. States have a great deal of control over the direction of future research: they can encourage certain technologies – by direct grants to researchers, by tax breaks to industry, and so on – and discourage others, and they can justifiably do so on grounds that are wider than those mandated by the harm principle. The harm principle tells us what we *cannot* do; it doesn't tell us how to choose among the options which it does not rule out. In order to make such choices, we can appeal to wider moral principles than those of political liberalism. If we were to find that a life which used memory alteration or erasure techniques was likely to be impoverished, then we could choose not to fund the development of the technology, even if we would not be permitted to forbid its use were it developed without our help. So ethical assessment of its worth remains relevant. And of course individuals may look to such assessments in deciding whether to make use of these technologies. It is one thing whether something should be banned; it is quite another question whether we should use it.

MODERATING TRAUMATIC MEMORIES

So far in this chapter, we have been exploring the possibility of inserting false memories into the minds of people, and we have considered the possibility, and the desirability, of erasing memories. Most of the current research on memory manipulation, however, has a rather different focus: the possibility of reducing the power of unwanted memories. In particular, this research focuses on the traumatic memories that give rise to post-traumatic stress disorder (PTSD). PTSD is a very serious and debilitating condition, affecting millions of people worldwide. Following exposure to a traumatic event, around 8.1 percent of men and 20.4 percent of women develop PTSD, yielding a lifetime prevalence rate of 5 percent for males and 10.4 percent for females in the United States (Kessler *et al.* 1996). The costs of PTSD are high, for the sufferer, his or her family and for the wider community. Quite apart from the direct suffering the disorder causes, costs include a burden on the health-care system, the failure of relationships, increased rates of reactive violence, and suicide. Any means that can be discovered to prevent PTSD, or to lower its incidence significantly, might therefore prove extremely valuable.

Obviously, the best way to reduce the incidence of PTSD is to reduce the incidence of the traumatic incidents that are likely to trigger it. Fewer wars, terrorist attacks and violent assaults would mean fewer cases of PTSD. Given, however, that these kinds of violence are unlikely ever to disappear entirely, and given that, even in the best of possible worlds, accidents will occasionally happen, we must seek alternative means of responding to PTSD.

The next best response to PTSD is to prevent its occurrence, even when people are exposed to potential triggers. There is some promising research that suggests that prevention of PTSD is possible. PTSD is believed to be based on an over-consolidation of memories of traumatic events. Trauma stimulates the release of endogenous epinephrine, which facilitates memory consolidation (via the effect of the stress hormone on the amygdala); this is probably an adaptive mechanism, since emotional significance is usually correlated with importance for survival and reproduction (in the environment of evolutionary adaptation, a mechanism that ensured that our ancestors never forgot the location of dangerous animals or other risks helped their survival). PTSD represents this adaptive mechanism gone awry: the event is recalled with a power and an intensity sufficient to retraumatize the individual; moreover, the memory is intrusive and constantly recalled. Pitnam and Delahanty (2005) suggest that a vicious cycle of memory consolidation in response to stress hormones underlies PTSD: the over-consolidated memory intrudes so powerfully into the thoughts of the subject that it triggers the stress hormones that facilitate consolidation once more, ensuring that the next time it will be recalled even more powerfully and more stressfully.

If PTSD is caused by the over-consolidation of memories, and this over-consolidation is facilitated by stress hormones, PTSD might be prevented by blocking the effect of the hormones. There is independent evidence that emotional arousal facilitates better recall, both in humans and in rats, and that this effect can be abolished by administration (*after* the arousing event) of a beta-adrenergic antagonist (a "beta blocker"), which blocks the effect of the stress hormones (McGaugh 2000; Cahill *et al.* 1994). Building on these results, Roger Pitman and colleagues (Pitman, *et al.* 2002; Pitman and Delahanty 2005) have produced encouraging results using propranolol for the prevention of PTSD. Pitman and his team administered propranolol, a beta-blocker, to car accident victims in the hours following their trauma. Pitman hypothesized that propranolol would interrupt the cycle of memory over-consolidation; as a consequence memory of the traumatic event would not be as vivid or as emotionally laden, and PTSD would be prevented. Clinical trials of propranolol are still in their relatively early stages, but the results so far are promising (similar work is being carried out in France; see Vaiva, *et al.* 2003).

Given the obvious benefits of preventing PTSD, this is important work. Nevertheless, some ethicists have expressed serious concerns about it. As we shall see, these concerns may be well founded. Nevertheless the parity thesis gives us reason to think that these concerns are no more pressing with regard to the prevention of PTSD pharmacologically than with regard to various other, generally and rightly accepted, current practices.

Consider, for instance, the response of the President's Council on Bioethics to these drugs. The council worries that the use of drugs to attenuate painful memories might interfere with a process that is normally adaptive. Since the greater impact upon us of traumatic memories reflects the (typically) greater importance of traumatic events to our lives, interfering with this process might be unwise. By taking the edge off traumatic memories, we might prevent people from learning from them, and from undergoing the process of personal growth that normally follows from misadventure. Even worse, we might encourage risky or even downright immoral behavior. Normal people experience guilt and often shame after they have harmed others (and especially if they have been detected in wrongdoing); these are powerfully aversive emotions, and discourage repetition of the wrongful action. But a drug capable of attenuating these feelings, by dampening the emotions experienced when the action is recalled, would ensure that their corrective effect is correspondingly weaker. As Leon Kass, the then chair of the President's Council, put it, such a drug would be a "morning-after pill for just about anything that produces regret, remorse, pain, or guilt" (Baard 2003). Kass may well be right to think that drugs that allow people to avoid powerfully aversive emotions can be abused, and therefore might allow agents to commit crimes against others with relative impunity. But it is worth stressing the several ways in which the danger here is not unprecedented; we face similar threats from existing ways of encouraging wrongdoing and discouraging the growth of conscience.

There are, for instance, already lower-tech ways in which people currently seek to avoid the consequences of their actions, including aversive emotions: the use of alcohol is the most obvious.

It is at least sometimes quite effective (Khantzian 1997). Moreover, there are also a range of techniques for facilitating immoral actions already available, some of which work on a very large scale. One such technique is as old as mankind: the demonization of the members of others groups and their consequent expulsion from the moral community. Jonathan Glover, in his *Moral History of the Twentieth Century*, details some of the "techniques for switching off respect and sympathy," used to manufacture efficient and remorseless torturers (Glover 1999: 37). Even without the aid of the contemporary sciences of the mind, such techniques are powerful and effective. Indeed, mere exposure to a racist and murderous ideology like Nazism can be effective in eroding moral responses. Glover notes that twenty percent of Nazi soldiers involved in mass executions experienced severe psychological problems as a result; "the fact that eighty percent did *not* report these problems is grim testimony to the power of psychological mechanisms of adjustment" (1999: 345). Further, and as the parity principle would lead us to expect, methods of manipulating agents' moral judgments without directly intervening into their brains currently exist. Dienstbier and colleagues (Dienstbier and Munster 1971; Dienstbier 1978) provided subjects with alternative explanations of the emotional arousal they felt when contemplating an immoral action (for example, by telling them that the arousal was due to a drug – actually a placebo – they had taken). They found that college students were more likely to cheat on an exam if they attributed their arousal to the drug, and not to contemplation of the wrongful action. This technique could, it seems, be used to manipulate subjects into reassessing actions they would otherwise consider immoral, thereby disposing them to perform these actions.

If, however, propranolol gives us a low-risk and side effect free means of moderating moral emotions, then its ease of use, and perhaps its effectiveness, seem sufficient to ensure that the problems it presents, when used deliberately to prevent pangs of conscience, are of a greater magnitude than anything we have seen before. It is unprecedented inasmuch as it is a technique available to individuals, to use at will and without the side effects associated with alcohol. Thus, the possible misuse of drugs like propranolol to deliberately avoid pangs of conscience may present problems that are genuinely novel. It is not clear, however, whether Kass is right in thinking that the effect of this intervention would be to encourage repetition of immoral acts. The scenario he envisages seems to be this: the wrongdoer deliberately seeks to avoid the aversive emotions typically associated with harming others in order to engage in serious wrongdoing with impunity. This is indeed a worrying possibility. However, there is an alternative possibility to consider: it may be that having engaged in a single act of wrongdoing substantially raises the probability of reoffending, precisely because the agent feels they have nothing more to lose, in terms of the state of their moral character or the pangs of guilt they experience. Seeing themselves as "stuck" with these feelings, as having, by a single foolish action, turned themselves into an outlaw in their own eyes as well as others', their inhibitions against reoffending may be substantially weakened. Might as well be hung – or haunted by guilt feelings – for a sheep as for a lamb. Given the opportunity to relieve these feelings, however, they may be able to restore themselves, in their own eyes, to the status of full moral agent, and thereby reduce their disposition to reoffend. This is, in important part at least, an empirical question: further research on the role of emotions in recidivism is urgently needed to settle it.

However this issue pans out, it must be stressed that of course the mere fact that a drug can be abused in pursuit of immoral ends is just one factor we must take into account when considering the advisability of making it available. If propranolol, or successor drugs, proves effective at combating PTSD, then its benefits probably outweigh its costs.

I now want to turn to another, apparently novel, problem which might arise from the use of drugs like propranolol. If neuroscience is enabling us to develop new techniques to battle old problems, it is also increasing our understanding of the way in which the mind works, and this new knowledge itself gives us reason to be cautious in how we use beta-adrenergic antagonists. Though the research upon which the following section relies is still somewhat undeveloped, what we know, or at least think we know, about moral judgment itself suggests that using beta-adrenergic antagonists risks temporarily disrupting moral judgment, at the same time as it works to prevent PTSD.

MORAL JUDGMENT AND THE SOMATIC MARKER HYPOTHESIS

The somatic marker hypothesis (SMH), most closely associated with Antonio Damasio, is a theory of the role of emotion and bodily states in judgment and decision-making. There is a long tradition in Western thought of opposing emotion and the body, on the one hand, to rationality, on the other. This tradition continues to influence both academic reflection and popular culture (think of the ultra-rational robots of many science fiction films, or Mr. Spock in *Star Trek*). We continue to think that emotions disrupt rationality. This is, obviously enough, sometimes true (and confirmed by contemporary work in the sciences of the mind: we know that stress hormones can interfere with good judgment, for instance). But the SMH suggests that precisely the opposite is true as well: in many circumstances, emotional arousal actually facilitates good decision-making.

The SMH is so-called because it holds that decision-making is often mediated by emotional response, and somatic states play an important role in such responses. The SMH proposes that emotions are expressed, in important part, as neural representations of bodily states (Damasio 1996). Bodily states may be involved directly or indirectly in emotional processing: directly, when an actual bodily state is signalled to the brain, or indirectly, when an 'as if' loop is used, with the amygdala and prefrontal cortices forming virtual representations of somatic states (Damasio 1994). More recent work has suggested that there may be two distinct and dissociable somatic marker systems, one involved in processing basic stimuli, the other involved in processing associated and more complex stimuli (Bechara *et al.* 2003). Somatic markers can operate overtly or covertly. They operate overtly to make a stimulus salient for an organism, and covertly to bias responses (Damasio 1996). Via both routes, they can lead to better decisions.

Somatic markers seem, for instance, to facilitate prudential decision-making. One well-known study (also mentioned in an earlier chapter) monitored the performance of subjects on the Iowa Gambling Task. In this task, subjects choose cards from one of four decks, two of which give large payoffs but also frequent large punishments, and two of which give smaller payoffs and smaller punishments. Normal subjects learn to favor the smaller payoff decks, which give a small but steady payoff, over the larger payoffs, which prove disadvantageous over time. Bechara, *et al.* (1997) discovered that normal subjects actually begin to favor these decks *before* they have understood the payoff structure. They suggest that somatic markers facilitate these responses, and may also facilitate learning the payoff structure. Subjects began to generate anticipatory skin conductance responses (SCRs) immediately before choosing from the disadvantageous decks. The SCRs preceded explicit knowledge of the payoff structure by a significant time. Only subsequently did subjects develop a "hunch" about the decks, a hunch that gradually became explicit knowledge. But advantageous *choice* predated knowledge. Bechara *et al.* (1997) suggest that consideration of the disadvantageous decks generated a somatic marker that biased response toward the advantageous decks.

Conversely, patients with bilateral damage to the ventromedial prefrontal cortex failed to generate anticipatory SCRs to the disadvantageous decks (though they did generate SCRs when they turned over a punishment card). Ventromedial patients failed to develop a hunch about the disadvantageous decks; moreover, though some of the brain damaged subjects attained explicit knowledge of the payoff structure, all the patients chose far more disadvantageously than the normal controls (Bechara *et al.* 1997). Somatic markers apparently improve prudential decision-making (at least in some circumstances) by covertly biasing responses, and the absence of these somatic markers can prove disastrous. Ventromedial patients' pattern of bad decision-making extends outside the laboratory to everyday life (Damasio 1994); this despite the fact that their abstract decision-making skills remain intact (Damasio *et al.* 1994).

There is convergent evidence that moral judgments utilize somatic markers. Ventromedial patients do not generally exhibit a pattern of immoral behavior. However, if the damage occurred early, in early childhood or before, patients exhibit behavior and a neuropsychological profile similar to subjects diagnosed with psychopathy (Anderson *et al.* 2000). It seems that the lack of empathic emotional response that is characteristic of ventromedial patients prevents the development of moral knowledge. Moreover, the moral responses of normal subjects can apparently be manipulated by altering their somatic responses, or by altering their interpretation of these responses. The research by Dienstbier and colleagues (Dienstbier and Munster 1971; Dienstbier 1978) mentioned above seems to demonstrate just such manipulation. By providing subjects with alternative explanations of the emotional arousal they felt when contemplating immoral actions, the experimenters increased the probability that subjects would engage in them.

More recent research on moral cognition has been explicitly aimed at testing the somatic marker hypothesis. Batson and colleagues (1999) manipulated subjects' moral judgments by providing them with false physiological feedback. They found that false feedback had no discernible effect on subjects' rankings of various values, but did significantly affect specific decisions concerning these values. Batson and colleagues suggest that values are ranked using a "cold" (i.e., affectless) strategy of retrieving information about values from memory, whereas more specific decisions are guided, in part, by somatic markers. Wheatley and Haidt (2005) used posthypnotic suggestion to induce a disgust response to arbitrary words. They found that subjects rated moral transgressions as significantly more serious when the vignette contained the disgust primed word than when it did not; they even tended to disapprove of actions innocent of any possible moral violation when it was described using the primed word, sometimes confabulating reasons for disapproval. The authors of both studies take their findings to support the somatic marker hypothesis.

Apparently, then, somatic responses powerfully influence moral judgments; so powerfully that if subjects feel certain responses while contemplating an entirely innocent action, they will tend to regard it as wrong. Now, what does all this have to do with trauma and memory? There is good reason to suspect that the beta-adrenergic antagonists that block the effect of stress hormones, thereby preventing the over-consolidation of memories and hence the development of PTSD, will also attenuate somatic markers, and therefore (perhaps subtly) influence moral judgments. Propranolol acts to block the transmission of a neural signal by blocking adrenergic receptors in the amygdala – a region strongly linked with associative learning and emotion processing (Pitman and Delahanty 2005). But the amygdala is also one of the three key brain regions proposed to mediate somatic markers (Bechara et al. 2003). Given that the stress hormones blocked by propranolol also play a causal role in producing the somatic markers that guide moral judgment, moral judgment can be expected to differ in subjects under its influence.

What might the effects of propranolol on moral judgment be? Batson et al. (1999) suggest that moral judgment utilizes two independent strategies: a "cold" strategy, which relies upon memory retrieval, and a "hot" strategy that refers to somatic markers to gauge the wrongness of a contemplated action. This suggestion seems plausible: with regard to many moral problems ("Is it permissible to torture babies for fun?") we do not need to reflect to come up with an answer; we simply retrieve it from memory. There is no reason to think that beta-adrenergic antagonists will interfere with these common judgments; they attenuate the consolidation of new memories but do not influence old ones. However, they might well influence moral reflection which relies upon the second, hot, route (and therefore the results of reflection on novel moral problems).

Suppose, for instance, subjects in the laboratory were asked to contemplate novel, emotionally engaging, moral dilemmas. We might, for instance, use the scenarios deployed by Greene *et al.* (2001), in their fMRI study of moral judgments. These scenarios, which Greene himself adapted from a lively tradition of debate within moral philosophy, are interesting and puzzling because they present pairs of problems, which are apparently very similar in their morally salient features, but which provoke radically divergent moral judgments. Consider, for instance, the famous *Trolley Problem*:

(a) Imagine you are standing next to railway tracks, when you see an out-of-control trolley hurtling towards you. If the trolley continues on its current path, it will certainly hit and kill five workers who are in a nearby tunnel. You cannot warn them in time, and they cannot escape from the tunnel. However, if you pull a lever you can divert the trolley to a sidetrack, where it will certainly hit and kill a single worker. Assume you have no other options available to you that would save the five men. Should you pull the lever?

(b) Imagine that this time you find yourself on a bridge over the railway tracks when you see the trolley hurtling along toward a group of five workers. The only way to prevent their certain deaths is for you to push the fat man standing next to you into its path; this will stop the trolley but the man will die. It's no use you leaping into its path; you are too light to stop the trolley. Should you push the fat man?

Most people think that it is permissible, and perhaps even obligatory, to pull the lever in scenario (a), diverting the trolley and thus saving five lives at the cost of one. Most people – indeed, often the very same people – also say that it is impermissible to push the fat man into the path of the trolley in scenario (b). Yet there is a prima facie inconsistency between these predominant responses: pulling the lever in

(a) is justified because it saves five lives, at the cost of one; but failing to push the fat man into the path of the trolley involves passing up the parallel opportunity to save five lives at the cost of one.

There have been many attempts to show that these two responses are justified by some deeper principle, which would make them consistent despite appearances (Thomson 1976; Foot 1978). But there is no consensus, or even widespread agreement, that any of these explanations are plausible. One recent explanation is that these responses are the product of our evolutionary history, as it is reflected in the structure of our minds. Greene *et al.* (2001) scanned the brains of subjects as they contemplated these dilemmas and other, similarly structured, ones (as well as control questions). They found significant differences in the brain regions activated when processing dilemmas which are personally engaging (such as pushing the fat man off the bridge) versus dilemmas which are more impersonal (such as pulling the lever). When considering the former class of cases, regions of the brain associated with emotion were very active, but they were not active when subjects were considering impersonal dilemmas. In more recent work, Greene (2005; forthcoming) has speculated that this difference is the result of our evolutionary history: since we evolved in an environment in which distant, and technologically mediated, harms were not possible, we respond differently to such harms than to those which are more direct. We shall discuss Greene's speculations in a later chapter. What matters, for the moment, is simply that his results give us further reason to think that emotions, and therefore somatic markers, play an important role in the processing of moral dilemmas.

Suppose this is correct, and that propranolol does indeed attenuate somatic response. In that case, subjects under its influence who face novel ethical dilemmas – ones for which they do not already have a ready answer in memory – can be expected to give different responses to control subjects who are not affected by the drug. It may be that these differences will be relatively small, but just for that reason, they may be significant: whereas the gross impairments produced by alcohol and some other drugs are easily detected, and responses influenced by them appropriately discounted, the very subtlety of the alterations produced by propranolol will make them hard to guard against, both for the agent themselves and for those around them. If the differences are large enough to be morally significant, then the inability to monitor the changes will matter greatly.

How likely is the hypothesis that propranolol will affect moral judgment, and how significant might any effect be? There is already evidence that centrally acting (i.e., crossing the blood–brain barrier to act directly on the brain) beta-adrenergic antagonists affect non-moral judgment. Corwin *et al.* (1990) tested psychiatrically normal subjects, who were taking propranolol for the treatment of hypertension, on a short-term memory task. Subjects were asked whether a word shown to them had appeared on a list of words previously seen. Clinically depressed individuals exhibit a conservative bias on this task; they are more likely than controls to say that a word was not on the list, whereas sufferers from mania exhibit the opposite bias. Corwin *et al.* found that normal subjects on propranolol exhibited a conservative bias, similar to that characteristic of depressives. This result has been independently replicated (Callaway *et al.* 1991).

These studies suggest that propanolol has a biasing effect on behavior that is comparable to that seen in clinically depressed subjects. However, the subjects in these trials had been taking propranolol continuously for three months; its use in the prevention of PTSD would likely involve far fewer doses. For this reason, the biases exhibited by hypertension sufferers on propranolol might not show up in people treated for potential PTSD. However, there is evidence that even a single dose of the drug can influence decision-making. Rogers *et al.* (2004) studied the effect of a single dose of propranolol on the performance of psychiatrically normal subjects on a gambling task. They discovered that subjects administered the drug were relatively insensitive to the size of potential losses, when the probability of losing was high. Rogers *et al.* speculate that propranolol makes subjects less sensitive to punishment signals, thereby altering decision-making. As a result, subjects become less risk-averse than controls.

Neither of these studies focused on moral judgments specifically, though it is obvious that insensitivity to risks (in particular) could well have consequences, perhaps disastrous consequences, that fall squarely in the domain of morality (indeed, there is a case for saying that risk is a moral issue; financial loss is loss of a good that can be used for moral purposes, such as provision of essential services, and most risks can be translated into monetary terms). In fact, if responses to typical moral dilemmas are simply retrieved from memory, it may be that the effects on risk-aversion are more significant than the hypothesized effect on moral judgment, since most people will only rarely face novel dilemmas which require significant on-line processing. On the other hand, if our ordinary moral judgment relies upon a combination of memory retrieval and on-line processing, perhaps with the on-line processing helping us recall the relevant responses, then the effects of propranolol on moral judgment will be very significant. All of this requires further empirical work, to discover how great the effects of propanolol are, and how reliant we are upon on-line processing in everyday moral judgment.

If it should turn out that the effects are significant (something which I am hoping to discover in research currently underway with Nicholas Allen), then we need to exercise great care in using propranolol for the prevention of PTSD. In some settings, the drug might prove relatively unproblematic. If its effects wash out relatively quickly, then it might be possible to administer it in emergency wards, in the immediate aftermath of a traumatic event, or to instruct subjects to take it immediately before going to bed. In that case, subjects would not be called upon to make moral judgments while the drug is affecting their cognition. But in some settings, including some of those currently under consideration as prime circumstances for its use, the administration of propranolol could prove disastrous. It has been suggested, for instance, that propranolol could be administered to military personnel, *before* they go into battle (Baard 2003). The rationale is obvious: soldiers can be expected to witness traumatic scenes, and if the best way to prevent the development of PTSD involves administration prior to the event, then it makes sense to use the drug pre-emptively (even if the drug is just as effective administered within a few hours of the event, because it is often difficult to be sure when a military engagement is over it is equally difficult to be certain that individuals are no longer involved in the action at the time of administration). But if propranolol affects moral judgments, using the drug in this way risks creating soldiers with ethical standards that are unacceptably low. In the absence of the somatic signals that let him or her know that a contemplated course of action would be wrong, the soldier may lack not (as Kass fears) regret, but moral judgment.

CONCLUSION

The kind of radical memory alterations envisaged in films like *Eternal Sunshine of the Spotless Mind* or *Total Recall* are not imminent; indeed, they may even prove impossible for reasons both technical and conceptual. The holism of the mental ensures that inserting many kinds of important beliefs will prove impossible, or nearly so: either inserted beliefs will unravel or the subject will no longer be globally rational. Holism seems to present a significant obstacle to the erasure of beliefs and memories too.

But we may already have the means to moderate the emotional significance of memories, and thereby to weaken their hold over us. It is probable that this technique could be used to encourage agents to forget events more quickly than they otherwise would; over a few weeks, rather than months, or months, rather than years. More disturbingly, these drugs may weaken the pangs of conscience, and alter moral judgments. If such problems arise, their use will have to be carefully controlled.

End notes

1. The fact that memories are reconstructions and not necessarily veridical pictures of the past raises ethical issues of its own. We shall consider these problems later in this chapter, when we examine how memories can be distorted or implanted.

2. There is some suggestion that neuroscience itself might succeed where observation has failed: that is, it might be possible to develop some kind of brain scan that distinguishes true memories from false. Cabeza *et al.* (2001) asked subjects whether words on a list had appeared on one that was presented to them previously. False recognition was associated with a lower degree of activation of the parahippocampal gyrus than true. However, it is far from clear that this result could be used to distinguish genuinely recovered memories from false: first, the difference was relatively small, big enough to show up as a group difference, but too small to be reliably used to distinguish individual false recollection from true; second, the parahippocampal gyrus is involved in perceptual information processing; the result may reflect nothing more than the recovery of perceptual information, and therefore the difference may show up only for identical perceptual clues, and may thus be a one-off effect (i.e., it may not be possible to repeat the test; indeed, it might have to be done at the point of putative memory recovery – which will prove impossible if memory recovery is a gradual process).

3. Wilson apparently regards these kinds of cases as undesirable; for him, they represent a loss of autonomy on the part of one or both agents. I think this is mistaken. Autonomy does not require – indeed, it *never* involves – radical independence from others. We are all deeply dependent upon one another, physically and epistemically. I see no special reason to distrust the kind of interdependence that extended memory stores or extensive epistemic reliance upon others involves. For a consideration of the extent and kind of independence required by autonomy, see Mackenzie and Stoljar 2000.

6 The "self" of self-control

What is the self? There is no single or simple answer to that question. The term, which is a term of art (as a freestanding noun, the word "self" is hardly ever used in ordinary English) is used in a range of sometimes conflicting ways; so many that some philosophers despair at finding any unifying element underlying its disparate uses and therefore recommend that we discontinue using it at all as the name for a philosophical problem (Olson 1999). I suspect that these philosophers are right to this extent: there is no single sense or even a closely related set of senses, unifying all or even most of the central uses of the term. There is therefore no problem of the self. Nevertheless, there are a number of *problems* of the self. In this chapter, we shall consider just one.

The problem of the self upon which I want to focus is, briefly, this: why is the self *singular*? This is not the first problem that generally comes to mind when we consider the problem of the self. However, it is a problem that is especially pressing for us. Consider the evidence from neuroscience, reviewed in earlier chapters, that the mind consists of a multitude of discrete modules and mechanisms. Consider, too, the extended mind hypothesis, according to which mind can include or incorporate a set of tools external to the self. Given that the mind consists of a motley collection of tools and mechanisms, why is there a self at all? Why is this self experienced as singular, and is this experience veridical?

Even this question, why is the self singular, can be broken down into further, only tangentially connected, problems. We might enquire into the so-called *unity of consciousness*; that is, into the question of why our experience of our minds is of a single stream of consciousness. That's not the question I want to explore here, interesting though it is. Instead, I want to focus on human behavior: why, given the fact that our brains consist of many mechanisms, do we act in such a well-coordinated manner? Briefly, the puzzle is this: brains consist of many modules, each of which does its own thing; many of these modules drive behavior, directly or indirectly (indirectly: for instance, by producing desires or inclinations). Yet our behavior looks remarkably consistent. How is the coordination problem solved? And (more importantly from the point of view of neuroethics), what light does the problem and its solution shed on how we normally act, and on the range of pathologies of action to which we are subject?

Is there a problem here at all? It might be thought that any coordination problem would have been solved by evolution. After all, all the modules which together constitute my mind/brain are in the same boat: except in very rare circumstances, modules cannot behave in ways that benefit themselves, from an evolutionary point of view, without also benefiting the whole ensemble of modules. Defection from a cooperative strategy will be punished, almost always, by a lack of success at passing on the genes which promote such defection. Accordingly, we should expect the modules to work together. They may be analytically separable, and they may dissociate either as a result of brain injury or of clever laboratory manipulations, but in the real world they will always work together.

This line of reasoning has a lot going for it. We ought to expect that evolutionary pressures will ensure that the major coordination problems have been solved. Indeed, the brain itself has a number of mechanisms to ensure that discrete modules work together. There are identifiable sites within the brain where information and representations from diverse sources are integrated. For instance, very basic bodily information, from various sources, is integrated in the brain stem, providing the basis for what Damasio (1999) calls "the proto self" (Churchland 2003). There is also evidence that emotions play a neurobiological integrating role by coordinating brain plasticity (Ledoux 2003). Neuroscientists have made significant progress in recent years in identifying mechanisms which contribute to solving the so-called binding problem, the problem of how information from different sources – about the shape, the color and the position of objects, for instance – is integrated into a single complex perception. Temporal synchrony seems to play a role in binding representations together (Engel *et al.* 1999). Such representations enter, or are poised to enter, consciousness, and therefore can play a role in guiding behavior that is an intelligent response to information from many sources.

However, though some degree of unity is guaranteed by these mechanisms, there is strong evidence that the binding mechanisms do not provide us with the optimal degree of unity we need in order to pursue the kinds of lives which we value. The unity they provide us with is unity only over the briefest stretch of time, whereas the kind of unity we need, to pursue fully human lives, is long-term unity. I shall briefly sketch the reasons why we need such unity in order to pursue the best kind of life, before turning to the evidence that such unity can be lost, even in the absence of neurological injury.

What sense of "self" is at issue in the question concerning the unity of our behavior? The self in question is the self of self-control. Now, self-control is a puzzling idea. When we say that someone has lost self-control, we don't mean that someone *else* is controlling them. But if they are acting intentionally and voluntarily, and no one else is controlling them, then they must be controlling themselves – or so it seems. How should we make sense of this puzzle?

Consider an ancient paradigm of the loss of self-control, from Plato's *Republic*. Plato tells us the story of a certain Leontion, who was outside the city walls when he noticed a pile of corpses, the bodies of executed criminals. Leontion was fascinated by the corpses and drawn to look at them, but at the same time he was repulsed and disgusted, by the corpses and by his own desire:

> For a time he struggled with himself and covered his eyes, but
> at last his desire got the better of him and he ran up to the

corpses, opening his eyes wide and saying to them, 'There you
are, curse you – a lovely sight! Have a real good look!'

(Republic 440a).

Leontion lost his self-control. Yet his actions were not controlled by
another person; he acted, as Plato himself says, on *his* desire. It was
his desires that "got the better of him." Leontion's predicament
captures the essence of a loss of self-control. When someone loses
this kind of control, they act as they want to. However, their action
does not reflect their self-image.

That is not to say that conflict with one's self-image is sufficient
for loss of self-control: after all, one's self-image could be the product of
self-deception. Someone might regard themselves as trustworthy,
reliable and upright, and yet constantly behave in ways that are self-
interested, at the expense of the legitimate moral interests of others.
Such a person does not seem to suffer from a loss of self-control. In
addition to failing to cohere with one's self-image, behavior which
reflects a loss of control also fails to cohere with a person's values and
endorsed desires; values and desires that are actually in control of that
person's behavior for significant stretches of time. Just what proportion of my behavior must actually reflect a set of my values for those
values to count as mine I leave open; it seems likely, however, that at
least half of my behavior must be in accordance with my values or I am
wrong in thinking that they are *my* values.

I control myself, roughly, when my actions stem from my non-
self-deceptively endorsed values. Typical cases of loss of self-control
fit this mould: the woman who loses her temper and says something
she later regrets, the man who departs catastrophically from his diet
or from his vow to limit his drinking; the kleptomaniac who steals a
trinket they do not value or the heroin addict who feels powerless to
give up their drug; all these individuals control their actions, but
their behavior does not reflect their deepest values.

Now, why does it matter whether our behavior reflects our
deepest values? Why do we value self-control? As the examples of its

loss we have just reviewed make clear, self-control is *instrumentally* valuable to pursuing the kind of life we want. When we lack self-control, we may find ourselves at the mercy of passing fancies. If I cannot control myself, I cannot trust myself; to stop at one drink at the bar, to pass on dessert, to hold my peace when someone says something I find irritating. If my self-control is very badly damaged, I will be stimulus-driven, and unable to follow a coherent life-plan. Consider, first, some spectacular and pathological cases of loss of self-control. People who suffer from *utilization behavior*, a disorder caused by damage to the frontal lobes, respond compulsively to the affordances – the suggestions for use – of objects in their immediate environment. For instance, if a glass of water is placed in front of them, they will typically raise it to their lips; if spectacles are placed in front of them, they will put them on – and if a second pair is then offered, they will put those on as well, despite the fact that they are already wearing a pair. They will continue to respond in this way, even after they are instructed not to (Estlinger *et al.* 1991; Lhermitte *et al.* 1986). These patients seem literally unable to help themselves, as do sufferers from *imitation behavior*, a social form of utilization behavior. Patients with this condition will imitate an examiner's movements even when told not to and given negative reinforcement (Lhermitte 1983).

Utilization behavior may, if it is severe, be incompatible with a decent human life. Sufferers cannot count on their ability to carry out plans, without being distracted from them by extraneous features of their environment. But even when self-control is within the normal range, we may find its temporary loss a significant problem. In the contemporary world, the ideal of authenticity is extremely powerful. As a consequence, most of us believe it is very important to pursue our own conception of the good life: an overarching image of what it means, for us, to be human. We want to live a life that expresses *our* central values, and we want that life to make *narrative* sense: we want to be able to tell ourselves and others a story, which explains where we come from, how we got to where we are, and where we are going. Indeed, as Marya Schechtman (1996) has agued, human beings typically understand themselves and each other in narrative terms; our very identity (in one sense of that term) is constituted by the contents of a (largely true) narrative we tell about ourselves. But imposing narrative unity on our lives requires that we be able to shape our behavior, at least in its most significant respects, in the light of the values we want our narratives to reflect and express. Losing control over oneself threatens that ability; it may result in our narrative taking turns we cannot endorse, or in constant disruptions to its evolving arc.

A significant degree of self-control is also required for people to live together in harmony and for the achievement of the kinds of goods that human beings can only realize in society. I can only make promises to others if I am able to ensure that I am (usually) capable of behaving in the future as I *now* desire; in other words, if my present self can exert a significant degree of control over the behavior of my future self. If we are to coordinate our actions, and therefore if we are to be able to realize the goods which come from divisions of labor, then we must be able to trust one another to deliver on our word. If we are to engage in intimate relationships, then we must coordinate our activities, divide responsibilities and reliably be there for one another. All of these activities take a relatively significant degree of self-control.

Patients suffering from utilization behavior or similar disorders may have to engage in complex calculations to prevent their behavior disrupting their lives. They may have to carefully structure their environments to enable them to carry out complex activities without interruptions. Of course, the kind of inability to inhibit responses characteristic of the frontal lobe patient is well outside the range of ordinary experiences of loss of self-control; when you or I find ourselves acting against our own all-things-considered judgment, we do not experience ourselves as stimulus driven. However, it may be that at least some ordinary losses of self-control can be illuminated by these neurological disorders. Utilization behavior may be explained by a dysfunction of a specific inhibition mechanism: on this hypothesis, the initial response of sufferers to objects and their affordances is entirely normal. They, and we, respond to such affordances automatically; the difference between us and them is that in us the frontal lobe mechanisms which act to inhibit inappropriate responses are intact, whereas theirs are not (Archibald *et al.* 2001). It may be that losses of self-control within the normal range of human experiences also reflect losses of, or weaknesses in the mechanisms of, inhibitory control. Such losses could come about in a variety of ways: developmentally, either as a result of an environment which does not encourage its proper development or as a consequence of innate factors, or as a response to environmental stressors which temporarily overwhelm inhibitory resources. Some researchers have suggested that common self-control problems, such as ADHD, might be traced to dysfunctions in the same mechanisms that underlie utilization behaviour (Archibald *et al.* 2001).

THE DEVELOPMENT OF SELF-CONTROL

Though the elements of a solution to the problem of coordinating the various mechanisms that together constitute our minds is part of our evolutionary heritage, nevertheless the extent to which self-control is developed varies from person to person. We each need to learn to control ourselves, as part of normal development, and some of us learn the lesson better than others. Walter Mischel and his colleagues have been gathering data on the development of self-control for decades. Mischel's team developed an experimental paradigm to test children's ability to delay gratification. Children were offered a choice between two alternatives, one of which they valued more than the other (for instance, one marshmallow versus two). The experimenter left the room, telling them that if they waited until he or she returned, the child would get the more highly valued reward, but that they could call the experimenter back at any time (by ringing a bell) and receive the less highly valued reward at once. Children differed greatly in their ability to wait for the second reward (Mischel 1981).

Mischel's studies have demonstrated a number of important points. Perhaps most interesting is the discovery that ability to delay gratification at age four is strongly predictive of a range of desirable characteristics in adolescence and later: academic success, social competence, attentiveness, concentration, and the ability to form and execute plans (Mischel et al. 1989). This finding seems to confirm the claims made above, about the instrumental value of the ability to control oneself for the achievement of goods we value. The child, adolescent or adult who cannot exert a sufficient degree of control over him or herself cannot successfully pursue academic excellence (which is a project pursued over time and in which results gradually accumulate) or prevent themselves being distracted by immediate gratifications incompatible with success.

Mischel also found, more surprisingly perhaps, that the ability to delay gratification seemed to depend in very important part on the deployment of a set of skills. Rather than self-control simply depending upon a mysterious faculty of "will-power," the ability to delay gratification depends crucially on self-*distraction*. This finding was precisely the opposite of the experimenters' hypothesis: rather than focusing upon the reward for waiting, the good delayer thinks either about something else entirely, or focuses upon aspects of the reward that are not linked to the ways in which it is rewarding (for instance, rather than think of the sweetness of the marshmallows, the child thinks of them as fluffy white clouds). It seems that focusing on those aspects of the rewards that make them desirable ensures that self-control resources are overwhelmed relatively quickly (Mischel 1989). Moreover, children who are good delayers deploy these strategies spontaneously, and by the age of five understand the kinds of strategies which are effective. Self-control is, or depends upon, a set of skills and that suggests that it can be taught and learned. In any case, Mischel's work has shown clearly that the coordination problem is not solved for us; though we are each minimally unified simply by virtue of neurobiological mechanisms that ensure we can function as organisms, we do not achieve an optimal, or even (for living a decent human life) a sufficient level of unity of behavior without further effort and learning.

Further evidence for the all too grim reality of failures of self-control is provided by a range of problems to which people are subject, even in the absence of neurological damage. Most obviously, the disorders on the obsessive-compulsive spectrum (obsessive-compulsive disorder (OCD), kleptomania, trichotilliamania, and so on) can be understood as failures of self-control. Self-control in OCD, kleptomania or intermittent explosive disorder can be undermined in one or more of several ways. One possibility is that such disorders make the self-distraction strategies utilized by the children in Mischel's studies harder to deploy – perhaps by forcing the (subjectively perceived) desirable qualities of the objects of the compulsions or obsessions to the attention of the agent. If, as I shall shortly suggest, self-control is a depletable resource, and it is depleted by focusing on these qualities, then concentration on these qualities will quickly lead to its exhaustion. Alternatively, OCD and other disorders might impact directly on our reserves of self-control: on this hypothesis, agents' abilities to deploy self-control strategies is unimpaired, but because their self-control resources are already depleted, they cannot resist for long. Of course, both explanations might work in concert to produce failures of self-control. (Note, however, that neither explanation, nor a combination of both, can be a full explanation of these disorders. The hypotheses attempt to explain why sufferers give in to their desires; in addition, we need an explanation for the sometimes bizarre content of the desires: why do sufferers from trichotilliamania experience the urge to pluck out their hair? Why do many sufferers from OCD derive a brief respite from performing ritualistic actions?)

The other class of disorders of self-control to which human beings are all too prone involve failures appropriately to regulate consumption of rewarding substances, or engagement in rewarding activities: food, alcohol, sex, drugs. We often attempt to explain these disorders simply by invoking the notion of addiction, as though that put an end to all further questions. But, while it is clear that addiction genuinely exists, and that it plays a role in explaining the behavior of addicts, it is far from a complete explanation by itself. In fact, I shall argue, the same basic mechanism is at work in all failures of self-control, from disorders on the obsessive-compulsive spectrum to addiction, from inability to delay gratification to failures of will-power in dieting.

EGO-DEPLETION AND SELF-CONTROL

Let's begin with the reasons for the failure of the addiction hypothesis as a complete explanation for the behavior of addicts. The addiction hypothesis, in its most usual form, postulates that addictive desires are literally irresistible. On this view, addiction destroys agency itself: addicts do not choose to consume; they are impelled by their addiction. The only difference between the addict and, say, the man who, in Aristotle's example of non-voluntary behavior, is carried somewhere by the wind (*Nichomachean Ethics*, 1110a) is in the location of the force that acts upon them: the wind impels from without, while addiction impels from within. But in both cases, the person is carried away, regardless of their wishes or beliefs.

This is the picture of addiction so eloquently expressed by William James:

> The craving for a drink in real dipsomaniacs, or for opium or chloral in those subjugated, is of a strength of which normal persons can form no conception. 'Were a keg of rum in one corner of a room and were a cannon constantly discharging balls between me and it, I could not refrain from passing before that cannon in order to get the rum;' 'If a bottle of brandy stood at one hand and the pit of hell yawned at the other, and I were convinced that I should be pushed in as sure as I took one glass, I could not refrain:' such statements abound in dipsomaniacs' mouths.
> *(James 1890: 543)*

James wrote more than a century ago, but the view he espoused is still common. It dominates the common imagination, and it has many adherents among philosophers, bioethicists and psychologists. For Louis Charland, for instance, "the brain of a heroin addict has almost literally been hijacked by the drug" (Charland 2002: 43). For Carl Elliott (2002), the addict "is no longer in full control of herself. She must go where her addiction leads her, because the addiction holds the leash." For Alan Leshner (1999), the initially voluntary behavior of drug-taking gradually transforms into "involuntary drug taking, ultimately to the point that the behavior is driven by a compulsive craving for the drug." Even the *Diagnostic and Statistical Manual* of the American Psychiatric Association holds that addiction "usually" involves "compulsive drug taking behavior."

It is clear, however, that addictive desires are not literally compulsive; not, at least, if by "compulsive" we mean to refer to desires that either bypass the agent's will altogether, so that they act regardless of what they want, or to forces that the agent is literally unable to resist. There is plentiful evidence that addicts can and do resist their desires to consume their drugs, for shorter or longer periods. Indeed, if addictive desires were compulsive (in the sense alleged), it is difficult to see how addicts could give up voluntarily. But they do, in their thousands, largely without assistance from others (Sobell *et al.* 2000). There is plenty of direct evidence, in any case, that addicts exercise some degree of control over their consumption behavior. Consumption is price sensitive, in a manner that would be surprising if addictive desires were compulsive (Fingarette 1988; Elster 1999; Neale 2002). Neither cravings for the drug, nor the fear of withdrawal are so powerful as to overwhelm the volitional resources of addicts: the typical addict goes through withdrawal several, perhaps many, times. Indeed, some deliberately abstain for prolonged periods in order to lower their tolerance for the drug, and thereby decrease the dose they will need to achieve the high they want (Ainslie 2000). Addicts do indeed experience cravings – more intensely for some drugs than for others – and withdrawal is indeed a very unpleasant experience (though once again the extent to which this is so varies from drug to drug; cocaine addiction seems to be almost entirely a matter of craving and not withdrawal). But in no cases are these forces, singly or combined, sufficient to move the addict against their will.

In the face of this evidence, it is tempting to conclude that addiction is simply an excuse: that when addicts give in to their desires, they choose in the normal way we all choose, and that they therefore act as autonomously and as freely as you and I when we choose to consume chocolate ice-cream or bananas (Foddy and Savulescu 2006). But as all of us who have ever struggled with an addiction – whether to caffeine, tobacco or to heroin – know, that it is far too hasty. Addicts say that they use against their will, and there does seem to be some sense in which this is true. After all, not only is there the phenomenological evidence, to which many of us can attest, that breaking an addiction is difficult, there is also the evidence that comes from the fact that addicts slowly destroy their lives and the lives of those close to them. They engage in illegal, dangerous or degrading activities in order to procure their drug, they lose their jobs, their partners and their homes. If it was *purely* a matter of autonomous choice, we should not expect their lives to spiral out of control so dramatically. Addicts frequently say that they consume against their wills; I shall argue that there is a sense in which this is true.

Addictive behavior follows a characteristic temporal pattern. Addicts find it relatively easy to resist their desires in the short-term, but tend to give in to them over the longer term. Some addicts build their lives around an abstinence/binge cycle; for others, it is only when they attempt to give up permanently that the pattern is manifested. Addictive desires seem to be relatively easily resisted in the short-term, but in the long run consumption seems almost inevitable (especially if the addict relies upon sheer willpower to resist their desire). I suggest that it is by focusing on this temporal pattern that we can best understand the ways in which addiction impairs autonomy.

The most natural explanation for the way in which addiction impairs autonomy will invoke the features that make it addiction: craving and withdrawal. However, the temporal pattern mentioned is just the opposite of what we would expect if these features were doing most of the work in driving the behavior of addicts. It is relatively easy to get through withdrawal, as we have already seen, and though cravings are sometimes intense, they are intermittent and tend to reduce in strength as time passes. If the intensity of cravings and the pain of withdrawal explained addictive behavior, we should expect failures to occur more or less immediately, whereas if addicts were able to get through the first few days, we should expect the task to get easier. Instead, addicts attempting to give up regularly achieve short-term success, which may last for hours, days, or even months, followed by longer term failure.

I suggest that addiction sceptics – that is, those who deny that addiction impairs autonomy – are right to this extent: the mechanisms which explain the behavior of addicts are, as they suggest, also present in perfectly normal behavior. However, we should not conclude from this that addiction does not impair autonomy. Instead, we should recognize that autonomy can be impaired by persistent desires in cases which do not involve addictive substances.

In fact, there is now a considerable body of evidence showing that everyone has a hard time resisting persisting desires. Indeed, the evidence suggests that it may be *impossible* to resist a persistent desire for all that long. The evidence here comes from a series of studies on the phenomenon that has been dubbed *ego-depletion* (Baumeister *et al.* 1998; Baumeister 2002). In these studies, subjects are divided into two groups. One group is assigned a self-control task, such as resisting a desire; the control group is instead given a tiring task which does not require self-control to anything like the same extent. For instance, in a typical study the first group were ushered into a room filled with the smell of freshly-baked cookies, which were laid out on plates in full view. The subjects were told that they were to participate in a study on taste perception; one group of subjects would eat the cookies and another would eat radishes. They, they were told, were the radish group. They were then presented with plates of radishes, and left with instructions to eat several of them. The experimenters withdrew and covertly observed the subjects. They were observed to sniff and even handle the cookies, but despite the fact that they thought they were unobserved, all of them dutifully ate radishes and not the cookies. Meanwhile, the control group performed a task that did not require self-control, but which was tiring – a typical task was performing a series of three digit multiplications on paper.

Subjects from both groups were then tested on a common task, which does require self-control. Typical tests include squeezing a handgrip for as long as possible, persisting at an unsolvable anagram task, or keeping one's hand immersed in icy water. Subjects who have previously performed a self-control task – resisting the cookies, or watching a funny video while keeping a completely straight face – perform worse at the common task than do subjects in the control group, inasmuch as they persist at the task for a significantly shorter time. Moreover, their lack of self-control carries over to more naturalistic settings. For instance, dieters who are ego-depleted eat more after the tests than do non-dieters (Vohs and Heatherton 2000).

Ego-depletion experiments seem to show that self-control is a limited resource. The psychologists who have developed, tested and refined the ego-depletion hypothesis describe it as the muscle model of self-regulation (Schmeichel and Baumeister 2004). Self-control is like muscular strength: as we use it, it grows weaker, and can only be restored by rest. Just as the number of push-ups I can perform depends, importantly, on the tiredness of my arm muscles, so the length of time I can exercise self-control depends on how much of my self-control resources I have recently used. Self-control is depletable over the short term, but, like muscular strength, exercise seems to build it up over the longer term.[1]

Ego-depletion experiments have focused on the behavior of subjects, and have not produced much direct evidence as to the mechanisms which underlie the phenomenon. However, there is independent evidence, from PET and fMRI studies of the neural mechanisms involved in choice and deliberation, which seems to provide pointers to the mechanisms of self-control. We know that the anterior cingulate cortex and the prefrontal cortex are highly active when subjects are required to make choices and to exercise self-control, but are not activated when subjects engage in more mechanical, automatic or well-rehearsed behavior (Zhu 2004). There is also evidence that executive processes are sensitive to fluctuations in glucose to a far greater degree than automatic or routine processes (Fairclough and Houston 2004). New research by Gailliot et al. (2007) demonstrates that self-control tasks draw upon glucose to a greater extent than do other executive processes. This research showed that the degree of ego-depletion could be predicted from falls in blood glucose, and, moreover, that the effects of ego-depletion on self-control disappeared soon after subjects consumed glucose-rich food-stuffs. The authors cite independent evidence that problems assimilating glucose are linked to aggression and juvenile delinquency. Falls in glucose levels thus seem to explain ego-depletion. Gailliot et al. note the irony that dieters tend to lower their blood glucose, thereby reducing their own self-control resources.

Self-control is thus apparently especially depleting of glucose. There is some evidence to suggest, additionally, that the energy used in self-control comes from a store especially reserved for this purpose. Though subjects in ego-depletion paradigms report no more fatigue after their initial ego-depleting task than controls who performed a non-self-control task, after performing the common task, at which ego-depleted individuals persist for a shorter time, they report greater fatigue than controls who have persisted longer (Vohs et al. unpublished). It seems likely that fatigue is the mediating factor in explaining depletion of the executive function. The evidence seems equivocal between two interpretations of how this occurs: (a) it might be that the initial ego-depletion task fatigues the subject, though the fatigue is unconscious until is passes some threshold; or

(b) the initial task does not fatigue – subjects' report of tiredness is veridical – but it depletes a resource in the absence of which subjects tire more quickly. One possibility is that consciousness has no direct access to the modular resource drawn upon by the executive function, so that depletion does not give rise to any experience, but once reserves of this resource are depleted, the executive function draws upon general purpose energy supplies, depletion of which is consciously experienced. Perhaps the modular resource supplies energy to the frontal lobes, energy which is expended in the unconscious inhibition of impulses; once this supply is depleted the task of inhibiting the urges is taken over by consciously monitored mechanisms. In any case, once self-regulatory resources are depleted, self-control becomes harder and harder, and giving in to the temptation to stop the task, or consume the drug, becomes inevitable.

The ego-depletion hypothesis seems to explain the temporal pattern observed in drug addiction. Addicts find it relatively easy to resist their cravings at first, but continued resistance depletes their self-control resources making continued resistance more and more difficult. Typically, they eventually give in, which provides temporary relief from the craving and allows them to build up their self-control resources once more. Then the cycle begins again.

It might seem that if the ego-depletion hypothesis were true, and willpower is a finite resource, we would be unable to explain how addicts are ever able to give up their drugs. Doesn't the hypothesis predict that each of us will inevitably give in to our desires, sooner or later, thus making successful long-term abstinence impossible? No: the hypothesis predicts only that we inevitably give in to *continuously persisting* desires. If all desires were continuously persisting, then resistance would be impossible. Fortunately, we can take steps to make it less likely that our desires persist. Recall the evidence from Mischel and colleagues: the most successful technique here is simply to turn our attention away from the cues that trigger the desires. In the normal case, most of us can distract ourselves reasonably successfully most of the time. Addicts find this technique difficult to employ, since the cues that trigger their cravings tend to capture their attention. However, they can take steps to avoid encountering the cues in the first place. The evidence is very strong that addictive desires are strongly cue-sensitive (Loewenstein 2000).[2] The situations, places and people associated with drug use trigger the cravings, and avoiding these cues helps to keep the desires under control. If the desires persist, then addicts will consume, as their self-control resources are depleted. But if they can take steps to ensure that their cravings are only intermittent, addicts can significantly raise the probability that they will always have enough self-control to successfully resist on each occasion.

Addicts find it so hard to remain drug-free, then, because they are not able – or do not realize the need – to remove themselves sufficiently from the cues that trigger their cravings. If drug-taking is a habitual response to stress, or if the addict usually uses with their partner, then removing themselves from the relevant cues may be impossible or very costly. It is therefore not at all surprising that giving up an addiction is extremely difficult, in a wide range of circumstances. Since many addicts find themselves unable to structure their lives in such a manner as to avoid drug-taking – despite the fact that many of them genuinely desire to abstain permanently – their autonomy is impaired. They are not able to guide their behavior in the light of the values that, for most of the time, they endorse.

The ego-depletion hypothesis promises to explain a great deal: not only the cycle of consumption and abstention often observed in addicts, but also the behavior of sufferers from impulse-control disorders, and even many of the failures of self-control to which we are all ordinarily subject. Consider OCD. Along with other disorders on the impulsive-compulsive spectrum, OCD shares a great deal with addiction. In particular, these disorders exhibit the same temporal profile: inhibiting the urge to perform the act is relatively easy at first, but of increasing difficulty as time passes. This suggests that ego-depletion is part of the explanation of how these disorders impair autonomy; the self-control resources of the agent are inevitably exhausted by continued resistance. Unsurprisingly, sufferers from OCD often find themselves resorting to indirect self-control strategies, centered around redirection of attention. Just as addicts need to avoid the stimuli which beget craving, and set them down the path to ego-depletion, so OCD sufferers find themselves needing to withdraw from situations that trigger urges which are especially dangerous or inconsistent with their self-image and values (Leckman *et al.* 1999). They are aware that they will likely give in to these urges, if they allow them to continue unabated. Inevitably, their self-control resources will be exhausted.

Ordinary failures of self-control may be explained in precisely the same way: by depletion of the resources of self-control. This may seem a surprising claim, given that we do not normally *experience* ourselves as losing control. Our akratic actions feel entirely normal – they don't feel compelled or otherwise odd. But this fact does not differentiate them from the pathological actions of sufferers from disorders on the impulsive-compulsive spectrum. Even sufferers from Tourette's syndrome (TS), a paradigm of irresistible impulse, report that their actions feel normal (Leckman *et al.* 1999): as one TS sufferer puts it, "I do the tic" (Cohen and Leckman 1992). We know far too little about the mechanisms which underlie ego-depletion to do any more than speculate about why these actions feel voluntary, and whether the feeling is veridical. One possibility is that the depletion of the resources of self-control operates upon the desires of the agent: rather than experiencing themselves as unable to resist any longer, they experience judgment-shift (in Richard Holton's (2004) felicitous phrase). There is independent evidence that addicts experience such judgment-shifts; indeed, such shifts seem characteristic of losses of self-control (Ainslie 2001).

On this hypothesis, when they consume their drug the addict does what they want to do; nevertheless, on the account of autonomy I have briefly sketched, they act against their own values: whenever they are not under the preference-shifting influence of their desire, their claim that they do not want to consume the drug is sincere, and most of the time they are not under its influence. Their loss of control, and of autonomy, is a more dramatic version of the kind of loss to which we are all subject, when we find ourselves giving in to temptation: we want to eat the chocolate cake when we eat it, but our subsequent claim that we acted against our own will is, in some sense, true.

SUCCESSFUL RESISTANCE

One regrettable consequence of views that are blind to the role that external scaffolding plays in thought and behavior is that they overlook the role of the environment in guiding our actions, and therefore the ways in which autonomy can be weakened or strengthened by alterations external to the individual. Autonomy is *developmentally* dependent upon the environment: we become autonomous individuals, able to control our behavior in the light of our values, only if the environment in which we grow up is suitably structured to reward self-control. Some environments are more conducive than others to the acquisition of self-control resources which are, at least partially, internal. But self-control remains dependent upon the environment throughout the lifespan: our ability to bring to bear our self-control resources, and their sufficiency to the task at hand, depends upon the structure of the environment in which we attempt to control ourselves. This implies that others can attempt to control us by modifying our environment. It also implies that we can successfully control *ourselves* by modifying our own environments.

We have already glimpsed some of the ways that others might attempt to control us by modifying our environments. In an earlier chapter, we reviewed how work in social psychology might be adapted to encourage impulse buying: by ensuring that consumers' self-control resources are at a low ebb when they are offered the opportunity to purchase something they find (at least somewhat) tempting, we raise the probability of their making purchases they will later regret. Vohs and Faber's (2002) work on ego-depletion and consumption seems to offer great opportunities to marketers.

Of course, though the application of the ego-depletion framework to consumption patterns is a recent development, marketers have been engaged in the systematic application of social science for over a century. Supermarket shelves and malls are already carefully designed to encourage consumption. One example among literally thousands: Wansink *et al.* (1998) identified an "anchoring" effect in consumption behavior, according to which consumers decide how many units of a product to purchase by reference to the number they normally buy. They therefore suggest that retailers can increase sales by raising the number used as an anchor; for instance by pricing goods in multiples (e.g., three for $3), or (paradoxically) by placing limits on the numbers that can be purchased ("limit: twelve per customer"). In the search for ever more effective ways of selling, marketers have now turned to neuroscience (Zaltamn 2003). No doubt the new sciences of "neuromarketing" will produce new techniques for retailers to apply, but there is no reason to fear these new techniques any more than those which will stem, are already stemming, from social psychology.

If environmental manipulations can be used to weaken self-control, they can also be used, by others or by ourselves, to strengthen it. We saw above that self-control depends, in important part, upon a set of skills that children acquire as they mature; for example, skills of self-distraction. In other words, though each normal agent is minimally unified by virtue of the set of mechanisms that ensure that, for instance, the binding problem is solved and they can act as a single unit at a time, unification of the agent temporally, that is the acquisition of the ability to extend one's will across time so that one can begin a project *now* secure in the knowledge that one's future self will complete it, is an achievement that each of us must strive for individually. We must each learn to delay gratification, and to sacrifice immediate, smaller, rewards for later, larger, rewards. In so doing we unify ourselves. But successfully achieving this self-unification requires that the child's environment be structured appropriately.

Ainslie (2001) suggests we see selves as consisting of nothing more than constellations of interests competing for control of behavior; to the extent to which self-unification strategies succeed, some interests get swamped beneath others. The unified agent is then able to act on their own preferences and values, without fearing that their plans will be short-circuited when the opportunity for some more immediate reward presents itself. Unification is something we achieve in the process of intrapersonal bargaining, cajoling and coercing, through which each sub-agent attempts to secure the goals its seeks. When we begin the process of shaping ourselves, we do not seek coherence or agent-hood; there is no "I" coherent enough to seek these things. As the process continues, however, a self comes into being; it is built out of a coalition of sub-personal mechanisms and processes, but it has sufficient unity to pursue goals, to present a single face to the world, and to think of itself as a single being. It is now minimally unified. But unification typically does not cease at this point. From this point on, it – *we* – may continue more or less consciously to work on itself, shaping itself in the light of its values and ideals. Sub-agential mechanisms build the self that will then continue to shape itself.[3]

If the child is to successfully bring themselves to the point where they have a sufficiently unified self to engage in the project of further self-making, they will require help. At minimum, the child requires that caregivers ensure that there is the opportunity successfully to deploy basic self-unification strategies. Unlucky children find themselves in environments which do not reward delayed gratification (there is no point in holding off on eating that cookie now if one's father will simply take it away and eat it himself [Strayhorn, 2002]). Moreover, the child needs to be confronted with opportunities to practice self-control that are neither too demanding – ensuring frustration and the development of learned helplessness – nor too easy, ensuring that the skills do not develop further.

How, precisely, do we engage in self-unification, if we are lucky enough to develop the basic skills necessary in early childhood?

What can the addicted agent do, for instance, to free themselves from their predictable preference shifts and reversals? There are a variety of tactics available, some of them quite mechanistic. The simplest strategy is an extension of the self-distraction technique spontaneously hit upon by the children in Mischel's study: directing one's attention elsewhere, or making efforts to avoid the cues that trigger desires. It is this technique we utilize when we choose a route from work that doesn't take us past the bakery, with its tempting smells. Addicts are generally too fragmented for normal attention-distraction techniques to have much chance of succeeding; instead they are more successful at self-control when they structure their environments so that the cues which remind them of their drugs are entirely absent. Hence the fact that most of the soldiers who returned from Vietnam addicted to heroin had relatively little trouble kicking the habit, whereas those who try to give up while surrounded by the same people with whom they have consumed find it so very difficult (Loewenstein 2000).

More spectacular techniques might deploy what we might call, following Elster (2000), the Ulysses technique (by analogy with Ulysses' actions in tying himself to the mast of his ship, so that he could listen to the song of the sirens without being lured to his death). Agents self-bind when they take steps either to ensure that they are physically unable to give into a later desire, or to significantly raise the costs of giving in. Techniques aimed at physical prevention include time-locks on drinks cabinets, or – far more simply and prosaically – purchasing small size chocolate bars, so that we will not be tempted today by the chocolate we mean to keep for tomorrow. Techniques aimed at raising the costs of giving in include telling friends that we are on a diet, so that having dessert involves a loss of face as well as figure. Several such methods of self-binding have been used in the treatment of addiction. In one treatment modality, cocaine addicts write letters confessing their most shameful secrets, to be mailed in the event they drop out of the program (Schelling 1992: 167). Alcoholics take the drug disulfiram ("Antabuse"), which makes them feel sick if they drink. Both methods aim at raising the cost of consumption, and thereby at strengthening mechanisms sensitive to these costs. All of these are obviously external manipulations: we alter our own behavior not by making an extra effort – though that may well *also* be required – but by changing the context in which we choose.

ADDICTION AND RESPONSIBILITY

Writers on addiction and responsibility typically take one of two equally simplistic contrary positions. Either they argue that addicts should simply stop taking their drugs – the "just say no" strategy – and that addiction is no excuse at all, or, perhaps more commonly, they argue that the addict is helpless in the face of their addiction (we saw some examples of this view earlier in this chapter, from writers like Charland and Elliott). In fact, there are some things addicts can do to resist, both in the short and the long-term, and to shake off their addiction altogether. But doing these things is difficult: it requires skills and opportunities, as well as some luck. For this reason, addiction should typically be seen not as entirely eliminating responsibility, but as reducing it.

It may be literally impossible for the addict to refrain from taking their drug (depending upon the drug and the degree of addiction) when it is immediately available and their self-control resources are depleted. However, they can take steps to avoid finding themselves in these circumstances: they can ensure that they do not have easy access to the drug, and they can avoid the cues that trigger cravings and therefore the depletion of their self-control resources. Taking these steps may not be easy. They depend upon the addict being able to exercise a sufficient degree of control over their environment – something which they will not be able to do if, for instance, they find themselves in a typical prison, where their movements and surroundings are regimented, but where their drug is easily available (and where the temptation to consume is great, given the harshness of the reality from which drugs represent a temporary

escape). Moreover, the costs to the addict of altering their environment in the relevant ways may be high. They may have to leave
friends and family, if they regularly consumed the drug with them;
they may have to leave their neighborhood and even their city. For
someone reduced to poverty by addiction, these steps are even more
daunting than they would be for us. Indeed, they may be near
impossible; the addict may simply lack the financial wherewithal
(and they may know that they will soon be reduced to the kind of
despair that will motivate them to find the drugs in a new city).

It is also worth pointing out how the view that the mind is
confined within the skull works against the addict. To the extent to
which we promote the view that giving up a drug, whether it is
tobacco or heroin, is all a matter of "will-power," we direct them
away from the kinds of environmental modifications they need to
make if they are to regain control. The extended mind hypothesis,
the view that the mental is not wholly contained within the skull,
but spills out into the world, is *useful*: it enables us to better control
ourselves (and others). I take its real-world success as further evidence of its truth. Knowledge is power: if the hypothesis were false,
then it would not yield successful strategies. But the extended mind
hypothesis is controversial and counterintuitive; we cannot blame
the addict for failing to take it into account.

Addicts have some responsibility for their behavior, insofar as
they can be expected to hold out against their desires in the short-term
(especially when the alternative is engaging in a seriously immoral
action, such as mugging someone in order to procure the money to
buy drugs), and (depending upon their resources, intellectual, financial and social), they can often be reasonably expected to take steps to
break free from their addiction, or at least to minimize its impact
upon others. But since doing these things is at least somewhat difficult, their responsibility is often reduced. The degree of reduction will
depend upon their circumstances. We shall consider the light that the
sciences of the mind can shed on the closely related questions of free
will and moral responsibility more generally in the next chapter.

End notes

1. It is worth pointing out that there may be more than an analogy between self-control and muscular exhaustion. Recent research seems to show that depletion of *physical* resources is also controlled by neural mechanisms: when athletes feel themselves unable to continue, their feeling is not a veridical reflection of the state of resources available to their muscles, but is instead a feeling produced by brain mechanisms designed to ensure that physical resources are preserved (Noakes *et al.* 2004).

2. Loewenstein notes that Vietnam veterans with heroin addictions found it relatively easy to kick the habit: since it was developed and maintained in a very different environment from that in which they attempted to give up, they rarely encountered the cues that triggered cravings.

3. This view of the self as an achievement has close affinities with the view advanced by Dennett (1991). However, whereas Dennett – in at least some of his moods – seems eliminativist about the self, I see no reason why the constructed self should not count as a *real* self. Dennett has used this account of the creation of selves to explain various pathologies of agency, such as (so-called) multiple personality disorder; on his view, one-self-to-a-customer is merely the typical case, not a fact about the kinds of beings we are. Perhaps some extreme cases of autonomy-impairing addiction result, not so much in a single agent who cannot extend their will across time, but in a fragmentation of the agent sufficient to call into doubt their existence as a single being.

7   The neuroscience of free will

Can neuroscience, and the other sciences of the mind, shed light on one of the oldest and most difficult of all philosophical problems, the problem of free will and moral responsibility?[1] Some scientists believe it can. In their popular writings, these scientists often express the opinion that the sciences of the mind have shown that free will – and therefore moral responsibility – is an illusion. They argue, roughly, as follows: the sciences of the mind demonstrate that our thoughts, intentions, and (therefore) our actions are the product of deterministic processes, in the following sense: given the initial conditions (say, our genetic endowment at birth and the environment into which we were born), we *had* to act as we did. But if we were determined to act as we did, then we were not free, or morally responsible. Richard Dawkins, the great evolutionary biologist, has recently compared our practices of praising, blaming and punishing to Basil Fawlty's behavior in flogging his car for breaking down, in the TV series *Fawlty Towers*:

> Doesn't a truly scientific, mechanistic view of the nervous system make nonsense of the very idea of responsibility, whether diminished or not? Any crime, however heinous, is in principle to be blamed on antecedent conditions acting through the accused's physiology, heredity and environment. Don't judicial hearings to decide questions of blame or diminished responsibility make as little sense for a faulty man as for a Fawlty car?
>
> *(Dawkins 2006)*

Of all the claims made by scientists, this is the one that probably annoys philosophers the most. Not because they regard it as wrong – most do, but some actually agree with the claim – but because it is made in apparent ignorance of literally thousands of years of debate on the question whether free will is compatible with causal determinism. There are powerful arguments for the claim that it is incompatible, but also powerful arguments on the other side.

Most philosophers today are compatibilists; that is, they believe that free will is compatible with determinism. The case for compatibilism has several strands. First, compatibilists argue that the view that free will is incompatible with determinism rests upon a confusion of *causation* with *coercion* or *control*. I am unfree, certainly, if my actions are controlled by another agent: if, for instance, my desires and beliefs are simply irrelevant to what I end up doing. If someone physically manipulates me, or holds a gun to my head, then my actions have their source in someone else, and I am not responsible for them. But the mere fact that determinism is true (if it is true) doesn't show that our actions are coerced or controlled by others. When I go get myself a cheese sandwich, I do so because *I want to*, and this remains true even if I am *determined* to want a cheese sandwich. No one forces me to get a cheese sandwich. Not even *determinism* forces me: to be determined to do something is nothing like being forced to do it. Once again, force is something that is applied to me in spite of what I want, by others or the external world, but determinism, if it is true, works through *me* and *my* desires. We rightly resent force, external control and coercion, but we are just confused if we assimilate determinism to these external powers. Even if determinism is true, rational agents are typically free: free to do what they like.

Second, compatibilists point out that if it is difficult, at least for some people, to see how free will could be compatible with determinism, it is apparently rather more mysterious how it could be compatible with *indeterminism*. Some scientists and laypeople who hope to rescue free will do so by appeal to quantum mechanics. Quantum mechanics is the science of subatomic particles, and is the foundation of modern physics. It is the most fundamental theory we possess for describing the physical world. Popular misconceptions to the contrary, the theory is well understood and well confirmed. However, it is highly controversial just what the world described by quantum mechanics is like, in the most basic sense. Quantum mechanics uses probabilistic rather than deterministic equations to describe the behavior of sub-atomic particles. On the so-called Copenhagen interpretation of quantum mechanics, these equations capture the nature of physical reality: the equations are probabilistic because the world is fundamentally indeterministic. This inter-pretation is the dominant one; rival interpretations attempt to save determinism by postulating hidden variables or limits on observa-tion. It is therefore controversial whether the universe is entirely deterministic. However, it is far from obvious that contemporary physics can come to the aid of the incompatibilist who wants to preserve free will.

First, even if the universe is indeterministic at a sub-atomic level, it may be that these indeterminacies get washed out at the macroscopic level. The behavior of everything we can observe with the naked eye, or even with ordinary microscopes, *seems* determi-nistic and predictable: sub-atomic indeterminacy may simply be washed out. In that case, sub-atomic indeterminacy can be ignored: the world is deterministic for almost all practical purposes. Suppose, second, that that's not the case; that sub-atomic indeterminacy can affect the behavior of complex macroscopic objects such as human beings. How will that help? If I am not free, despite the fact that I can do what I want when I want, how does the fact that sometimes – due to a random event – I *fail* to do what I want when I want to enhance my freedom? Just the opposite seems to be the case: indeterminacy would *reduce*, not increase, my freedom, since I cannot control the random behavior of sub-atomic particles.[2]

Incompatibilists generally accept that it is a mistake to assimilate determinism to coercion or external control. But they have other reasons for thinking that determinism is incompatible with free will. They point out that we can apparently fail to be free even when we do what we want: for instance, when others manipulate our wants (Kane 1996; Pereboom 2001). Determinism might render us unfree in an analogous way. But, compatibilists respond, there are salient differences between cases in which our wants are manipulated and cases in which they are merely *caused*. We are someone's puppet in the first scenario, but not in the second. Different varieties of incompatibilists part ways at this point, depending upon their beliefs about the causal structure of the world. Some incompatibilists are determinists, and therefore hold that there is no free will in our world (Pereboom 2001). Some deny that determinism is true; they therefore hold that some actions (at least) are free. These incompatibilists are known as libertarians (Kane 1996; Ekstrom 1999; O'Connor 2000).

Obviously, we cannot hope to settle the debate whether free will is compatible with determinism, a debate that is perhaps the most complex and difficult in all of philosophy, here. It should be clear, however, that those scientists who think that the revelation that the brain is deterministic is sufficient to show that free will does not exist, without further argument, are mistaken: they do not know whereof they speak. That is not, however, to say that the sciences of the mind may not have a bearing on free will and moral responsibility.

The rest of this chapter will consider two topics. First, I shall examine a global challenge to our free will and moral responsibility. Some neuroscientists have argued that we are not free, not because our actions are determined, but because we do not consciously cause our behavior. Having seen off this threat, I shall examine some of the ways in which our growing knowledge about the mind will help us to distinguish *between* individuals. Rather than neuroscience showing that no one is ever responsible, I shall argue, attention to its discoveries will help us to see who is responsible, and who is not.

CONSCIOUSNESS AND FREEDOM

Some recent results in neuroscience and in psychology have been seen, by some thinkers, to present us with a fresh challenge to freedom, independent of determinism. These results allegedly show that we do not consciously cause our intentions, decisions or volitions, and therefore our actions. If this is true, many believe, we do not act freely. As Robert Kane, one of the leaders of the recent revival of libertarianism puts it, "If conscious willing is illusory or epiphenomenalism is true, *all* accounts of free will go down, *compatibilist and incompatibilist*" (Kane 2005).

In what follows, I will outline the threat, in the two forms in which it comes; I will also briefly sketch some of the ways in which philosophers have responded to it. These responses are designed to show that the experimental evidence does not, in fact, establish the claim that we do not consciously cause our actions. I shall then develop a response of my own. My response differs from the existing replies inasmuch as rather than attempting to show that the experiments are flawed, it shows that *even if* they successfully establish that consciousness does not play a direct role in action-causation, we can still be free and morally responsible agents. The evidence I shall cite for this claim will itself be drawn from the sciences of the mind.

WHO DECIDES WHEN I DECIDE?

In essence, the claim made by both variants of the empirical challenge to moral responsibility is this: consciousness plays no direct role in decision-making or volition. We do not consciously decide or consciously initiate action. Consciousness comes on the scene too late to play any causal role in action. Two thinkers have attempted, independently, to demonstrate that this is the case: Benjamin Libet, a neuroscientist, and Daniel Wegner, a psychologist.

Libet's experiment is one of the most famous in recent neuroscience: Libet and his colleagues asked subjects to flick or flex their wrist whenever they wanted to, while the experimenters recorded the "readiness potential" (RP) in their brains, which precedes voluntary movement by up to one second or so (Libet *et al.* 1983). Subjects were also asked to watch a special clock face, around which a dot of light travelled about twenty-five times faster than a normal clock (with each "second" therefore being about 40 milliseconds). They were required to note the position of the dot on the clock face at the time at which they became aware of the wish to move their wrist. Controlling for timing errors, the experimenters found that onset of RP preceded awareness of the wish by an average 400 milliseconds. In other words, subjects became aware of their decision to act only after its implementation was underway.

Libet's experiment has widely been seen as an empirical demonstration that there is no such thing as free will (Spence 1996; Pockett 2004). Libet has shown, the argument goes, that consciousness of the decision to act or of the volition comes too late to be causally effective. Consciousness is *informed of* the decision; it does not *make* it. But the agent, the target of ascriptions of praise and blame, is, if not identical to consciousness, at least more properly identified with consciousness than with the subpersonal mechanisms that are, as a matter of fact, causally effective in action. It turns out that *we* do not make our decisions; they are made *for us*. But if *we* cannot control what we decide to do, then we cannot be responsible for our decisions (Zhu 2004).[3]

Philosophers and cognitive scientists have not been slow to find fault with Libet's claims. For instance, Flanagan (1996a) argues that it is consistent with Libet's results that we consciously initiate important or "big picture" decisions, merely leaving the details of the implementation of these decisions to subpersonal processes. Thus, having – consciously – decided to comply with Libet's instructions to flick their wrist when they felt like it, his subjects might have delegated the details to the unconscious mechanisms which Libet's experiment tracks. If that's right, then our big picture decision might after all be made consciously. As Richard Double (2004) has recently put it, this picture leaves plenty of space for a *distal cause* (compatibilist) or *distal influence* (libertarian) view of moral responsibility. Alfred Mele (2007) shows that it is reasonable to doubt whether Libet is right in identifying the subjective reports with the *intention* or the *decision* to flick, rather than with an *urge* or a *desire* to flick. Hence, Libet's experiment might not bear upon the role of consciousness in decision-making at all. Haggard (Haggard and Libet 2001) has argued that though Libet is right in thinking that we do not consciously initiate actions, our conscious intention may coincide with the *specification* of action. Our decision *to* act may not be conscious, but the choice of how *precisely* to act (whether, for instance, to use our left hand or our right) might nevertheless be made consciously. Finally Dennett (1991; 2003) has shown that there are deep problems with relying upon subjective judgments of simultaneity, as a consequence of which we cannot rely upon Libet's results. In any case, Dennett argues, it is a mistake to think that there is a precise moment at which anything enters consciousness: the idea that there is any such moment is a hangover from the notion of the Cartesian Theatre, where everything comes together and is viewed by the self. Such a notion, Dennett points out, has rightly been discarded by philosophers and neuroscientists, since its truth requires that the self be an extensionless point – in other words, a Cartesian immaterial ego. Yet we all too easily fall back into modes of thought that commit us to it. Once we reject the notion of the Cartesian theatre finally and decisively, we shall recognize that consciousness is temporally smeared; not a moment, but a process with fuzzy edges.

Libet's is not the only threat to the role of consciousness in action, however. Before we assess his challenge and these responses to it, let's set out Wegner's version of the threat.

In his book *The Illusion of Conscious Will*, Wegner (2002) presents a wealth of evidence for essentially the same conclusion advanced by Libet: that consciousness does not initiate action. Wegner distinguishes between what he calls the phenomenal will – our experience of our will as causally effective – and the empirical will; the actual causal mechanisms of behavior. The eponymous "illusion of conscious will" arises when we mistake the first for the second; when we take our experience of causation to be a direct readout of the reality. In fact, our experience is a belated and unreliable record of action; it is neither itself a causal force, nor is it a direct reflection of the actual causal forces.

Wegner argues that, far from being the cause of our actions, the phenomenal will is itself caused by the mechanisms that actually produce actions. The real causal springs of our actions are subpersonal – and therefore unconscious – mechanisms. These mechanisms produce the action, but they also produce a mental preview of the action. So long as certain conditions are satisfied, agents take this mental preview to be the real cause of the action. As Wegner (2002: 64) puts it, "*People experience conscious will when they interpret their own thought as the cause of their action.*" We fall victim to this illusion when three conditions are satisfied: the mental preview of action occurs at the right time (prior to the action, but close to the moment of its initiation), the preview is consistent with the action and the agent is unaware of other potential causes of the action. Wegner calls these three conditions of the experience of conscious will the *priority, consistency* and *exclusivity* principles. Since his account explains why we think that our preview of the action causes it, Wegner calls it the theory of *apparent mental causation.*

In defence of his claim that conscious will is an illusion, Wegner offers us evidence that conscious will is subject to a *double dissociation*: its presence is not an infallible guide to our agency, and its absence is not an infallible guide to our passivity. Consider the second claim first. In a number of situations, both inside and outside the laboratory, people sincerely deny that they have acted, when in fact they have. Some kinds of paranormal experiences are good illustrations of this phenomenon. For instance, the phenomenon of table turning, which amazed so many Victorians, can be parsimoniously explained via Wegner's theory. In table turning, a group of people sit around a table, each with his or her hands flat on its surface. If they believe or hope that it will begin to turn on its own, it often, miraculously, will. The phenomenon was often interpreted as evidence for the existence of supernatural beings. Of course, the participants were themselves making the table turn; the real mystery is why they sincerely denied their own agency. Wegner suggests that when many agents each contribute to the causation of an action – in other words, when the exclusivity principle is not satisfied – we may easily overlook our own contribution. The movements of the pointer on the Ouija board can be explained in precisely the same way. So, sadly, can the phenomenon of facilitated communication, in which facilitators take themselves to be merely helping profoundly disabled people to communicate, but in which the "facilitator" is themselves the source of the message (2002: 195–201). It seems that absence of the feeling of will is not proof of absence of agency.

Whereas evidence for the second dissociation can be collected "in the wild," Wegner needed to design experiments to demonstrate the possibility of the first. Most convincing here is the "I-Spy" experiment (Wegner 2002; Wegner and Wheatley 1999). Briefly, the experiment placed subjects in a situation in which the degree of their causal contribution to an action was unclear, due to the presence of an experimental confederate. Wegner and Wheatley found that when the confederate caused an action in this situation, the subject would over-attribute it to themselves if they were primed in accordance with the priority principle. The feeling of conscious will can be produced by priority and consistency in the absence of exclusivity, and in the absence of genuine agency.

Philosophers have responded to Wegner's claims in ways that are closely analogous to the manner in which they have responded to Libet: they have denied that Wegner has shown that consciousness does not play a direct role in action. They have pointed out that the demonstration of a double dissociation does not show anything about the *normal* case. Consider perception: sometimes people fail to see an object in front of them – because of a more or less spectacular dysfunction in their visual system, or because it is disguised – and sometimes they claim to see what is not there (as in many visual illusions). Perception, too, is subject to a double dissociation. But it does not follow that our impression that our percepts are caused by objects in the world is generally false (Nahmias 2002; Metzinger 2004; Bayne 2006).

How strong are these responses to Libet and to Wegner? I shall not attempt to evaluate them in any detail. For what it's worth, I suspect they are (at minimum) successful in pointing out severe problems in their arguments and experimental designs. Neither has demonstrated, anywhere near conclusively, that consciousness does not initiate action or make decisions. However, though these philosophers have won this battle, I suspect they will lose the war: consciousness does not, in fact, play the kind of role in action that Libet and Wegner believe to be required in order for us to be morally responsible. We should therefore get on with assessing whether, and how, moral responsibility might be compatible with the finding that consciousness does not initiate actions or make decisions.

CONSCIOUSNESS AND MORAL RESPONSIBILITY

Prima facie, consciousness seems required for moral responsibility. Indeed, the claim that agents must be conscious of their actions (decisions) seems to be built into our legal system, and to drive our intuitions about praise and blame. Consider the legal doctrine of *mens rea*. Someone is guilty of a crime (strict liability aside, which is in any case rare in the criminal law) only if they were in the requisite state of mind, where "being in a state of mind" seems to require consciousness. In order to be liable for the highest degree of criminal responsibility, an agent must have performed a wrongful action *purposefully* and *knowingly*. A somewhat lower degree of moral responsibility can be imputed if the agent acted *recklessly*, which might be understood as having been conscious of the risks of one's conduct, but nevertheless having failed to take due care. These grades of moral responsibility seem to require consciousness: of intentions, of risks and possible consequences. To be sure, negligence does not seem to require consciousness, but it is the lowest grade of responsibility. For all grades above negligence, consciousness seems required for responsibility. And, precisely because negligence can be imputed in the absence of consciousness, some philosophers regard negligence as a legal fiction.

The notion that consciousness is required for moral responsibility seems therefore to be central to the criminal law. It also seems to be at work in explaining our assessments of responsibility in exotic cases, such as cases of automatism. Recall (from the introduction) the case of Ken Parks. In 1987, Parks drove the twenty-three kilometres to the Ontario home of his parents-in-law, where he stabbed them both. He then drove to the police station, where he told police that he thought he had killed someone. Only then, apparently, did he notice that his hands had been badly injured. Parks was charged with the murder of his mother-in-law, and the attempted murder of his father-in-law. He was acquitted, on the grounds that he had performed the act while sleep-walking. The court found, and on appeal the Canadian Supreme Court agreed, that he had committed the act in a state of automatism (Broughton *et al.* 1994). Now, I think it is clear that the best explanation of the widely shared intuition that Parks was not responsible for his actions is that he was not conscious of what he was doing (Levy and Bayne 2004).[4] Why consciousness should matter is not clear; *that* it matters seems obvious.

It seems, therefore, that agents can be responsible for their actions only if they were conscious of them. But why is consciousness necessary for moral responsibility? Libet and Wegner seem to think that demonstrating that consciousness lags behind decision-making shows that agents do not genuinely *control* their actions. It is for this reason that they are supposed not to be morally responsible for them. Conscious control is, as Wegner (2004) puts it, an illusion, but if we do not control our actions, we cannot be responsible for them. Libet argues that we ought not to hold agents responsible for actions performed "without the possibility of conscious control" (Libet 1999: 52). But if consciousness lags behind decision-making, *none* of our actions is consciously controlled. We should all be excused, just as we currenlty excuse those who suffer from automatism.

Wegner and Libet advance two independent arguments for the claim that the alleged lag demonstrates lack of control. Wegner (2004) suggests that given that the experience of conscious will is not always veridical, we ought to assume that authorship is always illusory. In other words, the dissociations he demonstrates threaten nothing less than the dissolution of the self. Since the feeling of willing can dissociate from the reality of willing, we ought to assume that both will and the accompanying experience are produced by the same mechanism, and not by the self. However, it is clear that this argument fails: nothing Wegner says gives us any reason to identify the self with the *experience* of the self. As we saw in the previous chapter, we can identify the self with a much broader network of states and mechanisms; if these states and mechanisms cause our actions, then *we* cause them. Actions so caused are, at least typically, caused by our beliefs and our desires. if my actions are caused by my beliefs and my desires, and I have no contrary beliefs or desires, then it seems plausible to maintain that I control them (Dennett 1984).

Nevertheless, Wegner and Libet have another, and more inter- esting, argument for the claim that the lag between consciousness and decision-making is evidence that we lack control over our decisions, an argument which focuses on *control* rather than on the *controller*. If we are not conscious of our decisions at the precise instant we make them, they seem to think, then we do not fully control them. It is caused by our beliefs and our desires, to be sure, but we have no choice over *whether* our actions are caused by our beliefs and desires. Instead, our actions are *passively* caused by our beliefs and desires. If we are fully and actively to control our actions, we require an *active causal power* to intervene in the decision-making process. We are properly free, they seem to suggests, only if we possess the power actively to intervene in our decision-making right up to (quite literally) the very last microsecond, thereby altering its course. Call this, the alleged requirement that we able to exercise such an active causal power in decision-making, the *decision constraint*. Libet and Wegner seem committed to denying that the decision constraint is ever satisfied, while most of the philosophical responses to them seem aimed at showing that it might be satisfied after all. I suggest that this is wasted effort. The decision constraint is highly unlikely to be satisfied. And that's a *good* thing. We dont't want an active causal power, capable of playing the kind of role that Libet and Wegner aim to show consciousness cannot play. The exercise of any such an active causal power, conscious or not, would not increase our freedom. Instead, it would likely *reduce* it.

Consider what decision-making would be like if we possessed such an active causal power. Suppose, for the sake of concreteness, that you are faced with some momentous choice: for instance, whether or not to accept a job in another city. There are many reasons in favor of your accepting the job (new and exciting challenges; better pay; more recognition, and so on) and many reasons against (your friends and family would be far away; the work raises moral qualms in you; you worry that you may have too little autonomy, and so on). Given the importance of the choice, you deliberate carefully before you make up your mind. This deliberation is, of course, carried out consciously: that is, you are aware that you are deliberating, and the considerations for and against accepting the job occupy your mind.

But look closer; what role might consciousness, as an active power, actually play? Let's approach this question by thinking about the process of decision-making. There are, it seems, two ways we could go about making decisions: either we could *weigh* our reasons, or we could *weight* them (Nozick 1981).[5] We *weigh* reasons when we try to find out how significant they are for us, given our beliefs, values, plans, goals and desires. We *weight* reasons when we assign them a weight and thereby a significance for us, either ignoring any pre-existing weight they might have had, or varying it. For instance, if when you deliberate about the job offer, you try to discover how important its relevant features are for you, you are weighing the reasons. You might try to think about the importance of family in your life, for example: how much will you miss your parents and siblings?

Will regular telephone conversations be able to replace day-to-day contact? How great will the loss to you be, and how much will the greater pay compensate for them? On the other hand, if you ignore or vary the weight that (say) proximity to family has for you – thinking, for instance, that though family has been very important to me up till now, I shall decide to assign it very little weight in my decision – *and* nothing about your other reasons explains the new significance you assign it, then you are engaged in weighting your reasons.

It is, I think, quite obvious that when we engage in deliberation, we take ourselves to be weighing reasons, and not weighting them. We try to discover how much things really do matter to us, not decide to make them matter to us – not, at least, in the way we would if were weighting them. We do, of course, sometimes try to make things matter more (or less) to us than they do: a man who finds himself absorbed in his work might regret the fact that his family doesn't weigh more heavily with him than it does, and he might take steps to increase the weight that family has in his decision-making (including, for instance, turning down a job offer that will take him far away from them). But (at least typically) this isn't weighting at all, but instead an indirect way of weighing. If the man wants to give a greater weight to family in his decision-making for *reasons* – because, for instance, he thinks that he will be happier if he makes more time for family, or because he thinks that it is morally wrong to spend so little time with them – than he is engaged in indirect weighing. He attempts to discern how much weight family *should* have for him, given what he believes and desires, and given what his values and goals really are. He is like the addict who desires to consume their drug but wants to be rid of the desire because it does not reflect their values. Properly weighting reasons, in the sense at issue here, is not indirect weighing: it is not trying to give greater weight to a reason in the light of the weight of *other* reasons. Instead, weighting a reason is assigning a weight to a consideration for no reason at all.

The power to weight reasons, to reiterate, is the power to assign them a weight which is at variance with the weight they would have for us if we weighed them; that is, the weight they have for us in the light of our beliefs and desires, goals, plans and values. Now, why would anyone want a power like *that*? This is a power to make something matter to us more, or less, than it should, given what we believe and want. Some philosophers have argued that we need such a power because in its absence our decisions could only turn out one way (McCall and Lowe 2005). It may well be that the only choice I can make, consistent with my values and beliefs, is for me to turn down the job. But, these philosophers argue, if my decisions can only go one way, they are determined, and therefore they are not free. We have already seen that there are reasons to doubt the claim that the mere fact that someone's actions are determined entails that they are not free; the claim seems even weaker when, as here, the worry is that our decisions are determined by *our own values and beliefs*. I shall not revisit this question here. Instead, I shall confine my attention to asking how the alleged power to weight reasons could enhance our freedom.

If you make decisions by assigning weights to your reasons, varying the weight that they would have for you were you instead to weigh them, you make your decision *arbitrarily*. Nothing, by hypothesis, can explain why you assign the weight you do – at least, nothing rational. But a decision that is arational, or irrational, is not a free decision.[6] If you assign weights to your reasons, either your assignment is caused (deterministically or indeterministically) by the weights they have independently of the act of deliberation (in which case we are really weighing reasons) or your assignment is arbitrary, and the arbitrariness of the assignment of weight transfers to the subsequent decision. A power to vary the weight your reasons would have for you, were you to weigh them, introduces an element of chance into your decision-making. It does not enhance freedom; it actually *reduces* it.

If we are to be capable of making free decisions, then, we do not need, or want, the power to weight our reasons. Instead, we need the power to weigh them: to discover how much weight we *should* give to them, given our beliefs and values. If that's right, though, we do not need an *active causal power* at all. Free decision-making can instead be a passive process: it can proceed by way of a mechanism that, like a set of scales, simply aggregates the weight of our reasons and measures which set is the weightier. An active causal power, conscious or not, that intervened at any stage of the weighing process would reduce our freedom, not enhance it. If satisfying the decision constraint requires that consciousness – or, indeed, anything else – must play such an active causal role in decision-making, then we had better hope that the decision constraint is unsatisfied.

Once we recognize that we do not need or want an active causal power, the claim that consciousness does not learn of the agent's decisions until after they are already underway no longer seems threatening. Given that we have no reason to want consciousness (or anything else) to play an active causal role in producing the decision, the fact (if indeed it is a fact) that consciousness might sometimes be out of the loop oughtn't to worry us. So long as our decisions are made rationally – which means by a process of weighing, and not weighting – precisely when consciousness learns of them doesn't much matter.

There are two possible objections to the forgoing, so far as I can see. First, it might be pointed out that people frequently choose in defiance of their reasons; they suffer from weakness of the will and find themselves choosing against their own better judgment. Second, it might be held that though we must decide in light of our reasons, we can nevertheless take them as mere guides, rather than as determinants of what we must do: perhaps the weights that our reasons have for us are reported to consciousness, or at any rate to an active causal power that is intrinsically conscious, which then decides whether or not to vary them. Let's consider these objections in turn.

It would be odd, to say the least, to think that weak-willed actions are, alone of all actions, free. In any case, these actions no more satisfy the decision constraint than any other kind. Though it is true that when we suffer from weakness of will, we decide, in some sense, in defiance of our reasons, the sense in which this is true is irrelevant here. There is a wider and a narrow sense of "reason;" the sense in which I choose against my reasons in weakness of the will is the narrow sense, while the sense in which my actions are always caused – deterministically or indeterministically – by my reasons is the wide sense. To say that when I act against my all-things-considered judgment I act against my own reasons is to say, roughly, that I allow myself to be moved by considerations that I do not reflectively endorse. To say that my weak-willed action is nevertheless caused by my reasons is to say, roughly, that it was caused by considerations that exert some causal power over my decision-making mechanisms in light of their attractiveness for me. I do not reflectively endorse my desire for a third beer; in that sense if I drink it I act in defiance of my reasons. But that third beer is nevertheless reason-giving for me; it exerts causal power over me because it satisfies some of my desires.

The second objection, that my decision can be guided by my reasons without being *caused* by them, seems to me hopeless. To the extent to which my decision departs from the course that the weight my reasons have for me recommends, it does so arbitrarily. The greater the role for consciousness, if we follow this route, the greater the chanciness of our decisions. If consciousness has the power to vary the weights our reasons have for us – and I don't see how it could have this power, in any case – then our decisions are less rational than we hoped, and we have less freedom-level control. We find a role for consciousness at the expense of responsibility.[7]

Decision-making is a response to weights which reasons have independently *of* the decision. Decision-making is not something performed by any kind of active causal power; instead, we simply see – *recognize*, are *struck by*, *grasp*; the metaphors are revealing – how weighty the reasons are, and our decisions follow from them. Indeed, the very phenomenology of decision-making reflects the extent to which it is a paradoxically passive phenomenon. As Dennett points out, decisions are in some sense things that happen *to us*:

> From some fleeting vantage points, they seem to be the preeminently voluntary moves in our lives, the instants at which we exercise our agency to the fullest. But those same decisions can also be seen to be strangely out of our control. We have to wait to see how we are going to decide something, and when we do decide, our decision bubbles up to consciousness from we know not where. We do not witness it being *made*; we witness its *arrival*.
>
> *(Dennett 1984: 78)*

Decision-making by deliberation is something that I do, and that I control inasmuch as I can cease to engage in it or persist in it, but I do not and cannot actively control its course or its upshot, by way of deciding how weighty my reasons are. If I could, it would not be deliberation – the weighing of reasons – but something else entirely; something non-conducive to moral responsibility.

No matter what the faults of their experimental designs, therefore, and for reasons entirely independent of their arguments, Libet and Wegner must be right. Decision-making is not a task of consciousness, as an active causal power. We cannot control our decision-making, for a simple reason: decision-making is, or is an important element of, our control system, whereby we control our activity. If we were able to control our control system, we should require another, higher-order, control system with which to exert that control. And if we had such a higher-order control system, the same problems would simply arise with regard to it. The demand that we exercise conscious will seems to be the demand that we control our controlling. And that demand cannot be fulfilled.

MORAL RESPONSIBILITY WITHOUT THE DECISION CONSTRAINT

Where does that leave us? Should we simply conclude that satisfying the decision constraint is unnecessary, because in fact consciousness has no role to play in responsible agency? At least one philosopher has suggested just that. According to David Rosenthal (2002), it does not matter whether or not our actions are caused consciously; what matters is whether our actions fit with the conscious picture we have of ourselves and of our ends. As we have already seen, however, there are good reasons to think that consciousness has some more direct role to play in moral responsibility. Parks was excused responsibility for his actions because he wasn't conscious at the time of action, not because his actions failed to fit with his conscious view of himself and his ends (which view could, in any case, be quite mistaken). How, then, might consciousness matter to moral responsibility, if the decision constraint cannot be satisfied, and if mere consciousness of decision turns us into spectators of our actions? I suggest that Rosenthal is right to this extent: what matters is indeed whether our actions reflect ourselves and our ends. Consciousness matters, however, because its presence (typically) brings it about that our actions reflect who we are and what our ends are.

Here is not the place to defend a particular account of consciousness. However, recent years have seen something of a convergence on, if not an account of consciousness, at least an account of something that consciousness *does*: it is, or facilitates, or results from (depending on the account) a global workspace, as Bernard Baars calls it (Baars 1988, 1997; Dehaene and Naccache 2001; Jack and Shallice 2001).[8] A global workspace is a space in which information, accessed from many different sources – from modular brain systems and from the environment – becomes accessible to many different parts of the brain simultaneously. Consciousness serves the function of allowing parts of the brain that are otherwise relatively isolated from each other to communicate. Consciousness is or at least facilitates what Dennett (2001) calls "fame in the brain," or "cerebral celebrity;" in the terms made famous by Ned Block (1997), phenomenal-consciousness facilitates access-consciousness. The contents of consciousness are globally available for behavior control; it is for this reason that consciousness is necessary for moral responsibility.

To say that information in consciousness is globally available is not to say that it is available *to consciousness*. Of course, it *is* available to consciousness; that much is tautologically true. What matters is that information is globally available to the subpersonal mechanisms; the actual causal mechanisms of behavior. As cases of automatism show, we do not need much in the way of consciousness for intelligent action. Subpersonal mechanisms can get along surprisingly well without it – which is to say without each other. But we have good reason to think that without consciousness agents are not morally responsible, because they act only on a subset of the information that normally guides them, and this subset is likely to be inadequate.

The picture I am urging is this: even though the decision constraint cannot be satisfied, even though consciousness doesn't *make* our decisions, consciousness matters for moral responsibility because conscious deliberation – typically – greatly improves the quality of the decisions the subpersonal mechanisms ultimately cause. Deliberation, the turning over in our minds of all the considerations that seem relevant to a decision, puts our decision-making mechanisms in contact with one another, and thereby with more, and more relevant, information: information about our values, about moral standards, about the world, about other people, about our plans and policies. As we deliberate, more and better information "comes to mind;" that is, is broadcast by the modular mechanisms to us and to each other (broadcasting to each other *is* broadcasting to us; broadcasting to us *is* broadcasting to each other, since we are nothing over and above the set of mechanisms). Moreover, the likelihood is that this information is somehow tagged or prioritized by deliberation, so that information about what matters most to us is broadcast more often, or more forcefully, to the *right* mechanisms (Baars 1997: 307). Deliberation is also a process of putting questions to ourselves; considering problems so that our subpersonal mechanisms can go to work on them, and broadcast the solutions back to us – and therefore to each other. Hence, the longer we deliberate, the better informed, the more intelligent, our actions, and the greater the extent to which they reflect our deepest values.

High-quality deliberation will therefore greatly increase the likelihood that the resulting actions reflect our real selves. Under responsibility-conducive conditions, actions will still be made by subpersonal mechanisms, but they will be controlled by *us*, in the fullest sense; by our real selves, for these mechanisms are us. It is this fact, the fact that deliberated-upon action is deeply reflective of our deepest values, that best explains the legal typology encapsulated in the doctrine of *mens rea*. Murder "in cold blood" is worse than unpremeditated killing, because a planned action better reflects my settled convictions, my sense of what really matters, my values, whereas a spontaneous action reflects only a part of my self, and perhaps a relatively inessential part at that.

The global workspace idea also explains why agents who act in a state of automatism are not responsible for what they do. Agents like Parks act only on a small subset of their action plans, policies, desires and goals. Their actions do not reflect their deepest selves, their settled convictions. Since the agent was not even conscious, we have good reason to think that their action is less reflective of their identity as practical agents than even the spontaneous and immediate actions of the agent who acts (for instance) under provocation, or who acts negligently. Thus, an action performed in a state of automatism is not attributable to the agent as an individual. Of course, it might be *reflective* of the agent; a thoroughly bad agent is as susceptible to entering the state of automatism as a good. But when a bad action performed in a state of automatism is reflective of the agent, it is only by chance that this is so. The bad agent did not have the opportunity to think twice, and therefore cannot be blamed for their action.[9]

The decision constraint cannot be satisfied. But it doesn't matter. When our subpersonal mechanisms make decisions, *we* make decisions. Though the mechanisms out of which our minds are built are dumb, when they act in concert the decisions they make are – or can be – intelligent. They are not random or arbitrary; they are rational responses to the environment, made in the light of *our* beliefs and *our* values. Indeed, this is how things *must be*: we *are* the set of our subpersonal mechanisms, and nothing else, and our intelligence just *is* the product of the successful combination of these dumb machines. They are us: they reflect our uniqueness, our differences from one another. My decisions reflect my history, my learning, my experience; I choose in ways that would be entirely inexplicable if what I thought did not heavily influence everything that I do. The mechanisms that make my decisions are, in fact, *me*. As Dennett (2003: 242) puts it, Libet has not shown that we are out of the loop: we *are* the loop. Decision-making cannot be conscious – that is, caused by consciousness – but that needn't matter, for the mechanisms that make the decision are nevertheless ours, us; they have our values, they have our beliefs, our goals (we have them *by* them having them), and when they decide, *we* decide.

That doesn't mean, however, that any and all decisions made by the subpersonal mechanisms and modules that populate my mind are *my* decisions, or that they are (by my lights) good decisions. It is only when the mechanisms work together that *I* decide, and that my decision is the one I want to make. Since consciousness (typically) allows this condition to be satisfied, by making information globally available, and putting the mechanisms in contact with one another, consciousness is after all a necessary condition of moral responsibility.

LESSONS FROM NEUROSCIENCE

The forgoing pages were devoted to resolving (to my own satisfaction, at least) the problem of how we can be free even if – even though – consciousness does not cause our actions: in other words, to seeing off a threat from neuroscience. I now want to turn to some more positive lessons from neuroscience, and related fields; lessons we can and ought to apply in our practices of blaming and holding to account, including our practices of punishing wrongdoers. I shall argue that our growing understanding of the brain and its pathologies is directly relevant to our moral and legal treatment of one another. Some agents who we would currently punish for wrongdoing ought to be excused from all blame; others ought to be punished less severely. In both kinds of cases, we ought to reduce sentences or mitigate censure because these agents do not (fully) meet the conditions properly laid down for moral responsibility, and they do not meet these conditions due to brain abnormalities.

Some thinkers deny that neuroscience should have an impact on our responsibility ascriptions. Gazzaniga (2005), for instance, argues that responsibility is a moral notion, and that morality is one thing and science another. Morse (2004, 2006) argues that those who believe that psychopathology can diminish moral responsibility confuse *abnormal* causation with *excuse*. Both of these writers are mistaken, as a brief investigation of the rationale underlying our practice of blaming and excusing shows.

Philosophers investigating moral responsibility have usually sought to reveal the underlying logic of responsibility ascriptions. They have typically done this by trying to discover what factors lead us to excuse others of responsibility for actions they have performed. There is a range of situations in which it is uncontroversial that agents ought to be excused, even though they have performed a wrongful act. Excusing conditions that are generally recognized include coercion, compulsion and certain kinds of ignorance. Why do these conditions excuse? The fundamental rationale seems to be this: in these cases, it would be *unfair* to blame me, because I do not exhibit any ill will in performing my action. In cases of compulsion, my action does not exhibit any ill will because I had no control over whether I performed it; I literally could not refrain. Since I could not prevent myself from performing that action, we cannot make any inferences from the fact that I performed it to the quality of my will. In cases of coercion, I chose (what I took to be) the morally best action from among those available to me. If I harmed you (say, by handing over your money to a thief who would otherwise have stabbed me), it is not because I wish you any ill, but because I believed that your losing the money was a lesser harm than my death. Finally, when I am (non-culpably) ignorant of the nature of my act, I do not intend the harm that arises; once more, it does not reflect badly on my moral character. In all these cases, it would be grossly unfair to blame me for what I did.

Once we understand the logic of excuses, we see that our practices of praising and blaming reflect facts about the nature of moral reality, as we perceive it. Justifications and excuses are not invented, as Gazzaniga thinks, but *discovered*: we rightfully blame another when, and only when, he or she performs a wrongful action that expresses ill will towards others. But if that's right, if blame requires the satisfaction of a set of conditions, we can blame wrongfully. We cannot, contra Gazzaniga, simply invent a moral practice. If, for instance, we decide to blame babies for their actions, say in soiling their nappies, and inflict punishment on them accordingly, we shall be guilty of moral wrong-doing: we blame them for something (a) over which they do not exercise appropriate control and (b) which does not reflect any ill will toward us. Our moral practices are not mere constructs, but instead reflect *facts* about the world, and about the nature of agents in the world: Do they really know what they're doing? Do they control their actions?

The underlying logic of moral ascriptions is recognized in legal practice, as well as philosophical theories. Most jurisdictions in the Western world acquit defendants if they fail a test based on the famous *M'Naghten Rules*, introduced in the mid-nineteenth century in England. These rules state that defendants are to be found not guilty if it is proved that:

> at the time of the committing of the act, the party *ACCUSED* was laboring under such a defect of reason, from disease of mind, as not to know the nature and quality of the act he was doing; or if he did know it, that he did not know he was doing what was wrong.

The M'Naghten Rules are a test of non-culpable ignorance: defendants are to be acquitted if they lack knowledge, factual or moral, concerning what they are doing. If I believe that hitting you is actually swatting a fly, I show you no ill will; similarly, I do not show you ill will if I think you enjoy being hit.

M'Naghten is a *cognitive* test: agents fail it by failing to possess the relevant knowledge. In addition to M'Naghten, or something like it, many jurisdictions also recognize a *volitional* defence. M'Naghten excuses only if the agent did not understand what he or she was doing, but what if they *understood* perfectly well, but were nevertheless unable to prevent themselves from acting wrongfully? What, in other words, if they were compelled? Irresistible impulse tests recognize this class of excuse. If the agent was compelled, say by kleptomania, to steal, they do not exhibit any ill will.

Morse (2004, 2006) argues that *abnormal* causes are not *excusing* causes. He is surely right that we can't infer that an abnormal cause excuses *just because* it is abnormal. But he is mistaken in thinking that no abnormal cause *could* be excusing. That depends upon the details of the cause. Morse seems to believe that the sciences of the mind cannot provide us with this kind of information; they can tell us whether or not the causes of an agent's behavior are normal or abnormal, but nothing beyond that. However, there's every reason to believe that neuroscience can provide us with detailed knowledge that bears, precisely, on the cognitive and volitional arms of tests for moral responsibility. We can acquire new knowledge, from neuroscience and allied fields, about whether agents understand (in the relevant fashion) what they are doing when they perform a morally wrongful action, and about whether they possess relevant control over what they do. Neuroscience can therefore expand our knowledge of when the excusing conditions apply.

NEUROSCIENCE AND THE COGNITIVE TEST

Most morally relevant defects of reason are not hard to detect. Those people most frequently acquitted of serious wrongdoing on the grounds that they fail the cognitive test suffer from florid psychosis and are quite obviously deluded. Recently, however, we have acquired the ability to detect more subtle ignorance.

From a very young age, normal children distinguish two categories of wrongdoing: *moral* and *conventional* transgressions (Turiel 1977, 1983; Nucci 1989; Smetana and Braeges 1990). Conventional transgressions are *authority* or *rule* dependent; moral transgressions are not. Children distinguish them in the following way: asked whether the transgression would still be wrong if a relevant authority permitted it, they answer "no" with regard to conventional transgressions, but "yes" with regard to moral transgressions. For instance, asked whether it would be wrong for a boy to wear a dress to school, children typically say "yes." But asked whether it would still be wrong if the teacher said it was alright, they say that it would be okay. They therefore implicitly categorize it as a conventional transgression. On the other hand, they remain adamant that, say, hair pulling is wrong, no matter what the teacher says about it. They categorize it is as a moral transgression, where moral transgressions are not authority or rule-dependent. Children are typically capable of categorizing transgressions in this manner by around thirty-six months of age.

Turiel and his coworkers (Turiel 1983; Turiel *et al.* 1987) argue plausibly that the difference between moral and conventional transgressions, the difference that children detect and which allows them to categorize them reliably, lies in the fact that the former alone are intrinsically harmful. Hitting someone or pulling their hair is painful, no matter what anyone says about it. But a boy wearing a dress harms nobody, or at least isn't *intrinsically* harmful (many people find conventional transgressions distressing, but their distress depends upon their viewing the act as wrongful, rather than the other way round). Children not only recognize that moral transgressions are different to conventional transgressions; they also recognize that they are less permissible: it is generally more wrong to violate a moral prohibition than a conventional prohibition.

In acquiring the ability reliably to distinguish between moral and conventional transgressions, children acquire *moral knowledge.*

If they lacked such knowledge, there would be a prima facie case for excusing them from responsibility for transgressions, or at least mitigating the blame they are due. Recent research indicates that one class of habitual wrongdoer does lack this knowledge: psychopaths.

The term "psychopathy" is usually applied to individuals who engage in antisocial, often seriously immoral, actions without any apparent sense of guilt, shame or remorse, or any sign of empathy for their victims. Psychopaths exhibit no obvious sign of mental impairment and may be above average in intelligence. They are stereotypically superficially charming, and use their charm to manipulate others. Psychopaths are believed to be responsible for over fifty percent of violent crimes, and a very large percentage of petty thefts, frauds and other relatively minor crimes (Reznek 1997: 136–40). Many psychopaths have long records of convictions for offences followed by short prison sentences and, often, stays at psychiatric institutions. But their deviant behavior is unresponsive to either punishment or psychiatric treatment.

Those who come into contact with psychopaths, laypeople and the psychiatric profession alike, usually regard them as bad, not mad. They seem perfectly in control of their actions; they do what they want to because they want to. They do not suffer from delusions; though they are habitual liars, they can distinguish between reality and their own fabrications. They know all too well how to manipulate people, how to feign contrition, how best to turn situations to their own advantage. In the absence of any clear sign of the traditional excusing conditions – ignorance, either of the nature of one's actions, or of the fact that they are wrong, and compulsion – juries typically hold them responsible for their crimes. Even psychiatrists generally hold them to be less deserving than other patients (Bavidge and Cole 1995).

In fact, however, psychopaths suffer from a deficit which should excuse them from (full) responsibility for their actions. Blair (1995, 1997) found that psychopaths, unlike children and control groups of convicted criminals, were unable reliably to distinguish between moral and conventional transgressions. They know the *rules* well enough: they know that (say) punching other people is prohibited. But when they are asked why this kind of action is wrong, they give explanations which refer only to the rules, unlike children and adult controls, who cite harm to others in justification of moral prohibitions.

Why do psychopaths lack the ability to distinguish moral from conventional transgressions? In recent work, Blair and colleagues (2005) suggest that the psychopath's difficulties can be traced back to problems with the amygdala. The amygdala is a central part of the emotional brain; the psychopath's amygdala dysfunction causes him or her (usually him) to have impaired representations of emotions. This leads to an impaired ability to recognize fearful and sad expressions in others; more crucially it interferes with the ability to categorize harms in terms of their effects on the emotional states of others. Hence the psychopath's inability to categorize transgressions into moral and conventional categories.

But should the psychopath's inability to categorize moral harms alter their degree of moral responsibility? Psychopaths apparently take harms to others to be wrong *only because* such harms are against the rules. For them, stealing from, or hurting, another is no more wrong than, say, double-parking or queue-jumping. But we distinguish these kinds of merely conventional harms from moral harms, and this distinction is reflected in the kind and amount of punishment we feel is appropriate for the two kinds of harms. Fines and other (relatively) minor penalties are the appropriate response to violations of conventional rules, because this kind of wrongdoing is relatively minor, and does not reflect very badly on the person who engages in it. Much more serious penalties like imprisonment are properly reserved only for serious offences, and only moral transgressions are sufficiently serious. For the psychopath, however, all offences are merely conventional, and therefore – from their point of view – none of them are all that serious. They just cannot see any reason why we should be more worked up about the one than the other; indeed, they don't even know

which is which. But since they don't grasp the justification for categorizing something as a moral transgression – that it causes a harm to
others – they don't express the same degree of ill will in committing a
moral offence as a normal individual would. For that reason, the
degree of responsibility is smaller, arguably much smaller, than it
would be for a comparable harm committed by you or me.

If all we knew about psychopaths was that their brains are
somewhat different from ours, then Morse would be right: this
knowledge would not be morally relevant. But we know (roughly)
how their brains differ from ours, and (again, roughly) how these
differences affect their ability to judge the wrongness of actions. We
know that psychopaths lack knowledge that is relevant to moral
judgment and action. Given our knowledge, it would be wrong –
morally wrong – to blame them in exactly the same way and to the
same degree as unimpaired offenders.

NEUROSCIENCE AND THE VOLITIONAL TEST
Neuroscience (and, once again, allied fields) is also shedding a
great deal of light on agents' abilities to control their behavior. This
research reveals that control varies from person to person in systematic ways: some people, through no fault of their own, have a much
harder time controlling their impulses and emotions than others.
But if that's the case, then there are good grounds for thinking that
they are somewhat less blameworthy for losing control (other things
being equal) than agents who can control themselves more easily.

Some psychiatric conditions are classified as impulse-control
disorders. These disorders may make self-control more difficult in
ways that are illuminated by the ego-depletion hypothesis. Disorders
on the impulsive-compulsive spectrum typically involve the experience of a strong impulse to perform an action, often an action which
is ego-dystonic. Sufferers inhibit this impulse for a greater or lesser
period of time before giving in and performing the act (Skodol and
Oldham 1996). How should we assess their responsibility for their
actions? Let's consider a concrete case: Tourette Syndrome (TS).

TS is characterized by frequent tics, motor and phonic. Simple tics (eye twitching, throat clearing, and so on) may be completely involuntary – indeed, young children with simple tics are sometimes unaware of them (Leckman et al. 1999). But more complex tics are preceded by an urge, which may be described as mental, physical or both. This urge is persistent and continuous; it can be resisted but eventually sufferers succumb. When they give in to the urge, however, they report that the resulting tic is experienced as wholly or partially voluntary (Leckman et al. 1999). Moreover, complex tics look like actions, and are sometimes perversely appropriate to the situation – chosen, or so it seems, for maximum offense. Thus, the sufferer may shout "fatso" only at or in the presence of an overweight person (King et al. 1999). Because their actions feel voluntary, TS sufferers sometimes blame themselves for them (Leckman et al. 1999). However, as most people recognize, it would be morally perverse for others to blame them (other things being equal). Why?

The most natural explanation, I suggest, is that though the act feels voluntary to the sufferer, we recognize that the difficulty he or she has inhibiting it significantly mitigates or even entirely removes their blameworthiness. Continuous and persisting urges eventually overwhelm agents' resources for self-control: that's the lesson of ego-depletion. Self-control is a limited resource, and when it's gone the urge is irresistible. Exactly how the urge finally overcomes the resources of self-control is, as yet, an open question. Noakes et al. (2004) argue that the closely analogous phenomenon of giving in to muscular fatigue occurs when the agent experiences themselves as literally unable to continue. In fact, they claim, the perception is not veridical, but is created by brain mechanisms designed to conserve energy for emergencies. On this interesting view, volitional failure might be very like, perhaps even a species of, cognitive failure: the agent fails to hold out against fatigue because they believe themselves to be unable to succeed. On the other hand, there are reasons to doubt that an analogous mechanism is at work in ego-depletion: the phenomenology of giving in to an urge to perform a tic or to give up at a task requiring self-control seems to be quite different, inasmuch as it is typically experienced as voluntary. One possibility is that these cases should be understood in the model of coercion, with the costs of resistance (in terms of adversive experience) mounting steadily until the agent gives in.

How great are the costs of resistance? We get a clear sense of their size by considering the kinds of incentives which TS sufferers find insufficient to motivate resistance. One sufferer, for instance, would bang his head against surfaces, push his fingers up his nose till blood gushed out and hit his own face, sometimes breaking his nose (Cohen and Leckman 1999). Other patients report resigning from jobs, or contemplating moving away, in order to remove themselves from situations in which they experience impulses to inflict violence on themselves or others (Leckman *et al.* 1999). The amount of pain and suffering that TS sufferers will inflict on themselves, in order to satisfy the urge to perform the tic, suggests that resistance is highly aversive. Given this evidence, the case for assimilating the loss of control characteristic of TS to cases of coercion, and excusing or mitigating responsibility accordingly, is strong. Of course, this does not give TS sufferers a blanket excuse for *all* kinds of wrong-doing: just as in more ordinary cases of coercion, we sometimes expect people to put up with threats or pain rather than perform very seriously immoral actions. King *et al.* (1999) report the case of a man who stopped visiting his pregnant sister because he experienced the urge to kick her in the stomach. We rightly expect him to resist this urge, even at great cost to himself, and to remove himself from the situation if that is the only way to prevent his self-control resources from being overwhelmed.

It is likely that other volitional disorders on the impulsive-compulsive spectrum excuse or reduce responsibility in the same kind of way. TS has a high degree of comorbidity with other disorders on this spectrum (Skodol and Oldham 1996), all of which appear to involve similar neural mechanisms (Schultz *et al.* 1999). It is natural to suppose that the impulses characteristic of these disorders are ego-depleting in the same way as Tourettic urges. If this explanation of the mechanisms at work in these disorders is correct, then they overwhelm self-control – and therefore excuse – in *precisely the same way* as ordinary desires that are equally persistent and continuous. All of us, if we are unable to redirect attention from the stimulus, or withdraw from proximity with it, would experience the same loss of control. What is distinctive about TS, in this hypothesis, is the abnormal source and content of the urge; the path from urge to performance is itself normal.

Other disorders may work, not by giving subjects an abnormal urge, but by reducing their ability to resist normal urges. Utilization behavior may be one such disorder: there is evidence that the urge upon which sufferers act is experienced by all of us, in response to the affordances offered by objects (Archibald *et al.* 2001). In the normal case, the urge is inhibited by frontal systems that prevent it even from reaching consciousness, but in utilization behavior these systems are damaged or bypassed. Other disorders may weaken inhibition or control systems, leaving subjects perfectly capable of resisting ordinary urges, but at the mercy of stronger impulses. People who are subjected to environmental stressors early in life may have elements of their neuroendocrine system permanently altered, resulting in a heightened response to subsequent stressors including threats. The baseline for activation of their threat system is effectively lowered (Blair *et al.* 2005). Once again, it is not clear how this translates into loss of control though a likely hypothesis is that the response is automatic.

We could multiply examples of neurological abnormalities which reduce self-control, make it more difficult to achieve, or which result in behavior which apparently bypasses the mechanisms of control altogether. All of these impairments are relevant to assessments of agents' responsibility, not because the causes of the action are abnormal, but because the usual excusing conditions, enshrined in law and commonsense, apply to these cases. When agents find self-control difficult, through no fault of their own, we typically reduce the amount of blame due to them (though of course we may require them to take steps to improve their self-control or to avoid situations which predictably will challenge it). As we acquire more knowledge, from neuroscience and allied fields, we may learn that other conditions also reduce responsibility by making self-control more difficult. There is every reason for law and social policy to embrace this growing knowledge.[10]

End notes

1. Throughout this chapter, I make the following, common, assumption: free will is a property of actions that is a necessary, though not a sufficient, condition of moral responsibility (in addition to freedom, there are epistemic conditions upon moral responsibility, conditions I have explored in detail in other work). In other words, if an agent does not act freely, he or she cannot be responsible for their action, no matter what else is true of them.

2. Of course, that's not the end of the matter. There are some ingenious theories about how quantum level indeterminacy could enhance free will. Kane (1996) suggests that indecision might disrupt the thermodynamic equilibrium in the brain, thereby amplifying the indeterminacy from the sub-atomic level to the level of neurons, and making it truly undetermined how I shall act. Note, however, that even on Kane's account we are responsible for our actions *because we satisfy compatibilist conditions*: we do what we truly want to do. I develop this line of argument in Levy (forthcoming).

3. Note that Libet himself does not believe that his work shows that we lack free will or moral responsibility. He holds that though we do not consciously *initiate* our actions – and therefore do not exercise free will in initiating them – we do possess the power consciously to *veto* actions. Hence we remain responsible for our actions, inasmuch as we failed to veto them. However, the claim that we possess such a veto power is incredible: if an unconscious readiness potential must precede the initiation of an action, it seems that it must also precede the vetoing of an action (Clark 1999). When Libet's subjects reported that they had vetoed an action, they exhibited a distinctive readiness potential; I suggest

that we identify the initiation-and-veto with this readiness potential, rather than postulate an independent and neurologically implausible veto power which does not require causal antecedents.

4. More precisely, Parks was probably only minimally conscious of what he was doing. It may be appropriate to attribute a degree of consciousness to an agent in a state of automatism, insofar as they remain capable of responding to features of the environment. In what follows, I set this complication aside.

5. Here and in what follows, I use the term "reason" very broadly. A consideration is a reason in favor of a decision when it inclines the agent toward taking that decision. Thus, the fact that eating the slice of cake would be enjoyable is a reason in favor of deciding to eat it, even if the agent regards eating the cake as all-things-considered undesirable. In this sense, reasons are not necessarily rational.

6. The claim that arbitrariness is incompatible with freedom-level control has a long history in the free will debate; some version of it is accepted on all sides (libertarians are often willing to countenance a higher degree of arbitrariness than compatibilists). It underlies the demand for contrastive explanations, first pressed by C.D. Broad (1952), but now widely demanded of an adequate account of free will. Its most recent expression is in the form of the so-called luck objection to event-causal libertarianism, such as the account defended by Kane (1996). Representative versions of this objection include Mele (1999), Strawson (2000) and Haji (2002).

7. Mightn't a libertarian happily embrace this conclusion? Since libertarians demand that our decision-making processes be indeterministic, in order that agents possess genuine alternative possibilities (holding the past and the laws of nature fixed), it seems open to them to accept the claim that the intervention of consciousness in decision-making is arbitrary (they would prefer to say indeterministic), insisting that it is precisely *because* the process has this feature that we are free and responsible agents. Two points in response: first, this is a conclusion that can be accepted only by libertarians, and only some among them (those who are willing to concede that indeterminism reduces, at least in some ways, our freedom-level control over our actions). Second, though the proffered account indeed succeeds in finding a role for consciousness in responsible action, it is not *qua* consciousness that it performs this role. If

consciousness is necessary for responsible action only because consciousness makes the decision-making process indeterministic, then this is a role that could equally be played by an indeterministic subpersonal mechanism. To that extent, the account fails to accord with our intuition that there is something about consciousness *itself* that makes it necessary for responsible action.

8. A higher-order thought (HOT) account of consciousness constitutes an exception to this consensus. On such an account, global availability of states does not require phenomenal consciousness. However, phenomenal consciousness is nevertheless correlated with global availability, even on such accounts. Whether or not a HOT account of consciousness is correct, it is likely that global availability can dissociate from phenomenal consciousness; see further below.

9. This account of how automatism excuses owes a great deal to Schopp (1991). A caveat is in order: phenomenal-consciousness is unlikely to be a sufficient condition of access-consciousness; indeed, it may not be a necessary condition. If zombies are indeed possible, it is (by hypothesis) possible that access-consciousness can exist without phenomenality. Perhaps phenomenal-consciousness is a necessary condition of access-condition in ordinary human beings. In any case, it is clear that even for us as we are currently constituted, it is not a sufficient condition. There are a number of conditions, from pathological states to ordinary dreaming, in which there seems to be phenomenality without global access (if our beliefs were on line when we dreamt, our dreams would not have the bizarre, logic-defying, content that is characteristic of them). Nevertheless, if – as I claim – phenomenal-consciousness is highly correlated with access-consciousness, and access-consciousness is a necessary condition of moral responsibility, the absence of phenomenal consciousness is a reliable indicator that the action is not deeply reflective of the agent, and therefore that they are not responsible for it.

10. It may be that these conclusions, that psychopaths, sufferers from impulse-control disorders and some other classes of agent, ought to have their degree of moral responsibility significantly reduced in some circumstances, are routinely resisted because it is believed that these people represent a high risk of reoffending. The conclusion may be easier to accept when we recognize that excusing someone of moral responsibility for an action does not commit us to leaving them free to

reoffend. Just as we may rightly sequester or even incarcerate people with infectious diseases, we may rightly sequester or otherwise limit the movements of the dangerous. We may not *punish* them, but that fact only constrains how we may treat them; it does not commit us to setting them free.

8   Self-deception: the normal and the pathological

In the previous chapters, I have argued that neuroscience (and allied fields) can shed light on some of the perennial questions of moral theory and moral psychology: the nature of self-control and the degree to which agents should be held responsible for their actions. In this chapter, I explore another puzzle in moral psychology: the nature and existence of self-deception.

Self-deception is a topic of perennial fascination to novelists and everyone else interested in human psychology. It is fascinating because it is at once puzzling and commonplace. The puzzle it poses arises when we observe people apparently sincerely making claims that seem obviously false, and against which they apparently possess sufficient evidence. The man whose wife suddenly has many mysterious meetings, starts to receive unexplained gifts and is reportedly seen in a bar on the other side of town with a strange man has every reason to suspect her of infidelity. If he refrains from asking her questions, or is satisfied with the flimsiest of explanations, and fails to doubt her continued faithfulness, he is self-deceived. Self-deception is, apparently, common in the interpersonal sphere, but it is also a political phenomenon. Western supporters of Soviet communism were often, and perhaps rightly, accused of self-deception, when they denied the repression characteristic of the regime.

We say that someone is self-deceived, typically, when they possess sufficient evidence for a claim and yet continue, apparently sincerely, to assert the opposite. Generally, self-deception seems to be emotionally motivated: we do not deceive ourselves about just anything, but only about things that are important to us and which we are strongly motivated to believe. The man who deceives himself about his wife's faithfulness might not be able to contemplate a single life; the woman who deceives herself about Soviet communism may have her narrative identity closely entwined with her political allegiances.

THEORIES OF SELF-DECEPTION

We often say that the self-deceived person really or "at some level" knows the truth. The formerly self-deceived themselves sometimes make this kind of claim, saying they "really knew all along" the truth concerning which they deceived themselves. Many theories of self-deception take this apparent duality of belief at face value, and therefore devote themselves to explaining how ordinary, sane, individuals are capable of contradictory beliefs. There is no puzzle, everyone acknowledges, with believing things that are mutually contradictory, when the conflict between them is not obvious. All of us probably have inconsistent beliefs in this sense: if we thought about each of our beliefs for long enough, and traced their entailments far enough, we could eventually locate a clash. But the self-deceived agent apparently believes two contradictory statements under the same description (or at least very similar descriptions). The husband in our example might believe both that *my wife is faithful* and *my wife is having an affair*, which is a bald contradiction, or perhaps, slightly less baldly, *my wife is faithful* and *all the evidence suggests my wife is having an affair*.

Some philosophers think that not only do the self-deceived believe inconsistent propositions, they are self-deceived because they have *deliberately* brought about their believing contradictory propositions. The best example here is the existential philosopher Jean-Paul Sartre. Sartre (1956) argued that self-deceivers *have to* know the truth, in order to set about concealing it from themselves. Just as a liar must know the truth in order to deliberately and effectively deceive others, so the self-deceiver "must know the truth very exactly *in order* to conceal it more carefully" (Sartre 1956: 89). Other thinkers who, like Sartre, take contradictory beliefs to be character-istic of self-deception also model it on interpersonal deception. Both kinds of lying – to others and to oneself – are supposed to be intentional activities. On what we might call the traditional conception of self-deception – defended by thinkers as diverse, and as separated from one another in time, as Bishop Joseph Butler (1970) in the eighteenth century, to Donald Davidson (1986) in the late twentieth century – self-deception is typically characterized by both these features: contradictory beliefs and intentionality of deception.

The contradictory belief requirement and the intentionality requirement are both extremely puzzling. How is it possible for someone to believe two blatantly contradictory propositions at one and the same time? How can anyone succeed in lying to him or herself; doesn't successful deception require that the deceived agent not know the truth? Defenders of the traditional conception of self-deception do not, of course, think that we succeed in lying to ourselves in precisely the same manner in which we might lie to another. Instead, they take self-deception to be an activity engaged in with some kind of reduced awareness. Moreover, they do not assert that the self-deceived believe their claims in precisely the same way that we generally believe our normal beliefs. Instead, they typically hold that the contradictory beliefs are somehow isolated from one another. Perhaps, for instance, one of the beliefs is held unconsciously. If the husband's belief that his wife is having an affair is unconsciously held, we may be able to explain how he is able to sincerely proclaim her faithfulness. We might also be able to explain the rationalizations in which he engages to sustain this belief: they are motivated, we might think, by mechanisms that are designed to defend consciousness against the unconscious belief.

More recently, however, philosophers have begun to advance *deflationary* accounts of self-deception. These philosophers point out that the traditional conception is quite demanding: it requires the existence of a great deal of mental machinery. It can be correct only if the mind is capable of being partitioned, in some way, so that contradictory beliefs are isolated from one another; moreover, typical traditional accounts also require that *both* beliefs, the consciously avowed and the consciously disavowed, are capable of motivating behavior (the behavior of engaging in rationalization, for instance). Given that the traditional conception is demanding, we ought to prefer a less demanding theory if there is one available that explains the data at least as well. These philosophers thus invoke Occam's razor, the methodological principle that the simplest theory that explains the data is the theory most likely to be true, in defence of a deflationary account.

Deflationary accounts of self-deception have been advanced by several philosophers (Barnes 1997; Mele 1997, Mele 2001). These accounts are deflationary inasmuch as they attempt to explain self-deception without postulating any of the extravagant mental machinery required by the traditional conception. They dispense with the extra machinery by dispensing with the requirements that necessitate it, both the intentionality requirement and the contradictory belief requirement. By dispensing with these requirements, deflationary accounts avoid the puzzles they provoke: we need not explain how agents can successfully lie to themselves, or how they can have blatantly contradictory beliefs. Of course, we still need to be able to explain the behavior of those we are disposed to call self-deceived. How are we to do that?

Deflationists argue, roughly, that the kinds of states we call self-deception can be explained in terms of motivationally biased belief acquisition mechanisms. We can therefore explain self-deception invoking only mechanisms whose existence has been independently documented by psychologists, particularly psychologists in the heuristics and biases tradition (Kahneman *et al.* 1982). Heuristics and biases typically work by systematically leading us to weigh some kinds of evidence more heavily than other kinds, in ways that might be adaptive in general, but which can sometimes mislead us badly. Thus, people typically give excessive weight to evidence that happens to be vivid for them, will tend to look for evidence in favour of a hypothesis rather than evidence which disconfirms it, are more impressed by their more recent experiences than earlier experiences, and so on. Deflationists argue, and cite experimental evidence to show, that these biases can be activated especially strongly when the person is appropriately motivated. Thus, when someone has reason to prefer that a proposition is true, the stage is set for the activation of these biasing mechanisms. For instance, the anxious coward will test the hypothesis that they are brave, and therefore look for confirming evidence of that hypothesis (setting in motion the confirmation bias); as a result evidence which supports this hypothesis will be rendered especially vivid for them, while evidence against it will be relatively pallid.

If this is correct, then self-deception is not intentional: it is the product of biased reasoning, but there is no reason to think the agent is always aware of their bias (neither in general, nor of the way it works in particular cases). Nor is there any reason to think that the agent must have contradictory beliefs. Because the agent is motivationally biased, they acquire a belief despite the fact that the evidence available to them supports the contrary belief: they cannot see how the evidence tends precisely *because* of their bias.

Deflationists claim that their less extravagant theory explains self-deception at least as well as the traditional conception. We have, they argue, no need to invoke elaborate mental machinery, because there is no reason to believe that the intentionality or contradictory belief requirements are ever satisfied. Mele (2001), the most influential of the deflationists, argues that his theory, or something like it, is therefore to be preferred unless and until someone can produce an actual case of self-deception in which the agent has contradictory beliefs, or in which they have intentionally deceived themselves.[1] In what follows, I shall attempt to meet Mele's challenge: I shall show that there are cases of self-deception in which the self-deceived person has contradictory beliefs. The evidence comes from the study of delusions.

ANOSOGNOSIA AND SELF-DECEPTION

Anosognosia refers to denial of illness by sufferers. It comes in many forms, including denial of cortical (i.e., caused by brain lesion) deafness, of cortical blindness (Anton's syndrome) or of dyslexia (Bisiach *et al.* 1986). Here I shall focus on anosognosia for hemiplegia: denial of partial paralysis (hereafter "anosognosia" shall refer only to this form of the syndrome). As a result of a stroke or brain injury, sufferers experience greater or lesser paralysis of one side of their body (usually the left side), especially the hand and arm. However, they continue to insist that their arm is fine. Anosognosia is usually accompanied by unilateral neglect: a failure to attend, respond or orient to information on one side (again usually the left side) of the patient, often including that side of the patient's own body (personal neglect). Anosognosia and neglect usually resolves over a period of a few days or weeks. However, both have been known to persist for years.

It is worth recounting some clinical descriptions of anosognosia, in order to give a flavor of this puzzling condition. Asked to move their left arm or hand, patients frequently refuse, on grounds which seem transparent rationalizations: I have arthritis and it hurts to move my arm (Ramachandran 1996); the doctor told me I should rest it (Venneri and Shanks 2004); I'm tired, or I'm not accustomed to taking orders (Ramachandran and Blakeslee 1998); left hands are always weaker (Bisiach *et al.* 1986). Sometimes, the patients go so far as to claim that they have complied with the request: I *am* pointing; I can clearly see my arm or I *am* clapping (Ramachandran 1996); all the while their paralyzed arm remains at their side.

It is tempting to see anosognosia as an extreme case of self-deception. It looks for all the world as if the excuses given by patients for failing to move their arms are rationalizations, designed to protect them from an extremely painful truth: that they are partially paralyzed. However, most neurologists deny that anosognosia should be understood along these lines. They point out that it has some features which seem puzzling on the psychological defence view.

In particular, a motivational explanation of anosognosia fails to explain its asymmetry: it is rare that a patient denies paralysis on the right side of the body. Anosognosia is usually the product of right hemisphere damage (most commonly damage to the inferior parietal cortex) that causes denial of paralysis on the left (contralateral to the lesion) side of the body. Most neurologists therefore argue that it must be understood as a neurological, and not a psychological, phenomenon (Bisiach and Geminiani 1991).

Clearly, they have an important point: any account of anosognosia must explain the observed asymmetry. Anosognosia is indeed a neurological phenomenon, brought about as a result of brain injury. Most other kinds of paralysis or disease, whether caused by brain injury or not, do not give rise to it. However, it may still be the case that anosognosia is simultaneously a neurological *and* a psychological phenomenon. Perhaps, that is, neurological damage and motivation are jointly necessary conditions for the occurrence of anosognosia.

V.S. Ramachandran is one prominent neuroscientist who interprets anosognosia along these lines. Ramachandran (1996; Ramachandran and Blakeslee 1998) suggests that the observed asymmetry can be explained as a product of hemispherical specialization. The left hemisphere, he argues, has the task of imposing a coherent narrative framework upon the great mass of information with which each of us is constantly bombarded. If we are not to be paralyzed by doubt, we need a consistent and coherent set of beliefs that makes sense of most of the evidence available to us. In order to preserve the integrity of this belief system, the left hemisphere ignores or distorts small anomalies. Since any decision is usually better than being paralyzed by doubts, ignoring anomalies is generally adaptive. However, there is a risk that the agent will slip into fantasy if the left hemisphere is allowed to confabulate unchecked. The role of keeping the left hemisphere honest is delegated to the right hemisphere. It plays devil's advocate, monitoring anomalies, and forcing the more glaring to the agent's attention.

There is a great deal of independent support for Ramachandran's hemispherical specialization hypothesis. In particular, evidence from cerebral commissurotomy ("split-brain") patients is often understood as supporting this view. On the basis mainly of this evidence, Gazzaniga (1985; 1992) has suggested that the left hemisphere contains an "interpreter," a module which has the task of making sense of the agent's activities using whatever sources of information are available to it. When it is cut off from the source of the true motivation of the behavior, the left hemisphere confabulates an explanation. Many researchers have followed or adapted Gazzaniga's suggestion, because it seems to explain so many observed phenomena.

For our purposes, the hemispherical specialization hypothesis is attractive because it neatly explains the asymmetry characteristic of anosognosia. When the right hemisphere is damaged, the left hemisphere is free to confabulate unchecked. It defends the agent against unpleasant information by the simple expedient of ignoring it; it is able to pursue this strategy with much more dramatic effect than is normal because the anomaly detector in the right hemisphere is damaged. But when the right hemisphere is intact, denial of illness is much more difficult. On the other hand, when damage is to the *left* hemisphere, patients tend to be more pessimistic than when damage is to the right (Heilman et al. 1998). Ramachandran suggests that this pessimism is the product of the disabling of the protective left hemisphere confabulation mechanisms.

I do not aim to defend the details of Ramachandran's account of anosognosia here. However, I suggest that it is likely that the best account of the syndrome will, like Ramachandran's, explain it as simultaneously a neurological and a psychological phenomenon. Only a combination of neurological and psychological mechanisms can account for all the observed data. Non-motivational theories of anosognosia cannot do the job alone, as I shall now show.

Some theorists suggest that anosognosia is the product of an impairment which makes the disease difficult for the patient to detect (Levine *et al.*, 1991). A syndrome like neglect is, for its subject, relatively difficult to discern; absence of visual information is not phenomenally available in any immediate way. Somewhat similarly, anosognosia for hemiplegia may be difficult to detect, because the patient may have an impairment that reduces the amount and quality of relevant information about limb movement. There are several possible impairments that could play the explanatory role here. Patients may experience proprioceptive deficits, they may experience an impairment in feedback mechanisms reporting limb movement (Levine *et al.* 1991), or they may experience impairments in "feedforward" mechanisms, which compare limb movements to an internally generated model predicting the movement (Heilman *et al.* 1998).

These somatosensory explanations of anosognosia face a common problem: the mechanisms they propose seem far too weak to explain the phenomenon. Suppose it is true that anosognosics lack one source of normally reliable information about their limbs, or even that they take themselves to continue to receive information that their limb is working normally via a usually reliable channel; why do they nevertheless override all the information they receive from other reliable sources, ranging from doctors and close relatives to their own eyes? After all, as Marcel *et al.* (2004) point out, the impairments produced by hemiplegia are not subtle: it is not just that patients fail to move their arms when they want to. They also fail to lift objects, to get out of bed, to walk. It is extremely difficult to see how lack of feedback, or some other somatosensory deficit, could explain the failure of the patient to detect these gross abnormalities.

More promising, at first sight, are theories that explain difficulty of discovery as the product not of somatosensory deficits, but of cognitive or psychological problems. On these views, anosognosia might be the product of confusion, (another) delusion or of neglect itself. In fact, however, these explanations do not suffice. It is true that some patients are highly delusional (Venneri and Shanks 2004) and anosognosics exhibit greater cognitive dysfunction, on average, than other stroke victims (Jehkonen *et al.* 2000). However, the degree of confusion is rarely sufficient to explain the anosognosia, and some patients exhibit no confusion at all (Jehkonen *et al.* 2000). Nor does anosognosia always co-occur with other delusions. Neglect accounts fare no better. Cocchini *et al.* (2002) report the case of a young male with anosognosia, who became aware of his paralysis when his left limbs were moved into the right half of his visual field. However, not all patients with neglect also suffer from anosognosia, indicating that neglect is not a sufficient condition for the latter; moreover, not all anosognosics suffer from neglect, indicating that it is not a necessary condition (Bisiach *et al.* 1986; Jehkonen *et al.* 2000).

Neither somatosensory impairment nor cognitive impairment is by itself sufficient to explain anosognosia. Might they nevertheless be *jointly* necessary? This seems to be the view of Davies *et al.* (2005). They advance a "generic" two-factor theory to explain anosognosia, where the first factor is an unspecified neuropsychological anomaly, and the second factor is some kind of cognitive impairment. It is difficult to assess this proposal, since it is more a programmatic statement setting out directions for future research then a serious attempt at an adequate explanation; it is therefore deliberately left empirically underspecified. However, to the extent to which the account is assessable, there are good reasons to think that it is unpromising, at least as it currently stands.

One reason Davies *et al.* refuse to pin their account to any particular first factor is that they are well aware that the impairments of sufferers differ from case to case. As we have already seen, a range of impairments could play a role in the aetiology of anosognosia, since many different impairments could make the degree of difficulty of discovery greater. We also saw, however, that these impairments on their own are rarely or never sufficient to explain anosognosia. The second factor therefore needs to carry a great deal of explanatory weight. And Davies *et al.* are a little more forthcoming on the second factor than on the first. They suggest that it is likely to be a memory deficit.

Though anosognosics often do have memory problems, previous studies have claimed to demonstrate a double dissociation between memory impairment and anosognosia (Berti *et al.* 1996). Davies *et al.* argue that these studies overlooked some very subtle memory impairments: examining nine patients with persisting unilateral neglect they revealed a range of memory impairments, some subtle. Despite previous negative findings, Davies *et al.* therefore believe that memory impairments might explain anosognosia, when such impairments are paired with a neuropsychological anomaly which makes discovery of hemiplegia more difficult.

There are, I suggest, several problems with the suggested model of anosognosia. First, if the memory deficits Davies *et al.* point to are to do the work of explaining the delusion, they ought to be relatively severe. A subtle deficit cannot explain how sufferers manage to overlook glaring anomalies in action and control. But it is surely subtle deficits that must be in question, if Davies *et al.* are right in claiming that previous studies that explicitly examined memory overlooked the deficits in question. Second, even in their own small study, degree of memory impairment was not predictive of presence nor degree of anosognosia. Finally, it is difficult to see how memory impairments explain the *concurrent* failures of anosognosics; how, for instance, does a memory impairment explain a patient's claim that they are *currently* clapping and can hear the sound?

These considerations do not demonstrate that a two-factor model cannot succeed. Davies *et al.* have not committed themselves to any first or second factors, and it may be that an alternative second factor will succeed where memory impairment has failed. Indeed, I suspect that a two- or possibly a three-factor model will eventually succeed in explaining anosognosia. However, I suggest we need to look to motivational factors, as a second or a third factor in explaining the syndrome. Anosognosia is *motivated* denial of illness; in other words, anosognosics are self-deceived.

If anosognosics meet the following three conditions, I suggest, then anosognosia is a kind of self-deception:

(1) Subjects believe that their limb is healthy.

(2) Nevertheless they also have the simultaneous belief (or strong suspicion) that their limb is significantly impaired and they are profoundly disturbed by this belief (suspicion).

(3) Condition (1) is satisfied *because* condition (2) is satisfied; that is, subjects are motivated to form or retain the belief that their limb is healthy because they have the concurrent belief (suspicion) that it is significantly impaired and they are disturbed by this belief (suspicion).

The conjunction of conditions (1) and (3) yields contradictory belief if anosognosia is self-deception, and anosognosics satisfy these conditions then there are cases of self-deception in which agents have contradictory beliefs. Condition (3) is not, however, meant as an intentionality requirement. Intentionality is *consistent* with (3): if agents intentionally self-deceive because they satisfy (2), then (3) is satisfied. But it is also satisfied if (2) primes mechanisms that bias the agent into self-deception. To that extent, satisfaction of all three conditions does not entirely rehabilitate the traditional conception of self-deception. Nevertheless, it comes close, inasmuch as it requires contradictory beliefs of the self-deceived. Finally, these are not intended as necessary conditions for self-deception. Nevertheless, they are plausibly taken to be sufficient conditions. I shall consider them in turn.

Do patients sincerely believe that their limb is healthy? Ramachandran and Blakeslee (1998) set out to test this belief. First, Ramachandran asked anosognosics, as well as non-anosognosic hemiplegic controls, to lift a tray upon which were placed six plastic glasses each half full of water. Non-anosognosics raised it by placing their good hand under the middle of the tray and lifting. But anosognosics attempted to lift it by placing their right hand on the right side of the tray and lifting, despite the fact that the left side remained unsupported. Of course, the glasses immediately fell to the ground.

In a second series of experiments, Ramachandran (1996) offered anosognosics and a control group of non-anosognosic hemiplegics the choice between two tasks, one of which required one hand while the other required both. The patient was told that they would receive a small reward ($2, a small box of chocolates, and so forth) for successful completion of the unimanual task or a larger reward for successful completion of the bimanual ($5, a larger box of chocolates, and so forth). Non-anosognosics always chose the unimanual task. But almost all anosognosics chose the bimanual task. They spent minutes attempting to complete the task – trying to tie shoelaces, for example – without showing any sign of frustration. When offered the same choice ten minutes later, they chose the bimanual task once more. This experimental evidence, coupled with the patient's apparent unshakeable conviction, gives us sufficient evidence to impute to them the belief that their arm is fine. They are disposed to assent to the proposition, and to use it as a premise in reasoning, short and long-term (patients often speak of returning to old jobs or hobbies that require both hands). Now, what of proposition (2)? Given their confidence that their arm is fine, what evidence is there that they *also* believe that it is in fact paralyzed?

Hirstein (2000; 2005), the only philosopher who has so far considered the implications of anosognosia for theories of self-deception, argues that we ought to take anosognosics at their word: their belief that they are fine is sincere and whole-hearted. Hirstein (2000) suggests that the conflicting doxastic states characteristic of ordinary self-deception (as he understands it, in the traditional manner) are located in one hemisphere each (the confabulatory belief in the left hemisphere and the unwanted knowledge in the right); more recently, he has suggested that the beliefs are represented in different ways, so as to avoid direct conflict between them (Hirstein 2005). In one or other of these ways, ordinary self-deceivers satisfy the dual-belief requirement. However, Hirstein argues that anosognosics do not satisfy the dual-belief requirement, because the part of the right hemisphere which specializes in anomaly detection is out of action (Hirstein 2000), or because the checking processes which normally monitor beliefs are out of action (Hirstein 2005). Hence anosognosics are entirely sincere when they claim that their paralyzed limb is healthy: the knowledge that something is amiss is not available to them. If their brain can nevertheless be said to represent the damage to their limb, this representation is subpersonal and inaccessible to personal consciousness.

However, contra Hirstein, there is evidence that anosognosics do believe that something is very wrong with their paralyzed limb. There are several such pieces of evidence, none of which is indisputable on its own. Together, however, they build a compelling case.

Before turning to the evidence, let me say a few words about what conditions must be satisfied before we can attribute a belief or a belief-like state to an agent. Hirstein holds, plausibly enough, that it is not enough to show that an information state is somehow represented in the brain to show that the agent believes the corresponding proposition. In addition, the proposition must be available, personally (where "personally" is the antonym of "subpersonally") to the agent. But availability comes in degrees, ranging from entirely unavailable, to available only to encapsulated modules, available only in forced-choice situations, available for effortful recall, all the way through to pathologically over-available (as in intrusive thoughts). Just how available is available enough? It is far from obvious just what degree of availability to the agent is sufficient to attribute the corresponding belief to them. This is a deep issue, and one I cannot aim to resolve here. Suffice it to say that the higher the degree of availability, the better the case for attribution of the belief. We have seen that the proposition that their arm is fine is highly available to the agent: immediately available to consciousness in response to queries about their arm. The higher the degree of availability to them of the proposition that their arm is paralyzed, the better the case for attribution of doxastic conflict. In what follows, I shall adduce evidence for progressively greater degrees of availability.

First, there is overwhelming evidence that the fact of paralysis is represented in the brains of anosognosics. The evidence comes from some ingenious and surprising experiments. Strangely, anosognosics can be brought to acknowledge their paralysis by the simple expedient of pouring cold water in their left ear (Cappa *et al.* 1987)! This procedure, known as vestibular stimulation, is hypothesized to "arouse" the parts of the right hemisphere normally engaged in anomaly detection and attention to the left side of the patient's personal space. Now, the interesting discovery for our purposes is that not only does vestibular stimulation lead to a temporary remission of anosognosia, it also results in the patient acknowledging frankly that their arm has been paralyzed ever since the stroke! It is apparent that awareness of their injury had been registering somewhere in their brains all along.

Second, there is (indirect) evidence that the relevant proposition has (at least) the lowest degree of *personal* availability to the anosognosic. The lowest degree of personal availability is availability only in forced-choice situations. It is the degree of availability of visual information to blindsight patients (Weiskrantz 1986). Blindsight is a fascinating condition, caused by damage to the visual cortex. Depending upon the extent of the damage, sufferers lose part or all of their sight. They are blind, on every common measure. But blindsight patients are able, in some circumstances, to use visual information. They may, for instance, be able to post a card through a slot whose angle changes from trial to trial, or be able to point to objects. They experience themselves as guessing, but they guess at well above chance. The blindsight patient cannot use visual information from their blind field in their everyday life, but they are able to use it in experimentally induced forced-choice situations. Similarly, there is evidence that anosognsosics can access information they normally deny in forced-choice situations. The evidence comes from experiments upon neglect. Neglect patients are blind to extrapersonal space as well as to the left side of their own bodies. They may, for instance, locate the midpoint of a line drawn on a sheet of paper well to the right of the actual halfway mark, since they see only part of the line. Similarly, they may not consciously register the left side of a drawing. Marshall and Halligan (1988) showed neglect patients drawings of houses, placed so that the leftmost part of the houses fell in their neglected field. The patients reported that the houses looked identical. What they could not – consciously – see was that one house was in flames on its left side. However, when they were asked which house they would prefer to live in, they picked the other – non-burning – house. Even though the houses looked identical to them, they preferred one to the other.[2]

Third, there is observational evidence that the explicitly denied knowledge guides some of the behavior of anosognosics, including their verbal behavior, indicating that it has a degree of availability somewhat above that of visual information in blindsight. Ramachandran reports evidence of what he (following Freud) calls "reaction formation": the expression of a thought antithetical to the denied proposition, which betrays its motivated nature by its very vehemence. For instance, a patient who opted for the shoelace-tying task when offered the choice between a unimanual and a bimanual task later reported (falsely) that they had tied the laces "with both my hands" (Ramachandran and Blakeslee 1998: 139); another patient claimed that her paralyzed left arm was actually *stronger* than her right (1998: 150). Moreover, though anosognosics may be resolute in their denial of illness, nevertheless they generally do not spontaneously attempt tasks which require both arms (Bisiach and Geminiani 1991; Venneri and Shanks 2004). (Conversely, some patients who admit paralysis nevertheless regularly attempt bimanual tasks such as knitting.) Moreover, anosognosics sometimes "displace" disorders, complaining of ailments that affect their left side, but claiming that they are on the right (Bisiach and Geminiani 1991). This displacement sometimes even concerns the paralyzed limb.

Fourth, there is strong evidence that the denied knowledge is dispositionally available to anosognosics, if not easily accessible. It is not necessary to resort to vestibular stimulation to get anosognosics to acknowledge paralysis. As Ramachandran and Blakeslee (1998: 149) note, they can be gently prodded into eventually admitting that their left arm is weak, or even paralyzed. Taken together, this evidence seems to constitute a strong case for attributing to anosognosics the belief, or at least the strong suspicion, that their limb is significantly impaired. (It would be interesting to repeat Ramachandran's unimanual versus bimanual task experiment, this time with much higher – though still significantly differential – rewards for successful completion of both tasks, or even with punishments for failing at the tasks, in order to see whether the bimanual task is still selected. It may be that the selection of this task is itself confabulatory behaviour, engaged in when the costs of failure are low.)

In this context, it is important to note a significant difference in the way in which information is processed in blindsight, on the one hand, and in the implicit processing demonstrated in neglect, on the other. Blindsight is a visuomotor phenomenon: it is manifested in the visual guidance of action in the absence of conscious experience. Visuomotor control is accomplished by what has come to be known as dorsal-stream processing. But implicit processing is a *ventral stream* phenomenon: it is subserved by the system that also subserves conscious experience (Goodale and Milner 2004). Whereas dorsal-stream phenomena cannot become conscious (except indirectly; insofar as agents become aware of how their actions are guided by such phenomena), ventral-stream phenomena are often conscious. Perhaps this explains the greater degree of availability of visual information in the neglected field of anosognosics than in blindsight sufferers.

So far, we have focused on showing that the belief (suspicion) that their arm is paralyzed can be attributed to anosognosics. Satisfying condition (2) requires, in addition to this doxastic component, the demonstration that patients are disturbed by the belief (suspicion). Intuitively, of course, the suggestion that suspicion of paralysis is disturbing is overwhelmingly plausible. In addition, there is observational evidence on this score. Patients sometimes experience a "catastrophic reaction" – an uncontrollable anguished outburst – upon being prodded into admitting their paralysis (Ramachandran and Blakeslee 1998; Cocchini *et al.* 2002). Clearly, the knowledge is experienced as extremely threatening.

Now, what of condition (3)? Why think that denial of paralysis is motivated by strong suspicion or belief in it? I suggest that we are forced to postulate an affective motivation for anosognosia, given that none of the other theories are sufficient to explain it, alone or in combination. The confusion theory of anosognosia can account for only a subset of cases, since confusion is frequently insufficient to account for denial, and sometimes entirely missing. Cognitive ("cold") theories which hold that anosognosia is caused by the isolation of the left hemisphere from one or another source of information (visual information, feedback from attempting to move the limb or feedforward from failure to attempt movement) face a common problem: they must somehow account for the fact that other sources of reliable information (eyesight, the testimony of doctors and of close relatives, inability to complete tasks requiring both hands, and so on), do not compensate for the missing channel. Hirstein's (2000: S422) claim that the left hemisphere "is unable to receive information about the left side of the body and its nearby space" is simply false; though it is certainly true that this information is disrupted, most especially in neglect, in ways that are difficult to understand, it has not disappeared from the patient's awareness altogether (Sacks (1985) recounts a case of a woman who would swivel her chair to the right, until a portion of the left side of her dinner plate came into view; by repeating the procedure several times, she managed to finish most of her food. This patient deliberately engaged in this behavior, because she knew that there was more food on her plate than she could currently see).

It is equally true, however, that a motivational explanation of anosognosia is insufficient by itself. Anosognosia is, as neurologists have rightly insisted, a neurological condition, though it is not *only* a neurological condition. Non-motivational explanations cannot account for it, but neither can motivational explanations by themselves. Instead, it is produced by a combination of motivational and neurological conditions. Exactly how they work together is still somewhat mysterious. Let me briefly sketch two hypotheses. First, it may be that as a result of the neurological damage, the information that the arm is paralyzed is relatively inaccessible to the patient. It may be indistinct ("dim," as Anton put it in his seminal 1899 paper). Availability, as we have already seen, comes in degrees; the lower the degree of availability, the less glaring the anomaly and the greater the corresponding ease for the patient to deny her paralysis. In this hypothesis, damage to the anomaly detection machinery plays no (direct) role in anosognosia. In the second hypothesis, damage to this machinery plays a direct role: representations concerning the limb have their normal degree of availability, but the machinery which is supposed to bring them to personal attention is unable to play its role properly. Of course, these hypotheses are not exclusive: it may be that representation is somewhat indistinct *and* the anomaly detector is damaged; perhaps neither factor is sufficient for denial of such a glaring anomaly by itself. In both hypotheses, neurological and affective conditions combine to produce anosognosia: patients deny paralysis because the idea is profoundly disturbing to them, but they are capable of successful denial only because neurological damage has resulted in relatively inaccessible representations, or a weakened anomaly detector, or both.

ANOSOGNOSIA AS SELF-DECEPTION

For our purposes, what matters most here is simply the fact that sufferers from anosognosia are plausibly interpreted as experiencing some kind of doxastic conflict. Though they confidently assert that their limb is healthy, the belief that all is not well is sufficiently available to them for us to be able to attribute to them (at least) the strong suspicion that they are paralyzed.

Anosognosia thus seems to present us with a real-life – indeed, clinically verified – case in which agents sincerely assert one thing, while nevertheless giving clear indications that they strongly suspect that the precise opposite is the case; and in which their assertion seems to require (*inter alia*) a motivational explanation. The demonstration that there really are cases of this kind goes a long way toward rehabilitating the traditional conception of self-deception. One of the major attractions of a deflationary account, recall, was that it is more parsimonious than the traditional: it does not require any exotic mental mechanisms such as partitions in the mind or unconscious mental states. But the example of anosognosia shows that since there are cases of self-deception characterized by contradictory beliefs, the postulation of this extra mental machinery is motivated: we need it to explain the phenomenon.

A defender of a deflationary account of self-deception might argue that anosognosia is too extreme and unusual a condition for us to be able to draw any general lessons from it. After all, whereas self-deception is something to which normal agents are all too prone, anosognosia is a rare condition precipitated by lesions to the right hemisphere of the brain. Perhaps, therefore, it is explained by mechanisms radically different to those at work in common-or-garden self-deception. It is certainly *possible* that anosognosic (or otherwise pathological) self-deception is the only kind characterized by contradictory beliefs; perhaps this kind of self-deception requires a breakdown in normal brain processes. However, given what we know, and what we can plausibly speculate, about anosognosia, it is reasonable to suspect that the processes at work in anosognosia are also at work in less pathological cases. We suggested that self-deceptive anosognosia might arise in one (or both) of two ways: (1) as a result of the indistinctness or relative inaccessibility of a belief, or (2) as a result of the failure of the right hemisphere anomaly detector to flag a glaring inconsistency in the patient's explanation of events and actions. It is overwhelmingly likely that the brain lesion is part of the explanation for the occurrence of (1) or (2) in the case of anosognosics, but it is also likely that brain lesions are not a necessary condition of either. The representations of *normal* people, too, fall on a continuum of accessibility, from unavailable through to occurrently conscious; we have every reason to think that relative inaccessibility will characterize many non-pathological cases. On hypothesis (1) above, when that is the case, and the subject is appropriately motivated, self-deception may occur. It is also likely that normal anomaly detector strength varies from person to person, and across time. Probably anosognosics can deny such a glaring anomaly as their paralysis only because they have suffered neurological damage. But most cases of self-deception are nowhere near so spectacular. Non-pathological inaccessibility of representations, or weakness of anomaly detection, or both, are sufficient for non-pathological (ordinary) self-deception.

There is, therefore, good reason to conclude that anosognosia presents us with a case of self-deception, as it is traditionally conceived, and that the mechanisms at work in this pathological case are features of everyday life. Hence the existence of this kind of case has important implications for our understanding of garden-variety self-deception. It demonstrates that doxastic conflict, apparently sustained by motivational mechanisms, is a real feature of human psychology. It therefore places the burden of proof squarely back upon the shoulders of the deflationists. No longer can they argue that their view is less psychologically extravagant than that of their rivals.

CONCLUSION: ILLUMINATING THE MIND

For thousands of years, philosophers have speculated about the nature and structure of the mind. In the process they have developed a set of distinctions and of approaches which will prove indispensable to clear thinking in psychology. Today, however, philosophical reflection must be supplemented by empirical investigation. The mind is stranger than many of us could possibly conceive, in the absence of data from neuroscience and allied fields. We would not guess that there were two visual pathways, for instance, one conscious and one unconscious, and that these two pathways can dissociate. If we are to understand our behavior, we need to turn to these sciences.

Contemplating the mind/brain, the ways in which it works and the ways in which it can go wrong, is often disturbing. It is disturbing because when we peer into the brain, we glimpse our fragility: everything we value, everything that makes life worth living (sensual experience, art, literature and science) and everything that makes us valuable (consciousness, rationality, autonomy) is dependent on the continued integrity of this delicate and endlessly complex organ. But it is also disturbing for another reason: it induces, or at least ought to induce, a kind of humility. When we begin to understand the multiple pathways and procedures which filter external information as it impinges upon our brain; the many ways in which it is processed before it reaches conscious awareness, or before it guides behavior *without* reaching conscious awareness, we realize how little introspective access we have to our own inner depths. Much of what happens happens off-stage, and we cannot peer into the wings, not, at least, directly.

The humility induced by our knowledge of the limits of our introspective access ought to make us less trusting of experience and of memory. We ought to be aware of the many reasons for which neither can be taken as giving us unimpeded access to the nature of reality. Both are constructions, or reconstructions, as much as representations. But the genuine triumphs of neuroscience should also make us aware of how much we are capable of discovering: using the right methods, and relying upon the structure of science as a filter and check – which means relying upon many others, few of whom we shall ever meet – we can begin to understand ourselves. Neuroscience only warns us against complacent self-reliance; it is itself a practical demonstration of the extended mind in action.

End notes

1. The challenge is not to find a case in which someone has purposefully deceived themselves; the challenge is to find a case that looks like ordinary self-deception, and in which the agent has purposefully deceived

themselves. Everyone agrees that it is possible for someone to deceive themselves, using some kind of external manipulation. External manipulations range from hiring a hypnotist, to engaging in a pattern of behavior designed to bring about a belief that the agent currently takes to be false (in the manner in which, according to Pascal, engaging in the outward forms of Christian worship would eventually bring about religious belief), to deliberately writing down false information in a diary, relying upon one's bad memory to ensure that when one reads it one will be taken in. None of these cases look like the kind of thing we ordinarily call self-deception, though articulating the precise difference is rather difficult.

2. This particular result is as Fahle (2003: 230) notes, "not undisputed." However, the evidence for priming effects and other kinds of implicit processing in unilateral neglect is now overwhelming; see, for instance Doricchi and Galati 2000; Vuilleumier *et al.* 2001.

9 The neuroscience of ethics

.

In the preceding chapters, we considered difficult questions concerning the ethical permissibility or desirability of various ways of intervening into the minds of human beings. In examining these questions, we took for granted the reliability of the ethical theories, principles and judgments to which we appealed. But some thinkers have argued that the sciences of the mind are gradually revealing that we cannot continue to do so. Neuroscience and social psychology, these thinkers claim, show that our ethical judgments are often, perhaps even always, *unjustified* or *irrational*. These sciences are stripping away the layers of illusion and falsehood with which ethics has always clothed itself. What lies beneath these illusions? Here thinkers diverge. Some argue for a revisionist view, according to which the lesson of the sciences of the mind is that all moral theories but one are irrational; on this revisionist view, the sciences of the mind provide decisive support for one particular ethical theory. Some argue for an eliminativist view, according to which the sciences of the mind show that *all* moral theories and judgments are unjustified. In this chapter, we shall assess these twin challenges.

How is this deflation of morality supposed to take place? The neuroscientific challenge to ethics focuses upon our *intuitions*. Neuroscience, its proponents hold, shows that our moral intuitions are systematically unreliable, either in general or in some particular circumstances. But if our moral intuitions are systematically unreliable, then morality is in serious trouble, since moral thought is, at bottom, always based upon moral intuition. Intuitions play different roles, and are differentially prominent, in different theories. But no moral theory can dispense with intuitions altogether. Each owes its appeal, in the final accounting, to the plausibility of one or more robust intuitions. Understanding the ways in which the assault on ethics is supposed to work will therefore require understanding the role of intuitions in ethical thought.

ETHICS AND INTUITIONS

Many moral philosophers subscribe to the view of moral thought and argument influentially defended by John Rawls (1971). Rawls argued that we test and justify moral theories by seeking what he called *reflective equilibrium* between our intuitions and our explicit theories. What, however, is an intuition? There is no universally accepted definition in the literature. Some philosophers identify intuitions with *intellectual seemings*: an irrevocable impression forced upon us by consideration of a circumstance, which may or may not cause us to form the corresponding belief – something akin to a visual seeming, which normally causes a belief, but which may sometimes be dismissed as an illusion (Bealer 1998).

Consider, for example, the intuition provoked by a famous demonstration of the conjunction fallacy (Tversky and Kahneman 1983). In this experiment, subjects were required to read the following description:

> Linda is thirty-one years old, single, outspoken, and very bright.
> She majored in philosophy. As a student, she was deeply concerned
> with issues of discrimination and social justice, and also
> participated in anti-nuclear demonstrations.

Subjects were then asked to rank a list of statements about Linda in order of their probability of being true, from most to least likely. The original experiment used eight statements, but five of them were filler. The three statements of interest to the experimenters were the following:

(1) Linda is active in the feminist movement.
(2) Linda is a bank teller.
(3) Linda is a bank teller and is active in the feminist movement.

A large majority of subjects ranked statement (3) as more probable than statement (2). But this can't be right; (3) can't be more probable than (2) since (3) can be true only if (2) is true as well. A conjunction of two propositions cannot be more likely than either of its conjuncts (indeed, conjunctions are usually less probable than their conjuncts). Now, even after the conjunction fallacy is explained to people, and they accept its truth, it may nevertheless go on *seeming as if* – intellectually seeming – (3) is more probable than (2). Even someone as mathematically sophisticated as Steven Jay Gould was vulnerable to the experience:

> I know that the third statement is least probable, yet a little homunculus in my head continues to jump up and down, shouting at me–'but she can't just be a bank teller; read the description.'
>
> *(Gould 1988)*

In other words, the description provokes in us an intellectual seeming, an intuition, which we may then go on to accept or – as in this case, though much less often – to reject.

There is some controversy about this definition of intuitions, but it will suffice for our purposes. In what follows, I shall identify intuitions with *spontaneous* intellectual seemings. Intuitions are spontaneous in the sense that they arise unbidden as soon as we consider the cases that provoke them. They are also, typically, stubborn: once we have them they are relatively hard to shift. Intuitions may be given up as false after reflection and debate, but even then we do not usually lose them, not, at least, all at once.

In moral thought, intuitions are often characterized as "gut feelings." This is slightly misleading, inasmuch as it might be taken to suggest that intuitions are lacking in cognitive content. But it does capture the extent to which moral intuitions (especially) are indeed typically deeply affective. Contemplating (say) the events at Abu Ghraib, or the execution of a hostage in Iraq, the indignation I feel powerfully expresses and reinforces my moral condemnation of the actions. For many other scenarios, real and imaginary, which I judge to be wrong, the affective response is much weaker, so much weaker that I may not even be conscious of it. However, as Damasio's work on somatic markers indicates, it is likely that even in these cases my judgment is guided by my somatic responses: measurements of my skin conductance, heart rate and other autonomic systems, would probably indicate heightened activity, of precisely the kind involved in affective responses. Many, if not all, moral intuitions should be considered both cognitive and affective, with the affective component having a powerful tendency to cause or to reinforce the corresponding belief.

To intuit that an act is right (wrong) is not, however, necessarily to go on to form the belief that the act is right (wrong). It's quite possible for people to have moral intuitions which do not correspond to their moral beliefs (just as we can experience an optical illusion, in the full knowledge that it is an illusion). Nevertheless, moral intuitions are normally taken to have very strong evidential value. An intuition normally causes the corresponding belief, unless the agent has special reason to think that their intuition is, on this occasion, likely to be unreliable. Intuitions are usually taken to have justificatory force, and, as a matter of fact, typically lead to the formation of beliefs that correspond to them.

Intuitions play an important role in many, perhaps most, areas of enquiry. But they are especially central to moral thought. According to Rawls, we test a moral theory by judging the extent to which it accords with our intuitions (or our considered moral judgments – we shall consider possible differences between them shortly). Theory construction might begin, for instance, by simply noting our intuitive responses to a range of uncontroversial moral cases, and then making a first attempt at systematizing them by postulating an overarching principle that apparently explains them all. Thus, we might begin with judgments that are overwhelmingly intuitive, like the following:

It is wrong to torture babies for fun;
Giving to charity is usually praiseworthy;
Stealing, lying and cheating are almost always wrong.

What principle might explain all these judgments? One possibility is a simple *utilitarian* principle, such as the principle formulated by Jeremy Bentham, the father of utilitarianism. According to Bentham, it is "the greatest happiness of the greatest number that is the measure of right and wrong;" that is, an action is right when it produces more happiness for more people than any alternative. It is therefore wrong to torture babies because the harm it causes them is so great; giving to charity is right, on the other hand, because it tends to increase happiness.

Once we have our moral principle in hand, we can test it by attempting to formulate *counterexamples*. Typically, a good counterexample is a case, real or imaginary, in which an action is wrong – intuitively wrong – even though it does not violate the moral principle under examination. If we can discover such a counter-example, we have (apparently) shown that the moral principle is false. Our principle is not, after all, in harmony with our intuitions, and therefore we have not yet reached reflective equilibrium.

Are there counterexamples to Bentham's simple utilitarian principle? Plenty. There are many cases, some of them all too real, in which an action which maximizes happiness nevertheless seems to be wrong. Indeed, even actions like torturing babies for fun could turn out to be mandated by the principle. Suppose that a group of people is so constituted that they will get a great deal of pleasure out of seeing a baby tortured. The pain caused to the baby might be outweighed by the pleasure it causes the onlookers, especially if there are very many of them and they experience a great deal of pleasure. In response to counterexamples like this, we continue the search for reflective equilibrium by refining our moral principles to try to bring them into harmony with our intuitions. For instance, we might look to a more sophisticated consequentialist principle – that is, a principle that, like Bentham's, bases judgments of right or wrong on the consequences of actions. Alternatively, we might look to a *deontological* principle, according to which people have rights which must not be violated – such as the right to freedom from torture – no matter the consequences. Mixed theories, and character-based theories, have also been developed by many thinkers.

The search for reflective equilibrium is therefore the search for a principle or set of principles that harmonizes, and presumably underlies, our intuitions, in much the same way as the search for grammatical rules is (according to many linguists) the making explicit of rules that competent language users employ implicitly. However, though intuitions guide this search, they are not taken to be sacrosanct by proponents of reflective equilibrium. It may be that a moral principle is *itself* so intuitively plausible that when it conflicts with a single-case intuition, we ought to keep the principle rather than modify it. Moreover, intuitions may be amenable to change, at least at the margins; we may find that our intuitions gradually fall into line with our moral theory. Even if they don't, it may be that we ought to put up with a certain degree of disharmony. The conjunction fallacy is obviously a fallacy: reflection on it, as well as probability theory, confirms this. We should continue to regard it as a fallacy no matter the degree of conflict with our intuitions in cases like "Linda the bank teller." Similarly, it may be that the best moral theory will clash with some of our moral intuitions. Nevertheless – and this is the important point here – moral theory construction begins from, and continues indispensably to refer to, our moral intuitions from first till (almost) the last. The best moral theory will systematize a great many of our moral intuitions; ideally it will itself be intuitive, at least on reflection.

Some theorists seek to avoid reliance on intuitions. One way they have sought to do so is by referring, in the process of attempting to reach reflective equilibrium, not to intuitions but to "considered moral judgments" instead. This tack won't work: if considered moral judgments are something different to intuitions – in some philosophers' work, they seem to be much the same thing – then we can only reach them *via* intuitions. If they are not intuitions, then our considered moral judgments are nothing more than the judgments we reach after we have already begun to test our intuitions against our moral principles; in other words, when our judgments have already reached a (provisional) harmony with a moral principle. Some utilitarians, such as Peter Singer (1974), suggest that their preferred moral theory avoids reliance on intuitions altogether. They reject intuitions as irrational prejudices, or the products of cultural indoctrination. However, it is apparent – as indeed our first sketch of a justification for utilitarianism made clear – that utilitarianism itself is just as reliant upon intuitions as is any other moral theory (Daniels 2003). Singer suggests that we reject intuitions in favor of "self-evident moral axioms" (1974: 516). But *self-evidence* is itself intuitiveness, of a certain type: an axiom is self-evident (for an individual) if that axiom seems true to that individual and their intuition in favor of that axiom is undefeated. Hence, appeal to self-evidence just *is* appeal to intuition.

The great attraction of utilitarianism rests upon the *intuitiveness* of a principle like Bentham's, which rests, itself, on the intuitiveness of the claim that pains and pleasures are, respectively and *ceteris paribus*, good and bad. No moral theory seems likely to be able to dispense with intuitions, though different theories appeal to them in different ways. Some give greater weight to case-by-case intuitions, as deontologists may do, and as everyday moral thought seems to (DePaul 1998). Others, like utilitarianism, rest the justificatory case on one big intuition, a particular moral principle taken to be itself so intuitive that it outweighs case-by-case intuitions (Pust 2000). Whatever the role intuitions play in justifying their principles or their case-by-case judgments, all moral theories seem to be based ultimately upon moral intuition.

It is this apparently indispensable reliance of moral reflection upon intuition that leaves it open to the challenges examined here. In a sense, these challenges build upon Singer's (indeed, we shall see that Singer himself has seized upon them as evidence for his view): they provide, or are seen as providing, evidence for the claim that intuitions are indeed irrational. But in its more radical form, the challenge turns against consequentialism, in all its varieties, just as much as rival moral theories: if our intuitions are systematically unreliable guides to moral truths, if they fail to track genuine, or genuinely moral, features of the world, then *all* moral theories are in deep trouble.

THE NEUROSCIENTIFIC CHALLENGE TO MORALITY

There are many possible challenges to our moral intuitions, and thence to the rationality of moral judgments. They come, for instance, from psychology (Horowitz 1998) and from evolutionary considerations (Joyce 2001; 2006). These challenges all take a similar form: they adduce evidence for the claim that our intuitions are prompted by features of our mind/brain that, whatever else can be said for them, cannot be taken to be reliable guides to moral reality. Here I shall focus on two versions of this challenge to our intuitions, an argument from neuroscience, and an argument from social psychology. First, the argument from neuroscience.

In a groundbreaking study of the way in which brains process moral dilemmas, Joshua Greene and his colleagues found significant differences in the neural processes of subjects, depending upon whether they were considering personal or impersonal moral dilemmas (Greene *et al.* 2001). A *personal* moral dilemma is a case which involves directly causing harm or death to someone, whereas an *impersonal* moral dilemma is a case in which harm or death results from less direct processes. For instance, Greene and colleagues used variations on the famous trolley problem (also considered in Chapter 5) as test dilemmas. The first version of this problem is an impersonal variant of the dilemma, whereas the second is a personal variant:

(1) Imagine you are standing next to railway tracks, when you see an out-of-control trolley hurtling towards you. If the trolley continues on its current path, it will certainly hit and kill five workers who are in a nearby tunnel. You cannot warn them in time, and they cannot escape from the tunnel. However, if you pull a lever you can divert the trolley to a sidetrack, where it will certainly hit and kill a single

worker. Assume you have no other options available to you that would save the five men. Should you pull the lever?

(2) Imagine that this time you find yourself on a bridge over the railway tracks when you see the trolley hurtling toward a group of five workers. The only way to prevent their certain deaths is for you to push the fat man standing next to you into its path; this will stop the trolley, but the man will die. It's no use you leaping into its path; you are too light to stop the trolley. Should you push the fat man?

The judgments of Greene's subjects were in line with those of most philosophers: the great majority judged that in the first case it is permissible or even obligatory to pull the lever, but in the second it is impermissible to push the fat man. Now, from some angles these judgments are *prima facie* inconsistent. After all, there is a level of description – well captured by consequentialism – in which these cases seem closely similar in their morally relevant features. In both, the subject is asked whether he or she should save five lives at the cost of one. Yet most people have quite different intuitions with regard to the two cases: in the first, they think it is right to save the five, but in the second they believe it to be wrong.

Most philosophers have responded to these cases in the traditional way described by Rawls: they have sought a deeper moral principle that would harmonize their intuitions. For instance, the following Kantian principle has been suggested: it is wrong to use people as a means to others' ends. The idea is this: in pushing the fat man into the path of the trolley, one is using him as a means whereby to prevent harm to others, since it is his bulk that will stop the trolley. But in pulling the lever one is not using the man on the tracks as a means, since his presence is not necessary to saving the lives of the five. Pulling the lever would work just as well if he were absent, so we do not use him. Unfortunately, this suggestion fails. Consider the looping track variant of the problem (Thomson 1986). In this variant, pulling the lever diverts the trolley onto the alternative track, but that track loops back onto the initial track, in such a manner that were it not for the presence of the solitary worker, the trolley would end up killing the five anyway. In that case, diverting the trolley saves the five, but only by using the one worker as a means: were it not for his presence, the strategy wouldn't work. Nevertheless, most people have the intuition that it is permissible to pull the lever.

Greene and colleagues claim that their results cast a radically different light on these dilemmas. They found that when subjects considered impersonal dilemmas, regions of the brain associated with working memory showed a significant degree of activation, while regions associated with emotion showed little activation. But when subjects considered personal moral dilemmas, regions associated with emotion showed a significant degree of activity, whereas regions associated with working memory showed a degree of activity *below* the resting baseline (Greene *et al.* 2001). Why? The authors plausibly suggest that the thought of directly killing someone is much more personally engaging than is the thought of failing to help someone, or using indirect means to harm them.

In their original study Greene and his co-authors explicitly deny that their results have any direct moral relevance. Their conclusion is "descriptive rather than prescriptive" (2001: 2107). However, it is easy to see how their findings might be taken to threaten the evidential value of our moral intuitions. It might be suggested that the high degree of emotional involvement in the personal moral dilemmas clouds the judgment of subjects. It is, after all, commonplace that strong emotions can distort our judgments. Perhaps the idea that the subjects would themselves directly cause the death of a bystander generates especially strong emotions, which cause them to judge irrationally in these cases. Evidence for this suspicion is provided by the under-activation of regions of the brain associated with working memory. Perhaps subjects do not properly think through these dilemmas. Rather, their distaste for the idea of killing prevents them from rationally considering these cases at all (Sinnott-Armstrong 2006).

The case for the claim that Greene's results have skeptical implications for morality has recently been developed and defended by Peter Singer (2005) himself. For Singer, Greene's results do not merely *explain* our moral intuitions; they explain them away. Singer's case rests upon the overwhelmingly likely hypothesis that these responses are the product of our evolutionary history (echoing here Greene's (2005; forthcoming) own latest reinterpretation of his results). He suggests that it is likely that we feel a special repugnance for direct harms because these were the only kinds of harms that were possible in our environment of evolutionary adaptation. Understanding the evolutionary origins of our intuitions undermines them, Singer claims, not in the sense that we cease to experience them, but in the sense that we see that they have no moral force:

> What is the moral salience of the fact that I have killed someone in a way that was possible a million years ago, rather than in a way that became possible only two hundred years ago? I would answer: none.
>
> *(Singer 2005: 348)*

Since it is an entirely contingent fact that we respond more strongly to some kinds of killing than others, a fact produced by our evolutionary history and the relatively recent development of technologies for killing at a distance, these intuitions are shown to be suspect, Singer suggests. As Greene himself has put it "maybe this pair of moral intuitions has nothing to do with 'some good reason' and everything to do with the way our brains happen to be built" (2003: 848).

Singer suggests, moreover, that the case against the intuitions prompted by personal and impersonal moral dilemmas can be generalized, to cast doubt on moral intuitions more generally. If the neuroscientific evidence suggests that moral intuitions are the product of emotional responses, and it is plausible that these responses are themselves the product of our evolutionary history, and not the moral structure of the world, then all our moral intuitions ought to be suspect, whether or not we possess any direct neuroscientific evidence to demonstrate their irrationality. After all, the cognitive mechanisms we have as the result of our evolutionary history are not designed to track moral truths; they are designed to increase our inclusive fitness (where inclusive fitness means, roughly, our success in increasing the proportion of copies of our genes in the next generation). Evolution at best ignores moral truth, and at worst rewards downright selfishness. So we cannot expect our evolved intuitions to be good guides to moral truth.

Singer tasks himself to find further evidence of the irrationality of intuitions in psychology; specifically in the work of Jonathan Haidt, the source of the second challenge to morality we shall examine here. Over the past decade, Haidt (2001; 2003; Haidt *et al.* 1993) has been developing what he calls the social intuitionist model (SIM) of moral judgments. The model has two components: the first component centres upon the *processes* by which moral judgments are formed; the second centres on their *rationality*. The process claim is that moral judgments are the product of intuition, not reasoning: certain situations evoke affective responses in us, which give rise to (or perhaps just *are*) moral intuitions, which we then express as moral judgments. The rationality claim is that *since* moral judgments are the product of emotions, they neither are the product of rational processes nor are they amenable to rational influence.

Haidt takes the process claim to constitute evidence for the rationality claim. *Because* moral judgments are intuition driven, they are not rational. Haidt suggests that the processes which drive moral judgments are arational. Our judgments are proximately produced by our emotional responses, and differences in these responses are the product of social and cultural influences; hence moral judgments differ by social class and across cultures. We take ourselves to have reasons for our judgments, but in fact these reasons are *post hoc* rationalizations of our emotional responses. We neither have reasons for our judgments, nor do we change them in the face of reasons (Haidt speaks of the "moral dumbfounding" he encounters, when he asks subjects for their reasons for their moral judgments. They laugh, shake their heads, and express surprise at their inability to defend their views – but they do not alter them). Hence, moral judgments are not rational. On the contrary, our moral intuitions often conflict with the moral theories *we ourselves* endorse.

If Haidt is right, then the SIM provides powerful evidence in Singer's favor: it seems to show that our moral intuitions are rationally incorrigible, and that they frequently clash with our best moral theories. Of course, Singer only wants to go so far with the SIM. He wants to use it to clear the ground for an alternative, non-intuition-based, moral theory, not to use it to cast doubt on morality *tout court*. Haidt does not consider a non-intuition-based alternative; nothing he says therefore conflicts with Singer's claim that the SIM is a problem for his opponents, and not for him. We, however, have already seen that there are good grounds to doubt that the sceptical challenge can be contained in the manner Singer suggests. It is simply false to think that *any* moral theory, Singer's utilitarianism included, can dispense with intuitions. If the challenge to intuitions cannot be headed off, morality itself is in trouble.

RESPONDING TO THE DEFLATIONARY CHALLENGE

The challenge from neuroscience (and related fields) to morality has the following general form:

(1) Our moral theories, as well as our first-order judgments and principles are all based, more or less directly, upon our moral intuitions.
(2) These theories, judgments and principles are justified only insofar as our intuitions track genuinely moral features of the world.
(3) But our moral intuitions are the product of cognitive mechanisms which evolved under non-moral selection pressures, and therefore cannot be taken to track moral features of the world; hence
(4) Our moral theories, judgments and principles are unjustified.

This argument, whether it is motivated by concerns from psychology or from neuroscience, casts doubt upon our ability to know moral facts. It is therefore a direct challenge to our moral epistemology. It is also an indirect challenge to the claim that there are any moral facts to be known: if all our evidence for moral facts is via channels which cannot plausibly be taken to give us access to them, we have little reason to believe that they exist at all.

In this section, I shall evaluate the neuroscientific evidence against the value of intuitions; the argument that since our intuitions reflect the morphology of our brains, and that morphology developed under non-moral selection pressures, we ought to dismiss these intuitions in favor of those that are less affectively charged. I shall delay a consideration of the argument from social psychology, resting on Haidt's work on moral dumbfounding, until a later section.

Singer's strategy is to cast doubt, first, on a subset of our moral intuitions, and then to generalize the suspicion. Some of our intuitions, he argues, are irrational, as Greene's evidence demonstrates. Evolution gives us an explanation of why we have such irrational responses: our moral responses evolved under non-moral selection pressures, and therefore cannot be taken to be reliable guides to moral truth. But, Singer suggests, since all our intuitions are equally the product of our evolutionary history, the suspicion ought to be generalized. All our intuitions ought to be rejected, whether we have direct evidence for their irrationality or not. How strong is this argument? I shall argue that though Singer is surely right in thinking that some of the intuitions provoked by, say, trolley cases are irrational, and that evolutionary considerations explain why we have them, some of our intuitions escape condemnation. If that's right, then of course the generalization strategy must fail: some of our intuitions are (for all that Singer, Greene and Haidt have shown) reliable, and we can refer to them in good conscience.

Greene's claim, endorsed by Singer, is that because our differential responses to trolley cases are the product of our affective states, they are not rational, and therefore ought to be rejected as guides to action. As Singer puts it:

If, however, Greene is right to suggest that our intuitive responses are due to differences in the emotional pull of situations that involve bringing about someone's death in a close-up, personal way, and bringing about the same person's death in a way that is at a distance, and less personal, why should we believe that there is anything that justifies these responses?

Singer 2005: 347

Now, I suggest that two different arguments can be discerned here. First, it might be suggested that our intuitive responses in some of these cases should be dismissed as irrational *because* they are emotionally laden. Second, it might be suggested that our intuitions in these cases should be dismissed because they are a response to a feature of the situation – whether it was caused directly or indirectly – that is morally irrelevant. These two suggestions need to be considered separately. I shall, however, delay discussion of the second suggestion until we have developed a framework within which to discuss it.

The first claim, that because some of our moral intuitions are expressions of emotional responses, they ought to be disregarded, rests, obviously, on a particular view of emotions. It is a view that we have had reason to examine several times before; the traditional view that associates emotions with obstacles to rationality. As we have seen, this is a view that is rejected by most contemporary philosophers, who instead urge one or another *cognitivist* account of emotions. Emotions, these philosophers argue, are generally reliable guides to reality, including moral reality (Neu 2000; Nussbaum 2001; Jones 2004). Moreover, neuroscience itself provides independent support for some kind of cognitivism about emotions. We have already examined this evidence, but it's worth reviewing again.

Recall Damasio and colleagues' work (reviewed in Chapter 5) on the way in which somatic markers – which are usually perceived as feelings – guide prudential decision-making. Far from finding that our emotional responses mislead us, they found that they improved prudential decision-making. In one famous study, they studied performance on the Iowa Gambling Task (Bechara *et al.* 1997). In this task, subjects chose cards from one of four decks, two of which gave large payoffs but frequent large punishments, and two of which gave smaller payoffs, but also smaller punishments. Normal subjects learned to favor the smaller payoff decks, which, on average, gave a small but steady payoff, over the larger payoffs, which proved disadvantageous over time. Damasio's team discovered that normal subjects actually began to favor the advantageous decks *before* they understood the payoff structure. Subjects began to generate anticipatory skin conductance responses to the disadvantageous decks. These SCRs predated explicit knowledge of the payoff structure by a significant time. Only subsequently did subjects develop a "hunch" about the decks, a hunch that gradually became explicit knowledge. But advantageous *choice* predated knowledge. Thus the emotional response biased choice away from disadvantageous options and toward advantageous. Damasio has argued that psychopaths are disastrous decision-makers precisely because they lack the right *feelings* (Damasio 1994). They do not have the intuitive responses which allow us relatively easily to navigate the social and cognitive world.

The mere fact, then, that our moral intuitions are (partially) affective responses does not seem sufficient to discredit them; such feelings can after all be reliable guides for choice. Moreover, there is independent evidence that moral intuitions are produced, at least in important part, by the same systems that guide prudential choice. Somatic markers apparently play a role in ordinary moral reasoning (Batson *et al.* 1999; Wheatley and Haidt 2005). Now, it is surely *possible* that though emotions are a reliable guide in prudential decision-making, they systematically mislead moral reasoning; that if a moral response is emotionally laden, we ought to disregard it. But why should we believe that? Very powerful emotions can overwhelm people, and distort their reasoning, but given that emotions are apparently more usually helpful, we have no reason to distrust our normal emotional responses.

The evidence from neuroscience does not support Greene and Singer's claim: the mere fact that areas associated with emotions are differentially active in judging personal and impersonal dilemmas does nothing to show that either set of intuitions is suspect. We have no general reason to discount affectively colored judgments; such judgments can be reliable. Indeed, it might be argued that it is not the responses of ordinary subjects that ought to be disregarded as suspect, but the judgments of the minority who judge according to utilitarian standards. There is one class of naïve – that is, philosophically untrained – subjects who have consistently utilitarian intuitions in trolley problems and similar dilemmas. These are patients with damage to the ventromedial prefrontal cortex (VM patients) (Hauser 2006). VM patients have generally unimpaired reasoning, with intact intelligence and abstract moral reasoning. But they are disastrously bad at practical reasoning, both prudential and ethical. Like the famous Phineas Gage, the best-known VM patient, they often find themselves unable to hold down jobs, sustain relationships or save money. Damasio (1994) suggests that their problems are the result of impaired affective processing brought about by the VM damage. Now, the fact that VM damage can be shown, on *independent* grounds, to issue in faulty decision-making provides us with evidence of the kind that Singer lacks: evidence that the processes which issue in certain judgments are unreliable or distorting. The same lack of affective response that causes VM patients to choose badly in everyday life is also responsible for their consequentialist reasoning in trolley problems. Far from vindicating consequentialism as the uniquely rational, because unemotional, response, the fact that these judgments are caused by the very same deficit that can be shown to issue in a consistently disadvantageous pattern of choices seems to put them under a cloud of suspicion.

Let me address one possible objection from neuroscience to the claim I'm making here, that the mere fact that a judgment is affectively colored is no reason to discount its evidential value. Roskies (2003, 2006) has argued, on the basis of studies of VM patients, that moral judgments do not necessarily have an affective component. She believes that these patients are walking counterexamples to a philosophical thesis: the thesis known as internalism. Internalism (in this context) is the view that moral judgments are intrinsically motivating; that is, that an agent who sincerely judges that they ought to (or ought not to) perform a particular act will *necessarily* be (at least somewhat) motivated to act accordingly. Roskies argues that there is no reason to think that VM patients fail to make moral judgments. After all, they acquired their mastery of moral concepts in the normal way, prior to their lesion; why think they have suddenly lost these concepts, especially given that their judgments on most abstract moral reasoning tasks are normal? But, she argues, they are usually not at all motivated to act on their judgments. Hence, internalism is false.

Roskies' argument is controversial. Suppose, however, that it is correct. Mightn't Singer cite Roskies' work as evidence for his view? That is, mightn't he argue that Roskies has shown that, contra what I have claimed above, moral judgments do not have an affective element as an essential element, and that therefore the utilitarian – non-affectively motivated – judgment has the better claim to being moral? Singer could claim that the utilitarian, "cold," judgment is the truly moral judgment, since Roskies has shown that any affective component is extraneous to the essence of moral judgment. I think that in fact Roskies' work is unhelpful for Singer for two reasons. First, her work, assuming it is correct, establishes only that moral judgments do not necessarily have an affective component, not that when and if they have such a component they are less reliable than when they lack it. Roskies argues only that "cold" judgment deserves to be called "moral," not that it deserves a higher status than "hot." Second, it is compatible with her evidence that emotion does, after all, play an essential role in *the acquisition* of the ability to engage in moral judgment.

VM patients are in some ways remarkably similar, in behavior and judgments, to psychopaths; indeed, VM syndrome has been dubbed "acquired sociopathy" (Saver and Damasio 1991). One salient difference between them, however, is that psychopaths, unlike VM patients, are severely impaired in their moral judgments; specifically, they cannot reliably distinguish moral from conventional transgressions. The precise etiology of this impairment is still controversial, but there is growing evidence that the emotional impairments experienced by psychopaths are the proximate cause of their inability to master moral concepts (Blair *et al.* 2005). It is because they are insensitive to the fact that paradigm moral transgressions cause distress in victims, regardless of the system of rules in place, that they do not "get" the moral/conventional distinction. As Prinz (2004) points out, the failure of psychopaths to acquire such mastery is good evidence that understanding moral concepts requires appropriate affective responses.

VM patients are masters of moral concepts, then, only because they acquired them before their brain damage; at a time when they possessed normal emotional responses. Psychopaths do not master moral concepts because psychopathy is a developmental disorder; there was never a time at which the psychopath experienced normal emotional responses. Further, there is evidence that suggests that the earlier VM damage is suffered, the greater the degree of moral impairment (Anderson *et al.* 2000). But if it is true that emotional response is necessary for the acquisition of moral concepts – for the very *idea* of morality, as a system of prohibitions and prescriptions that is categorically different from conventional rules – then the claim that emotion enables, rather than distorts, moral judgment is greatly strengthened. It may be that a stronger thesis is defensible. Even if it is true that once acquired, moral judgments can be made in the absence of affect (as Roskies argues), it is possible that without an affective anchor, these judgments will tend to drift. Perhaps VM patients (for instance) will eventually lose their mastery of moral concepts (just as a once sighted blind person might conceivably gradually lose their mastery of color concepts). In that case, it would not only be the acquisition, but also the continuing application, of moral concepts that would require the appropriate emotions throughout the lifespan. This is an empirically testable proposition; here philosophy must give way to experimental method.

MORAL CONSTRUCTIVISM

Singer and Greene both suggest that if it is true that our moral intuitions are the product of our evolutionary history, we cannot see them as tracking moral truths, since evolution is indifferent to moral reality. Now, this argument seems to presuppose a particular, and controversial, view of moral facts. On the view presupposed, moral facts are *independent* of our responses and our interests. If this view is correct, then Singer and Greene would have a strong case, for if our moral responses evolved under non-moral selection pressures, we would have no reason to think them capable of tracking moral facts. We would have no more reason to trust them as guides to morality than we have to trust our hearing as a guide to infrared radiation; no reason to think that the faculty gets any grip on its supposed target.

But this particular conception of moral facts is not the only one on offer, nor is it the most plausible. Indeed, it is not a view that naturalists ought to profess. The view of moral facts as existing independently of us is non-naturalist: it takes morality to be some-how part of the furniture of the universe, in some manner indepen-dent of the kinds of entities science investigates. In some versions it is a Platonism, holding that moral facts belong to a *sui generis* category, equally (or more) real as the observable world, but irre-ducible to them; in others it is religiously motivated and takes moral facts to consist in laws laid down by God. Naturalists sometimes reject the existence of morality, because they cannot conceive how moral facts could exist once these non-naturalist alternatives are rejected. But moral skepticism and non-naturalism do not exhaust the available alternatives.

Among the meta-ethical rivals to non-naturalism, the many varieties of moral constructivism are, I suggest, especially attractive. Moral constructivism is the view that moral facts and properties are constituted by – constructed out of – the stances, attitudes, conventions or other states or products of human beings. Moral constructivism comes in many different flavors, depending upon the properties of actual or ideal human beings held to be constitutive of morality: contractualist (Scanlon 1998), ideal observer (Firth 1952), Kantian (Korsgaard 1986), relativist (Wong 1984; Levy 2002b) or dispositional (Lewis 1989), among others. If moral constructivism is true, moral facts are not independent of us, in the manner supposed by the non-naturalist. Instead, they are importantly the product of our (more or less idealized; that is, worked over in the manner suggested by reflective equilibrium) moral responses. But if moral facts are, in important part, the product of our responses, then there is much less danger that our intuitions will systematically fail to be responsive to moral facts. Instead, morality may be constructed out of our (idealized) intuitions.[1]

However, if moral constructivism builds morality out of intuitions, it does not commit us to the claim that *all* our moral intuitions are correct just as they are. Moral constructivists may – though they need not – be moral realists, at least in the sense that they believe that many moral questions have uniquely right answers. Insofar as they embrace realism, they are committed to thinking that some intuitions are unreliable, if for no other reason than different people have conflicting intuitions, which cannot *all* be right. The moral constructivist is willing to have their moral responses corrected, but they will not be persuaded that all their intuitions are unreliable by evidence of the kind that Greene and Singer adduce. There is no reason for the moral constructivist to fear that *the mere fact* that morality has evolved, and requires for its realization a particular and contingent set of brain structures, undermines it. The moral constructivist can regard discoveries about the neurological underpinnings of moral intuitions as telling us how moral judgments are *implemented*. Greene's evidence can help to explain morality, without explaining it away.

Consider, once more, the Greene/Singer claim that our moral intuitions are the product of an evolutionary history which was shaped by non-moral selection pressures. We have every reason to believe that this holds true for *all* our most fundamental moral intuitions: we have them because being disposed to respond in these kinds of ways increased the inclusive fitness of our very distant ancestors (Levy 2004). Many of these responses we have because they benefited primitive organisms, who possessed nothing like the cognitive sophistication of our recent primate ancestors. The earliest identifiable building blocks of morality consist, arguably, in the cooperative dispositions of creatures as primitive as predatory fish and the much smaller fish which clean them. These fish are often the right size to make a good meal for the predators. Yet the latter do not attempt to eat the cleaners; instead, they seek them out, and when they locate them go into a kind of trance while the smaller fish removes parasites from them. The small fish sometimes actually swim inside the mouths of the larger, and out their gills, in their search for the parasites, without being threatened. Why? The answer seems to be because ancestors of these predators who accepted cleaning services and then made a meal of the cleaners were outperformed by those who returned to the same spot many times, to have their parasites removed again. The benefits of regular parasite removal outweigh the benefits of a one-off meal (Trivers 1985).

It is likely that this cooperative disposition – technically, to play the tit-for-tat strategy in an iterated interaction – emerged relatively early in evolution, and was preserved in the lineage leading to us. Our primate relatives have it (de Waal 1996); our common ancestor with them presumably had it, and even much more distant relatives, like vampire bats, have it (Wilkinson 1990). We, too, have this disposition to cooperate with cooperators; we play the tit-for-tat strategy in a wide range of circumstances, ranging from the trivial (tipping for service in restaurants; Frank 1988) to the momentous (the development of the system of "live and let live" in the trench warfare of WWI; Axelrod 1984). Should we conclude that this disposition, to reward cooperation and punish betrayal or free-riding, should be rejected as not *truly* moral because we have it as a product of our evolutionary history? From the constructivist viewpoint, this history explains our intuitions, but it does nothing to show that they are unjustified. We respond in these ways because evolution disposed us to, but because we respond in these ways, morality exist for us: it is built out of these responses (among others).

Indeed, the intuitions that underlie utilitarianism, for instance the intuition that pain is bad whether it is experienced by oneself or by another, is almost certainly itself the product of our evolutionary history. Singer believes that ethics must be based on universal benevolence, and that as a matter of fact evolution has not, and could not, provide us with the feelings that could motivate such concern. The "unit of selection", he claims, is too large for natural selection to have endowed us with such a feeling (2005: 334). Hence, we must look elsewhere for its origin: to reason stripped of emotion. Now, if Singer is concerned with universal benevolence, from my constructivist viewpoint it is because *he* does feel the appropriate emotions. Does that conflict with the evolutionary standpoint? Not at all: such a universal concern for conspecifics is precisely (*pace* Singer) what we ought to expect from evolution, and what we in fact observe. Singer makes the common mistake of confusing the proximate mechanisms that motivate behavior with their distal explanations. Evolution does not seek the best solution to a problem; it seeks the most efficient, and therefore favors quick and dirty heuristics over slower and more accurate mechanisms. In the environment of evolutionary adaptation, pretty much everyone with whom we interacted was a relative; we therefore favored our relatives simply by favoring conspecifics. Hence, today, in a very different social environment in which we interact more often with strangers than with relatives, we have the feeling of universal benevolence.

Of course, the story I have just told is somewhat speculative. But the evidence that universal benevolence has evolved is plentiful. It consists, once again, in the proto-moral behavior of other animals. Other social animals exhibit a concern for conspecifics, independent of their degree of relatedness or of opportunities for reciprocity. Rhesus monkeys, for instance, will prefer a smaller reward to a larger, if they can only procure the larger at the cost of an electric shock to a conspecific (Masserman *et al.* 1964). Even rats will work to avoid distress to conspecifics (Rice and Gainer 1962). The likelihood is that, contra Singer, our ancestors in the environment of evolutionary adaptation were similarly concerned for conspecifics. Moreover, there is evidence that indicates that our own concern for others has its most primitive roots in this inherited response: even neonates react to the distress of others (Thompson 1998).

Just as the benevolence to which utilitarianism appeals is likely the product of our evolutionary history, and ought not be discounted for that, so our intuitions in trolley problems too are almost certainly the product of evolution, and *that fact alone* does nothing to discredit them. If moral facts were the kinds of things non-naturalists supposed – Platonic entities, or ideas in the mind of God, for instance – then morality would be vulnerable to Singer and Greene's objection. But if morality exists only for rational creatures capable of guiding their behavior by its demands, this is plausibly because it can be *identified* with the (suitably regimented) deliverances of our moral intuitions. If you accept that moral facts are natural facts, constituted by human needs, pains and pleasures, dispositions or whatever it may be, then whatever mechanisms track these natural properties and give rise to moral intuitions are moral mechanisms (whatever else they might be). That they evolved under non-moral selection pressures is irrelevant to their current function. Morality is constituted by the systematic reactions of moral beings; so long as we accept this, we have little reason to fear that the discovery of the mechanisms which underlie those reactions will undermine it.

I said above that two separate arguments could be discerned in Singer's challenge to the intuitions in the trolley problem. The first, the one upon which we have focused so far, is the argument directly from neuroscience: because our intuitions in personal moral dilemmas are emotionally laden, we ought to disregard them. This argument, as we now see, fails. Singer's second argument, however, is importantly different. It turns on the claim that our intuitions track morally irrelevant features of cases. We respond differently to cases which differ only in the directness of the means used to harm or kill. But surely the mere fact that one way of killing is close up and personal, and the other impersonal and technologically mediated, can't itself be morally significant. Hence our intuitions in these cases are suspect. This argument, I suggest, is much stronger than the first. However, it does not have the implications that Singer claims for it.

The claim that the degree of immediacy in causing harm or death is morally irrelevant is surely correct. It is also, almost certainly, correct that the explanation of why we have this differential response is evolutionary; the harm in the close-up-and-personal case is far more vivid for us because it taps into relatively primitive responses, and it does *that* because the harm was (as Greene and Haidt (2004) put it) of "a kind that a chimpanzee can appreciate." But neither of these facts does anything to discredit the other intuitions subjects experience in response to personal moral dilemmas, or the intuition-based approach to moral thought more generally. Let's consider these questions in reverse order.

The reason why the fact that we respond differently to cases depending upon the (surely morally irrelevant) directness of the means used to kill does not discredit the intuition-based approach is simple: the discrediting in question is an example of the method of reflective equilibrium in action, not an argument against it. Singer appeals, precisely, to our intuitions, in asking us to see that directness of harm is morally irrelevant. The argument from neuroscience plays *no* role at all in this part of his argument. Instead, he engages in normal philosophical argumentation, challenging us to say how distance could be morally significant, all by itself. We ought to agree with Singer's substantive conclusion, that distance is morally irrelevant, but his methodological point we should reject.

The reason why Singer's argument does not challenge all our intuitions in trolley cases and similar dilemmas is that distance seems to be only one factor at work in explaining our moral intuitions here. Other principles also appear to be at work. For instance, there is an important intention/foresight distinction that seems to play a role in some of these cases: people think that it is worse to intend harm, as a means of bringing about morally desirable consequences, than it is merely to foresee that harm will come about as an inevitable consequence of engaging in action that is otherwise morally justified. It is, at least arguably, this distinction that is at work in explaining our intuitions in some versions of the trolley cases. We see ourselves as intending the harm to the fat man when we push him, but merely foreseeing the harm to the man on the tracks when we pull the lever. Now, is the intention/foresight distinction morally relevant? It is far from obvious that it is not. Consider the difference between deliberately bombing civilians in war time, in order to demoralize the enemy, and bombing a military target such as a munitions factory, in the certain knowledge that civilians in the surrounding area will be killed as well. Even if we can be certain that the same number of civilians will die in the latter case as in the former, indeed, even if we have good reason to think that *more* civilians will die in the second case, they seem to be quite different, morally speaking. Intending the harm, in the first case, seems morally far less permissible than merely foreseeing it, as a regrettable consequence of legitimate military action, in the second.

This is not intended to be either a defense of the intention/foresight distinction, or an attack upon utilitarianism. At the end of the day, it may be that we ought to reject the distinction; perhaps some kind of consequentialism is the best normative theory. The point, rather, is this: *if* we are to reject the intention/foresight distinction, it ought to be because we believe that it cannot do the work demanded of it, perhaps because we find consequentialism too intuitive itself, or perhaps because as we survey the range of cases the distinction is supposed to explain, we find the pattern too ad hoc to think that it tracks genuinely moral properties. All this is to say that it will not be neuroscience that discredits the distinction, if it is discredited, but moral philosophy conducted as usual.

MORAL DUMBFOUNDING AND DISTRIBUTED COGNITION

Let us turn, now, to the evidence from cognitive psychology. Haidt's claim, endorsed by Singer, is that our moral intuitions are irrational, and our explanations for them nothing more than *post hoc* rationalizations. Singer believes he finds in Haidt support for the view that intuitions are emotional responses, and that *therefore* "reason can do no more than build the best possible case for a decision already made on non-rational grounds" (Singer 2005: 351). But Singer – and Haidt – pays insufficient attention to the actual content of the reported intuitions. Haidt's work on "moral dumbfounding" – the phenomenon when someone reports an intuition that an action is wrong, but is unable to justify that response – actually demonstrates that dumbfounding is in inverse proportion to the socio-economic status (SES) of subjects (Haidt *et al.* 1993). Higher SES subjects differ from lower not in the moral theories they appeal to, but in the content of their moral responses. In particular, higher SES subjects are far less likely to find victimless transgressions – disgusting or taboo actions – morally wrong than lower. Hence higher SES subjects can and do justify their responses by appealing to harm. Lower SES subjects also appeal preferentially to a harm-based moral theory, but since they also judge victimless transgressions to be wrong, they are unable to justify their responses. Now, this pattern of responses seems to be precisely the *opposite* of those Singer needs to support his case. Singer claims that our intuitive responses are immune to rational correction, but the differential responses of higher and lower SES subjects demonstrates that in fact moral intuitions are amenable to education. The greater the length of formal education, the less the likelihood of subjects holding that victimless transgressions are morally wrong (the effect of SES on the moral judgment of children is, accordingly, less than the effect on adults (Haidt *et al.* 1993: 620–2)).

Now, recall the method of reflective equilibrium. Applying it, we attempt to build our moral theories out of our intuitions, but we also expect that at least some of these intuitions will alter, or be rejected as misleading, as we refine our moral theory. It is apparent that the responses reported by Haidt cannot all be regarded as reliable guides to moral reasoning, simply because these responses conflict. Some of Haidt's subjects suggest that actions are permissible that others judge as impermissible. But this fact presents the friend of reflective equilibrium with no special problem. Indeed, they can claim Haidt's results as *confirmation* of their theory: intuitions are educable, just as they always claimed. Higher SES subjects have had better education, more time and opportunity to reflect on their intuitions and their moral theories, and – typically – exposure to a wider range of moral views. Their intuitions ought to be granted an accordingly greater weight.

DISTRIBUTED COGNITION: EXTENDING THE MORAL MIND

We began this book by examining the plausibility of the extended mind hypothesis. I advanced evidence that I took to support the hypothesis, but I also suggested that nothing of great moment depends, for our purposes, on whether it or its less radical rival, the embedded mind hypothesis, is true. No matter which wins this particular battle, we must recognize that high-level cognition, the cognition of which humans alone are capable and which may well be the most important factor in distinguishing us from other animals, is very heavily dependent on resources beyond the brain and body: cognitive tools, the stability of the environment used as epistemic scaffolding, language. We also sketched the way in which such distinctively human cognition is dependent upon its *social* embedding. Human knowledge is a community-wide enterprise. It is not produced by solitary geniuses, not, at least, for the most part, and even the occasional solitary genius does not produce anything of value unless he or she engages with the work of others. Science institutionalizes the production of knowledge as a collective enterprise: by demanding that only work that has been scrutinized by others – that is, published in peer-reviewed journals – is taken seriously, by demanding that methods are made publicly available so that they can be replicated, by encouraging mutual criticism of theories, it ensures that knowledge emerges from the interaction of thousands of different people across the world. The process of mutual criticism and correction ensures not only that knowledge production goes much faster than would otherwise be possible; like the introduction of tools and environmental resources for cognition, it also opens up entirely new ways of thinking that simply wouldn't be available to an individual.

Moral thought, too, should be thought of as a community-wide enterprise. Consider, once more, the ways in which high SES subjects differ, in their moral responses, to lower SES subjects. Both groups accept a harm-based moral theory, but higher SES subjects apply it more consistently (Haidt et al. 1993). Now suppose that moral thought is a community-wide enterprise, in the manner I suggest. In that case, we ought to give differential weight to the moral responses of different people, depending upon their role in the enterprise (just as we give differential weight to the views of different people concerning, say, climate change or evolution, depending upon their role in the distributed scientific enterprise). In a way somewhat analogous to (but also importantly different from) the way knowledge accumulates in the sciences, as a product of the interaction of many individuals, each possessed of special expertise, so morality is a community-wide enterprise, in which moral experts take a leading role.

There are two most important differences between morality, conceived of in this manner, and, say, physics. First, the gap between moral experts and the rest of the community, in terms of the possession of special expertise, is *much* smaller in morality than in physics; second, moral expertise is unlike expertise in physics in that it is transmitted at least as much outside the university and related institutions as inside. Moral expertise is not the exclusive preserve of moral philosophers; instead, it is a domain in which a multitude of thoughtful people outside the academy make important contributions. The arena in which moral debate occurs is, accordingly, not limited to the peer-reviewed journals. Instead moral debate also, and almost certainly more importantly, takes place in newspapers and on television; in novels and films: everywhere moral conflicts are dramatized and explored. Moral debate occurs on the television news, in current affairs programs, even in soap operas. It takes place largely, I suggest, through an implicit appeal to reflective equilibrium. That is, it takes place essentially through the appeal to consistency. These people (members of different races, with different sexual orientations) are just like us; why don't we treat them in the same way, or even: these animals are *relevantly* like us (they suffer pain, they become attached to their young); shouldn't we extend a measure of compassion to them?

Moral inquiry is like scientific enquiry in another way, too: the judgments of experts are gradually disseminated throughout their society. In this manner, innumerable people who are entirely unable independently to justify judgments come to possess them; moreover, to possess them as *warranted* beliefs. When knowledge is transmitted, justification can be transmitted as well. It is a mistake – a mistake generated by an excessive individualism about knowledge and about the mind, and therefore a mistake of the kind that radical externalism cautions against – to think that each individual is entitled only to the beliefs they can independently justify. Indeed, each of us would have precious few justified beliefs, if that were the case. Consider scientific beliefs. Right now, you are possessed of many scientific truths you cannot hope to justify. Can you explain why koalas aren't bears, why whales aren't fish, or how we know that the Earth is more than 6000 years old? Even if you can, even if you are very knowledgeable about science, indeed, even if you are yourself a practicing scientist, you are *still* possessed of many scientific truths you cannot justify. Much of the activity of working scientists depends upon simply accepting that, say, statistical algorithms work, even though they cannot justify these algorithms. Now, why should morality be any different?

Haidt, and Singer following him, takes moral dumbfounding – the inability of individuals to provide justifications for their beliefs – to be evidence against their rationality. All by itself, however, this inability is not evidence for any such conclusion. We ought not to expect ordinary agents, especially those who are unlikely to be possessed of much moral expertise, to be able to justify their moral responses. Warrant can be transferred by testimony from a community of experts to laypeople (Coady 1992); moral knowledge can be transferred in the same kind of way (Jones 1999). Morality as a social enterprise is amply vindicated if there is a gradual move toward greater consistency of moral response – if we are moving, however slowly, toward reflective equilibrium – and if the moral responses of experts gradually permeate society.

There is, I suggest, ample evidence to suggest that both of these processes are actually occurring. Recent history is plausibly seen as, *inter alia*, a story of moral progress, in which, first, a relatively small group came to believe that it was right to extend equal moral protection to people of other races, to women and to homosexuals, and to extend a degree of moral protection to non-human animals as well, and only subsequently did the rest of society fall into line with their views. No doubt this is an unevenly distributed process: certain social groups – those who have been exposed to the arguments more extensively, that is, higher SES groups – have made more moral progress than others. It is also, clearly enough, a process subject to setbacks, as contrary political and social forces fight back. But it is at least plausible to believe that it has played an important role in explaining the significant political changes in all Western, as well as many non-Western, societies over the past two centuries, from the abolition of (legal) slavery in the nineteenth century, to the enfranchisement of women in the twentieth and the gradual move toward the full recognition of the humanity of homosexuals.

It is also, I speculate, a process that is still underway. Recent research on the role of emotions in moral judgments continues to demonstrate their centrality. Of particular relevance here is the research based around the Harvard Moral Sense Test (http://moral.wjh.harvard.edu). This research asks people for their responses to many moral dilemmas, among them dilemmas similar to the trolley problem. It also asks subjects to *justify* their responses. An interesting pattern of responses has emerged (Hauser *et al.* 2007 Cushman *et al.* forthcoming; Young *et al.* 2006). Across all demographic groups, levels of education, ethnicities and both genders, people judge moral dilemmas similarly. For instance, this research replicated the findings of Greene *et al.* (2001), this time with a much larger sample, showing that people judge actions like pushing the fat man into the path of an oncoming trolley much less permissible than pulling a lever to divert a trolley, even though the consequences are apparently the same (89 percent judge actions like diverting permissible, compared to only 11 percent who judge actions like pushing the fat man permissible (Hauser *et al.* 2007)). The responses to this dilemma and to others indicate that subjects reason in accordance with the intention/foresight distinction, as well as other (putatively) moral principles. However, across all demographic groups subjects were remarkably bad at *justifying* their reasoning. Just as Haidt predicted, subjects often either confessed an inability to justify their response, or confabulated a justification, invoking irrelevant features. Even a majority of subjects who reported exposure to moral philosophy were unable to provide a sufficient justification of their actions. Is this bad news for the friend of reflective equilibrium?

Not necessarily. There are, in precisely the same studies, a few encouraging signs. First, though a majority of subjects who reported exposure to moral philosophy were unable to provide a sufficient justification of their reasoning, a significantly greater proportion of such subjects were able to provide sufficient justification than of subjects who did not report exposure to moral philosophy (forty-one percent versus twenty-seven percent). That seems to constitute evidence that reflection can improve the quality of one's reasoning. Presumably, the moral judgments of the former subjects are closer to reflective equilibrium with their moral principles than the judgments of naïve subjects.

For the practice of moral philosophy as an area of inquiry, both academic and across the wider culture, to be properly vindicated, however, something more is needed. We need to show not only that moral reflection enables people better to justify their *preexisting* judgments. We also need to show that moral reflection leads to better moral judgments. The research coming out of the Harvard Moral Sense Test is not designed to test this. In order to discover whether this is the case, a different study design would be needed, a long-itudinal study of subjects and their judgments. However, even in these studies there are some encouraging signs. Even as it reveals the difficulty that agents have in justifying their judgments, the Moral Sense Test also suggests that they are susceptible to rational pressures.

Subjects in the Moral Sense Test spontaneously, as well as in response to requests for justification, notice the apparent inconsistency between their responses. For instance, subjects exposed to pairs of dilemmas which differ only in whether a harm was intended or merely foreseen in the course of a single session notice the (apparent) inconsistency between their responses and this fact exerts pressure on their judgments. Only 5.8 percent of subjects who judged both kinds of scenario within a single session generated different permissibility responses (Hauser *et al.* 2007). In order to demonstrate that ordinary subjects judge in accordance with the intention/foresight distinction, the researchers had to use a between-subjects design, in which subjects were asked to judge the permissibility of *either* the first kind or the second kind of response. Subjects who become aware of the principles which are operative in their spontaneous judgments are capable of reflecting on these principles, and this affects their judgments.

Similarly, in a study on responses to what the experimenters call *the contact principle* – using physical contact to cause harm to another is morally worse than causing equivalent harm to another without physical contact (what we might call the chimp principle, recalling Greene and Singer) – subjects were unwilling to endorse the principle when they became aware that it was operative in their judgments (Cushman *et al.* 2006). They became aware of an apparent inconsistency between the principles actually operative in their judgment and the principles they are willing to accept. Now, noticing this inconsistency, and accordingly becoming hesitant in one's judgments, is precisely the first step down the road to reflective equilibrium. The next step consists in establishing a greater degree of harmony between one's judgments and one's moral principles. Singer has made a convincing case that we ought to reject the moral relevance of mere distance. The moral relevance of the intention/ foresight distinction is less certain. The way to ascertain its relevance consists not (or certainly not *only*) in reflection on neuroscience and psychology, but in considering a further range of cases, as well as arguments for and against the distinction. Lack of consistency of judgments with principles calls for further revision, not for abandoning the enterprise.

Moral argument and debate is an ongoing, distributed, enterprise. The Harvard Moral Sense Test shows how very far from reflective equilibrium our judgments still are. Nevertheless, the evidence, from Haidt, and from the last two centuries of (patchy, hesitant) moral progress, suggests that the rate of change is not inconsiderable. Under the pressure of argument, which includes the pressure which comes from asking us to consider our responses to cases which are apparently similar, yet which provoke divergent responses from us, we tend to revise our judgments. The best justified intuitions can then be disseminated, in the ways that knowledge usually is; when it is transferred not as blind dogma, but as the product, always somewhat tentative and open to revision, of a distributed cognitive enterprise, we also transfer the warrant for the belief. Most of us, most of the time, will be able to articulate very little in the way of explicit justification for most of our beliefs. They are none the worse justified, when we assert them, for all that.

Neuroscience and the related sciences may yet force a radical revision of our view of morality. Whether we are moral beings is, at least in important part, an empirical question: is there a discernible pattern to our moral responses? Do we systematically confabulate reasons for our judgments? Do our responses coincide in a suspicious manner with our self-interest? Perhaps future imaging studies will show, beyond reasonable doubt, that self-interest is our primary motivation in moral judgment (I'm skeptical, on empirical grounds, but given that it is an empirical question I can't rule it out a priori). But the evidence available to us so far gives us reason to be optimistic: there are, as yet, no grounds for concluding that morality is an illusion.

We humans are able to accumulate knowledge at a rapid pace because we engage in systematic divisions of labor. We extend – or, if you like, embed – our minds in the social scaffolding of tools and symbols, and allow our justifications for our beliefs to be distributed as well. For many of our beliefs, the justifications are spread across many groups of specialists, with no one person being in possession of all the relevant information. We are absolute reliant upon one another, not just materially, but also in what we can know. This is not a picture that fits comfortably with many of us: it is the very opposite of the culturally enshrined picture of the lone genius, and it clashes with widespread notions of individualism and authenticity. Nevertheless, it is a true reflection of the human condition, and taking it for granted is a necessary condition of the pursuit of knowledge; indeed, of the pursuit of a good life (we rely upon expert judgments not only in knowledge acquisition, but also in almost every aspect of everyday life: at the doctor's surgery, driving across bridges, eating our food). We cannot take it for granted as an implicitly accepted, but explicitly denied, picture anymore, however; not without distorting our understanding of our sciences and our society. When we engage in ethical reflection, especially concerning our minds, we need to understand its truth.

This book has aimed to illustrate the moral significance of the extended mind by exploring the ethics of the sciences of mind. If I am right, then grasping its truth will allow us to come to a better, more nuanced, understanding of how our minds are already technologically mediated and embedded, and therefore help us avoid knee jerk responses to technologies which ought neither to be celebrated uncritically, nor rejected hysterically, but assessed, one by one. Of course, however, I am committed to believing that this has been a contribution to a conversation, not the final word. If my arguments help to focus the debate, if they provide a spur to the engagement of many others, with different ranges of expertise and different view-points, if, in short, they become absorbed into the ongoing, socially distributed, project of the growth of knowledge and the slow pro-gression toward reflective equilibrium, I shall be content.

End note

1. Recently the appeal to intuitions in all areas of philosophy has come under fire from many directions (e.g., Nichols *et al.* 2003; Bishop and Trout 2005). I do not aim to defend the uses of intuitions across the board. Because moral constructivism is plausible, morality is especially well placed to see off threats of the kind sketched. Other areas are far more vulnerable, because the link between intuitions and their subject matter is much more tenuous. When we do metaphysics, for instance, we are interested in what the world is really like. But our intuitions, plausibly, do not track what the world is really like: they track our folk beliefs about the world. Since we know that our folk beliefs about such matters are often wrong, we should accord them relatively little evidential value. If we continue to formulate our theories in their light, we simply are not doing metaphysics at all. Instead, we are engaged in a branch of psychology: the description of a subset of our beliefs (Cummins 1998; Miller 2000). In other words, the view Goldman and Pust (1998) call *mentalism* is far more plausible with regard to morality than other areas of enquiry.

References

Adams, F. and Aizawa, K. (2001) The bounds of cognition. *Philosophical Psychology* **14**: 43–64.

Adams, F. and Aizawa, K. (forthcoming) Clark missed the mark: Andy Clark on intrinsic content and extended cognition. *Analysis*.

Aglioti, S., DeSouza, J. E. X. and Goodale, M. A. (1995) Size-contrast illusions deceive the eye but not the hand. *Current Biology*, **5**, 679–85.

Ainslie, G. (2000) A research-based theory of addictive motivation. *Law and Philosophy* **19**: 77–115.

Ainslie, G. (2001) *Breakdown of Will*. Cambridge: Cambridge University Press.

Alexander, M. P., Stuss, D. T. and Benson, D. F. (1979) Capgras' syndrome: a reduplicative phenomenon. *Neurology* **29**: 334–9.

Alloy, L. B. and Abramson, L. Y. (1979) The judgment of contingency in depressed and nondepressed students: sadder but wiser? *Journal of Experimental Psychology: General*, **108**, 441–85.

Alloy, L. B. (1995) Depressive realism: sadder but wiser? *The Harvard Mental Health Letter*, **11**, 4–5.

Anderson, S. W., Damasio, H., Tranel, D. and Damasio, A. R. (2000) Long-term sequelae of prefrontal cortex damage acquired in early childhood. *Developmental Neuropsychology*, **18**, 281–96.

Angell, M. (2004) *The Truth About the Drug Companies: How They Deceive Us and What to Do About It*. New York: Random House.

Anton, G. (1899) Über die Selbstwahrnehmung der Herderkrankungen durch den Kranken bei Rindenblindheit und Rindentaubheit. *Archiv für Psychiatrie und Nervenkranleheiten*, **32**: 86–127.

Archibald, S. J., Mateer, C. A., Kerns, K. A. (2001) Utilization behavior: clinical manifestations and neurological mechanisms. *Neuropsychology Review* **11**: 117–30.

Axelrod, R. (1984) *The Evolution of Cooperation*. New York: Basic Books.

Baard, E. (2003) The guilt-free soldier. *Village Voice*, January 22–8.

Baars, B. J. (1988) *A Cognitive Theory of Consciousness*. Cambridge: Cambridge University Press.

Baars, B. J. (1997) In the theatre of consciousness: global workspace theory, a rigorous scientific theory of consciousness. *Journal of Consciousness Studies* **4**: 292–309.

Bargh, J. A. and Chartrand, T. L. (1999) The unbearable automaticity of being. *American Psychologist*, **54**: 462–79.

Barnes, A. (1997) *Seeing Through Self-Deception*. Cambridge: Cambridge University Press.

Batson, C. D., Engel, C. L. and Fridell, S. R. (1999) Value judgments: testing the somatic-marker hypothesis using false physiological feedback. *Personality and social psychology bulletin* **25**: 1021–32.

Baumeister, R. F., Bratslavsky, E., Muraven, M. and Tice, D. M. (1998) Ego-depletion: is the active self a limited resource? *Journal of Personality and Social Psychology* **74**: 1252–65.

Baumeister, R. F. (2002) Ego depletion and self-control failure: an energy model of the self's executive function. *Self and Identity* **1**: 129–36.

Bavidge, M., and A. J. Cole. (1995) Is psychopathy a moral concept? In B. Almond, ed., *Introducing Applied Ethics*. Oxford: Blackwell, 185–196.

Bayne, T. (2006) Phenomenology and the feeling of doing: Wegner on the conscious will. In S. Pockett, W. P. Banks and S. Gallagher, eds., *Does Consciousness Cause behavior? An Investigation of the Nature of Volition*. Cambridge, Mass.: MIT Press, 169–86.

Bayne, T. and Levy, N. (2005) Amputees by choice: body integrity identity disorder and the ethics of amputation. *Journal of Applied Philosophy* **22**: 75–86.

Bayne, T. and Pacherie, E. (2005) In defence of the doxastic conception of delusion. *Mind and Language* **20**: 163–88.

Bealer, G. (1998) Intuition and the autonomy of philosophy. In M. R. DePaul and W. Ramsey, eds., *Rethinking Intuition: The Psychology of Intuition and its Role in Philosophical Inquiry*. Lanham, Md.: Rowman & Littlefield Publishers, 201–39.

Bechara, A., Damasio, A. R. and Damasio, H. (2003) Role of the amygdala in decision-making. *Annals of the New York Academy of Science* **985**: 356–69.

Bechara, A., Damasio, H., Tranel, D. and Damasio, A. R. (1997) Deciding advantageously before knowing the advantageous strategy. *Science* **275**: 1293–5.

Bechara, A., Damasio, H., Tranel, D. and Damasio, A. (2005) The Iowa Gambling Task and the somatic marker hypothesis: some questions and answers. *Trends in Cognitive Science* **9**: 159–62.

Berti, A., Làdavas, E. and Della Corte, M. (1996) Anosognosia for hemiplegia, neglect dyslexia, and drawing neglect: clinical findings and theoretical considerations. *Journal of the International Neurological Society* **2**: 426–40.

Bishop, M. A. and Trout, J. D. (2005) *Epistemology and the Psychology of Human Judgment*. Oxford: Oxford University Press.

Bisiach, E. and Geminiani, G. (1991) Anosognosia related to hemiplegia and hemianopia. In G. P. Prigatano and D. L. Schacter, eds., *Awareness of Deficit After Brain Injury: Clinical and Theoretical Issues*. New York: Oxford University Press, 17–39.

Bisiach, E., Vallar, G., Perani, D., Papagno, C. and Berti, A. (1986) Unawareness of disease following lesions of the right hemisphere: anosognosia for hemiplegia and anosognosia for hemianopia. *Neuropsychologia*, **24**: 471–82.

Blair, R. (1995) A cognitive development approach to morality: investigating the psychopath. *Cognition* **57**: 1–29.

Blair, R. (1997) Moral reasoning and the child with psychopathic tendencies. *Personality and Individual Differences* **26**: 731–9.

Blair, J. Mitchell, D. and Blair, K. (2005) *The Psychopath: Emotion and the Brain*. Malden, Mass.: Blackwell.

Block, N. (1997) On a confusion about a function of consciousness. In N. Block, O. Flanagan and G. Güzeldere, eds., *The Nature of Consicousness: Philosophical Debates*. Cambridge, Mass: The MIT Press, 375–415.

Bloom, P. (2004) *Descartes' Baby*. New York: Basic Books.

Blumenthal, J. A. *et al.* (1999) Effects of exercise training on older patients with major depression. *Archives of Internal Medicine* **159**: 2349–56.

Bourdieu, P. (1986) Forms of capital. In J. G. Richardson, ed., *Handbook of Theory and Research for the Sociology of Education*. New York: Greenwood Press, 241–58.

Bourtchouladze, R. (2002) *Memories Are Made of This: The Biological Building Blocks of Memory*. Frome: Weidenfeld & Nicolson.

Brasil-Neto, J. P., Pascual-Leone, A., Valls-Sole, J., Cohen L. G. and Hallett, M. (1992) Focal transcranial magnetic stimulation and response bias in a forced-choice task. *Journal of Neurology, Neurosurgery, and Psychiatry* **55**: 964–6.

Breen, N., Caine, D., Coltheart, M., Hendy, J. and Roberts, C. (2000). Delusional misidentification. *Mind and Language* **15**: 74–110.

Broad, C. D. (1952) *Ethics and the History of Philosophy*. London: Routledge and Kegan Paul.

Broughton, R., Billings, R., Cartwright, R. *et al.* (1994) Homicidal somnambulism: a case report. *Sleep* **17**: 253–64.

Buchanan, A., Brock, D. W., Daniels, N. and Wikler, D. (2000) *From Chance to Choice: Genetics and Justice*. Cambridge: Cambridge University Press.

Butler, J. (1970) *Butler's Fifteen Sermons Preached at the Rolls Chapel*. London: SPCK.

Cabeza, R. Rao, S. M., Wagner, A. D., Mayer, A. R. and Schacter, D. L. (2001) Can medial temporal lobe regions distinguish true from false? An event-related functional MRI study of veridical and illusory recognition memory. *Proceedings of the National Academy of Sciences* **98**: 4805–10.

Cahill, L., Prins, B., Weber, M. and McGaugh, J. L. (1994) Beta-adrenergic activation and memory for emotional events. *Nature* **371**: 702–4.

Callaway, E., Halliday, R., Perez-Stable, E. J., Coates, T. J. and Hauck, W. W. (1991) Propranolol and response bias: an extension of findings reported by Corwin *et al.* *Biological Psychiatry* **30**: 739–42.

Canli, T. (2006) When genes and brains unite: ethical implications of genomic neuroimaging. In J. Illes, ed., *Neuroethics: Defining the Issues in Theory, Practice, and Policy.* Oxford: Oxford University Press, 169–83.

Canli, T., Zhao, Z., Desmond, J. E., Kang, E., Gross, J. and Gabrieli, J. D. E. (2001) An fMRI study of personality influences on brain reactivity to emotional stimuli. *Behavioral Neuroscience* **115**: 33–42.

Canli, T., Sivers, H., Gotlib, I. H. and Gabrieli, J. D. E. (2002) Amygdala activation to happy faces as a function of extraversion. *Science* **296**: 2191.

Cappa, S., Sterzi, R., Vallar, G. and Bisiach, E. (1987) Remission of hemineglect and anosognosia during vestibular stimulation. *Neuropsychologia* **25**: 775–82.

Carruthers, P. (2005) Why the question of animal consciousness might not matter very much. *Philosophical Psychology* **18**: 83–102.

Caspi, A. McClay, J., Moffitt, T. E. *et al.* (2002) Evidence that the cycle of violence in maltreated children depends on genotype. *Science* **297**: 851–4.

Charland, L. C. (2002) Cynthia's dilemma: consenting to heroin prescription *American Journal of Bioethics* **2**: 37–47.

Churchland, P. S. (2003) Self-representation in nervous systems. *Annals of the New York Academy of Science* **1001**: 31–8.

Clark, A. (1997) *Being There: Putting Brain, Body, and World Together Again.* Cambridge, Mass.: The MIT Press.

Clark, A. (2002) Minds, brains and tools. In H. Clapin, ed., *Philosophy of Mental Representation.* Oxford: Clarendon Press, 66–90.

Clark, A. (2003) *Natural-Born Cyborgs: Minds, Technologies, and the Future of Human Intelligence.* Oxford: Oxford University Press.

Clark, A. (2005) Intrinsic content, active memory and the extended mind. *Analysis* **65**: 1–11.

Clark, A. (2006) Memento's revenge: The extended mind, extended. In R. Menary, ed., *The Extended Mind.* Aldershot: Ashgate.

Clark, A. and Chalmers, D. (1998) The extended mind. *Analysis* **58**: 7–19.

Clark, T. W. (1999) Fear of mechanism: a compatibilist critique of "the volitional brain". *Journal of Consciousness Studies* **6**: 279–93.

Coady, C. A. J. (1992) *Testimony: A Philosophical Study.* Oxford: Oxford University Press.

Cocchini, G., Beschin, N. and Della Sala, S. (2002) Chronic anosognosia: a case report and theoretical account. *Neuropsychologia* **40**: 2030–8.

Cohen, A. and Leckman, J. F. (1992) Sensory phenomena associated with Gilles de la Tourette's syndrome. *Journal of Clinical Psychiatry* **53**: 319–23.

Cohen, D. J. and Leckman, J. F. (1999) Introduction: the self under siege. In J. F. Leckman and D. J. Cohen, eds., *Tourette's Syndrome – Tics, Obsessions, Compulsions.* New York, John Wiley & Sons, Inc., 1–19.

Corwin, J., Peselow, E., Feenan, K, Rotrosen, J. and Fieve, R. (1990) Disorders of decision in affective disease: An effect of β-adrenergic dysfunction? *Biological Psychiatry* **27**: 813–33.

Cummins, R. (1998) Reflections on reflective equilibrium. In M. R. DePaul and W. Ramsey, *Rethinking Intuition*. Leuham Md.: Rowman & Littlefield Publishers, 113–27.

Currie, G. (2000) Imagination, delusion and hallucinations. *Mind and Language*, **15**, 168–83.

Cushman, F. A., Young, L. and Hauser, M. D. (2006) The role of conscious reasoning and intuition in moral judgments: testing three principles of harm. *Psychological Science* **17**: 1082–9.

Damasio, A. (1994) *Descartes' Error: Emotion, Reason and the Human Brain*. London: Picador.

Damasio, A. R. (1996) The somatic marker hypothesis and the possible functions of the prefrontal cortex. *Philosophical Transactions of the Royal Society Lond B* **351**: 1413–20.

Damasio, A. R. (1999) *The Feeling of What Happens*. New York: Harcourt Brace.

Damasio, H., Grabowski, T., Frank, R., Galaburda, A. M. and Damasio, A. R. (1994) The return of Phineas Gage: clues about the brain from the skull of a famous patient. *Science* **264**: 1102–5.

Daniels, N. (1985) *Just Health Care*. New York: Cambridge University Press.

Daniels, N. (2003) Reflective equilibrium. In E. N. Zalta ed., *The Stanford Encyclopedia of Philosophy*. http://plato.stanford.edu/archives/sum2003/entries/reflective-equilibrium/.

Darnton, R. (1985) *The Great Cat Massacre: And Other Episodes in French Cultural History*. New York: Vintage Books.

Dasgupta, N. (2004) Implicit ingroup favoritism, outgroup favoritism, and their behavioral manifestations. *Social Justice Research* **17**: 143–68.

Davidson, D. (1986) Deception and division. In J. Elster, ed., *The Multiple Self*. Cambridge: Cambridge University Press, 79–92.

Davies, M., Aimola Davies, A. and Coltheart, M. (2005) Anosognosia and the two-factor theory of delusions. *Mind and Language* **20**: 209–36.

Dawkins, R. (1983) *The Extended Phenotype: The Long Reach of the Gene*. Oxford: Oxford University Press.

Dawkins, R. (2006) Let's all stop beating Basil's car. *The Edge*. <http://www.edge.org/q2006/q06_9.html#dawkins>

DeGrazia, D. (1996) *Taking Animals Seriously: Mental Life and Moral Status*. Cambridge: Cambridge University Press.

DeGrazia, D. (2000) Prozac, enhancement, and self-creation. *Hastings Center Report* **30**: 34–40.

DeGrazia, D. (2005) *Human Identity and Bioethics*. Cambridge: Cambridge University Press.

Dehaene, D. and Naccache, L. (2001) Towards a cognitive neuroscience of consciousness: basic evidence and a workspace framework. *Cognition* **79**: 1–37.

Dennett, D. (1978) Brain writing and mind reading. In *Brainstorms: Philosophical Essays on Mind and Psychology*. London: Penguin Books.

Dennett, D. (1984) *Elbow Room: The Varieties of Free Will Worth Wanting*. Cambridge, Mass.: The MIT Press.

Dennett, D. (1990) The myth of original intentionality. In K. A. Mohyeldin Said, W. H. Newton-Smith, R. Viale and K. V. Wilkes, eds., *Modeling the Mind*. Oxford: Oxford University Press, 43–62.

Dennett, D. (1991) *Consciousness Explained*. London: Penguin Books.

Dennett, D. (1996) *Kinds of Minds*. New York: Basic Books.

Dennett, D. (2001) Are we explaining consciousness yet? *Cognition* **79**: 221–37.

Dennett, D. (2003) *Freedom Evolves*. London: Allen Lane.

DePaul, M. (1998) Why bother with reflective equilibrium? In DePaul and Ramsey, eds., *Rethinking Intuition*. Lanham, Md.: Rowman & Littlefield Publishers, 293–309.

DePaulo, B. M. (1994) Spotting lies: can humans learn to do better? *Current Directions in Psychological Science* **3**: 83–6.

de Waal, F. (1996) *Good Natured: The Origins of Right and Wrong in Humans and Other Animals*. Cambridge, Mass.: Harvard University Press.

Dickerson, F. B. (2000) Cognitive Behavioural Psychotherapy for Schizophrenia: A Review of Recent Empirical Studies. *Schizophrenia Research* **43**: 71–90.

Dijksterhuis, A., Bos, M. W., Nordgren, L. F. and van Baaren, R. B. (2006) On making the right choice: the deliberation-without-attention effect. *Science* **311**: 1005–7.

Dienstbier, R. A. (1978) Attribution, socialization, and moral decision making. In J. H. Harvey, W. J. Ickes and R. F. Kidd, eds., *New Directions in Attribution Research*, Vol. 2. Hillsdale, NJ: Lawrence Erlbaum, 181–206.

Dienstbier, R. A. and Munster, P. O. (1971) Cheating as a function of the labelling of natural arousal. *Journal of Personality and Social Psychology* **17**: 208–13.

Donald, M. (1991) *Origins of the Modern Mind*. Cambridge, Mass.: Harvard University Press.

Doricchi, F. and Galati, G. (2000) Implicit semantic evaluation of object symmetry and contralesional visual denial in a case of left unilateral neglect with damage of the dorsal paraventricular white matter. *Cortex* **36**: 337–50.

Double, R. (2004) How to accept Wegner's illusion of conscious will and still defend moral responsibility. *Behavior and Philosophy* **32**: 479–91.

Dunbar, R. (1996) *Grooming, Gossip, and the Evolution of Language*. Cambridge, Mass.: Harvard University Press.

Edwards, D. H. and Kravitz, E. A. (1997) Serotonin, social status and aggression. *Current Opinion in Neurobiology* **7**: 811–19.

Ekman, P. (2003) Darwin, deception, and facial expression. *Annals of the New York Academy of Sciences* **1000**: 205–21.

Ekman, P., O'Sullivan, M. and Frank, M.G. (1999) A few can catch a liar. *Psychological Science* 10: 263–6.

Ekstrom, L.W. (1999) *Free Will: A Philosophical Study.* Boulder, Co.: Westview.

Elliott, C. (1998) The tyranny of happiness: ethics and cosmetic psychopharmacology. In E. Parens, ed., *Enhancing Human Traits: Ethical and Social Implications.* Washington, D.C.: Georgetown University Press, 177–188.

Elliott, C. (2000) A new way to be mad, *The Atlantic Monthly* 286, No. 6, December.

Elliott, C. (2002) Who holds the leash? *American Journal of Bioethics* 2: 48.

Ellis, H.D. and Young, A.W. (1990) Accounting for delusional misidentifications. *British Journal of Psychiatry* 157, 239–48.

Ellis, H.D., Young, A.W., Quayle, A.H. and de Pauw, K.W. (1997) Reduced autonomic responses to faces in Capgras delusion. *Proceedings of the Royal Society: Biological Sciences,* B264, 1085–92.

Elster, J. (1999) *Strong Feelings: Emotion, Addiction and Human Behavior.* Cambridge, Mass.: The MIT Press.

Elster, J. (2000) *Ulysses Unbound.* Cambridge: Cambridge University Press.

Engel, A.K., Fries, P., König. P. Brecht, M. and Singer. W. (1999) Temporal binding, binocular rivalry, and consciousness. *Consciousness and Cognition* 8: 128–51.

Estlinger, P.J., Warner, G.C., Grattan, L.M. and Easton, J.D. (1991) Frontal lobe utilization behavior associated with paramedian thalamic infarction. *Neurology,* 41: 450–2.

Fahle, M. (2003) Failures of visual analysis: scotoma, agnosia, and neglect. In M. Fahle and M. Greenlee, eds., *The Neuropsychology of Vision.* Oxford: Oxford University Press, 179–258.

Fairclough, S.H. and Houston, K. (2004) A metabolic measure of mental effort. *Biological Psychology* 66, 177–90.

Farah, M.J. (2002) Emerging ethical issues in neuroscience. *Nature Neuroscience* 5: 1123–29.

Farah, M.J. (2005) Neuroethics: the practical and the philosophical. *Trends in Cognitive Sciences* 9, 34–40.

Farah, M.J. and Wolpe, P.R. (2004) New neuroscience technologies and their ethical implications. *Hastings Center Report* 34: 35–45.

Farah, M.J., Noble, K.G. and Hurt, H. (2006) Poverty, privilege, and brain development: empirical findings and ethical implications. In J. Illes, ed., *Neuroethics: Defining the Issues in Theory, Practice, and Policy.* Oxford: Oxford University Press, 277–87.

Farwell, L.A. and Smith, S.S. (2001) Using brain MERMER testing to detect concealed knowledge despite efforts to conceal. *Journal of Forensic Sciences* 46 (1): 1–9.

Fingarette, H. (1988) *Heavy Drinking: The Myth of Alcoholism as a Disease.* Berkeley: University of California Press.

First, M.B. (2005) Desire for amputation of a limb: paraphilia, psychosis, or a new type of identity disorder. *Psychological Medicine* 35: 919–928.

Firth, R. (1952) Ethical absolutism and the ideal observer theory. *Philosophy and Phenomenological Research* **12**: 317–45.

Flanagan, O. (1996a) Neuroscience, agency, and the meaning of life. In O. Flanagan, ed., *Self-Expressions: Mind, Morals, and the Meaning of Life*. New York: Oxford University Press, 53–64.

Flanagan, O. (1996b) I remember you. In *Self-Expressions: Mind, Morals, and the Meaning of Life*. New York: Oxford University Press, 88–98.

Flynn, J. R. (1994) IQ gains over time. In R. J. Sternberg, ed., *Encyclopedia of Human Intelligence*. New York: Macmillan, 617–23.

Foddy, B. and Savaluscu, J. (2006) Addiction and autonomy: can addicted people consent to the prescription of their drug? *Bioethics* **20**: 1–15.

Foot, P. (1978) The problem of abortion and the doctrine of the double effect. In *Virtues and Vices*. Oxford: Basil Blackwell.

Frank, R. H. (1988) *Passions Within Reason: The Strategic Role of the Emotions*. New York: Norton.

Freedman, C. (1998) Aspirin for the mind? Some ethical worries about psychopharmacology. In E. Parens, ed., *Enhancing Human Traits: Ethical and Social Implications*. Washington, D. C.: Georgetown University Press, 135–50.

Gailliot, M. T., Baumeister, R. F., DeWall, C. N., Maner, J. K. and Plant, E. A. (2007) Self-control relies on glucose as a limited energy source: willpower is more than a metaphor. *Journal of Personality and Social Psychology* **92**: 325–36.

Garland, B. (2004) *Neuroscience and the Law*. New York: Dana Press.

Gazzaniga, M. S. (1985) *The Social Brain*. New York: Basic Books.

Gazzaniga, M. S. (1992) *Nature's Mind*. New York: Basic Books.

Gazzaniga, M. S. (2005) *The Ethical Brain*. New York: Dana Press.

Gilbert, D. (1991) How mental systems believe. *American Psychologist* **46**: 107–19.

Gilbert, D. (1993) The assent of man: mental representation and the control of belief. In D. M. Wegner and J. Pennebaker, eds., *The Handbook of Mental Control*. New York: Prentice-Hall, 57–87.

Glannon, W. (2006a) Psychopharmacology and memory. *Journal of Medical Ethics* **32**: 74–8.

Glannon, W. (2006b) *Bioethics on the Brain*. New York: Oxford University Press.

Glover, J. (1999) *Humanity: A Moral History of the Twentieth Century*. London: Pimlico.

Goldman, A. and Pust, P. (1998) Philosophical theory and intuitional evidence. In M. R. DePaul and W. Ramsey, *Rethinking Intuition*. Lenham, Md.: Rowmam and Littlefield Publishers, 179–97.

Goodale, M. A. and Milner, A. D. (2004) *Sight Unseen: An Exploration of Conscious and Unconscious Vision*. Oxford: Oxford University Press.

Gould, S. J. (1988) The streak of streaks. *New York Review of Books* **35**: 8–12.

Greely, H. T. (2004) Prediction, litigation, privacy, and property: some possible legal and social implications of advances in neuroscience. In B. Garland, ed., *Neuroscience and the Law: Brain, Mind, and the Scales of Justice*. New York: Dana Press, 114–56.

Greene, J. Sommerville, R. B., Nystrom, L. E., Darley, J. M. and Cohen, J. D. (2001) An fMRI investigation of emotional engagement in moral judgment. *Science* **293**: 2105–8.

Greene, J. (2003) From neural "is" to moral "ought": what are the moral implications of neuroscientific moral psychology? *Nature Reviews Neuroscience* **4**: 847–50.

Greene, J. (2005) Cognitive neuroscience and the structure of the moral mind. In P. Carruthers, S. Laurence and S. Stich, eds., *The Innate Mind: Structure and Content*. New York: Oxford University Press, 338–52.

Greene. J. (forthcoming) The secret joke of Kant's soul. In Sinnott-Armstrong, ed., *Moral Psychology*.

Greene, J. and Haidt, J. (2004) How (and where) does moral judgment work? *Trends in Cognitive Sciences* **6**: 517–23.

Haggard, P. and Libet, B. (2001) Conscious intention and brain activity. *Journal of Consciousness Studies*, **8**: 47–63.

Haidt, J. (2001) The emotional dog and its rational tail: a social intuitionist approach to moral judgment. *Psychological Review* **108**: 814–34.

Haidt, J. (2003) The emotional dog does learn new tricks: a reply to Pizarro and Bloom. *Psychological Review* **110**: 197–8.

Haidt, J., Koller, S. H. and Dias, M. G. (1993) Affect, culture, and morality, or is it wrong to eat your dog? *Journal of Personality and Social Psychology* **65**: 613–28.

Haji, I. (2002) *Deontic Morality and Control*. Cambridge: Cambridge University Press.

Hamilton, A. (forthcoming) Against the belief model of delusion. In M. Chung, K. W. M. Fulford and G. Graham, eds., *The Philosophical Understanding of Schizophrenia*. Oxford: Oxford University Press.

Haugeland, J. (1998) Mind embodied and embedded. In *Having Thought*. Cambridge, Mass.: Harvard University Press, 207–37.

Hauser, M. D. (2006) The liver and moral organ. *Social Cognitive and Affective Neuroscience* **1**: 214–20.

Hauser, M. D., Cushman, F. A., Young, L., Kang-Xing Jin, R. and Mikhail, J. (2007). A dissociation between moral judgments and justifications. *Mind and Language* **22**: 1–21.

Haynes, J.-D., Sakai, K., Rees, G., Gilbert, S., Frith, C and Passnigham, R.E. (2007) Reading hidden intentions in the human brain. *Current Biology* **17**: 323–8.

Hazlett-Stevens, H. and Craske, M. G. (2004) Brief cognitive-behavioral therapy: definition and scientific foundations. In F. Bond and W. Dryden, eds., *Handbook Of Brief Cognitive Behaviour Therapy*. Chichester, UK: JohnWiley and Sons, Ltd, 1–20.

Heilman, K. M., Barrett, A. M. and Adair, J. C. (1998) Possible mechanisms of anosognosia: a defect in self-awareness. *Philosophical Transactions of the Royal Society of London* **B 353**: 1903–9.

Hirstein, W. (2000) Self-deception and confabulation. *Philosophy of Science* **67**: S418–29.

Hirstein, W. (2005) *Brain Fiction: Self-Deception and Confabulation.* Cambridge, Mass.: The MIT Press.

Holton, R. (2004) Rational Resolve, *Philosophical Review*, **113**: 507–35.

Horowitz, T. (1998) Philosophical intuitions and psychological theory. In M. DePaul and W. Ramsey, eds., *Rethinking Intuition.* Lanham, Md.: Rowmam & Littlefield Publishers, 143–60.

Hunt, E. (1995) The role of intelligence in modern society. *American Scientist* **83**: 356–68.

Illes, J. (2003) Neuroethics in a new era of neuroimaging. *American Journal of Neuroradiology* **24**: 1739–1741.

Illes, J., Racine, E. and Kirschen, M. P. (2006) A picture is worth 1000 words, but which 1000? In Judy Illes, ed., *Neuroethics: Defining the Issues in Theory, Practice, and Policy.* Oxford: Oxford University Press, 149–68.

Jack, A. I., and Shallice, T, (2001) Introspective physicalism as an approach to the science of consciousness. *Cognition* **79**: 161–96.

James, W. (1890) *Principles of Psychology.* New York: Henry Holt and Company.

Jehkonen, M., Ahonen, J.-P., Dastidar, P., Koivisto, A.-M., Laippala, P. and Vilkki, J. (2000) Unawareness of deficits after right hemisphere stroke: double dissociation of anosognosias. *Acta Neurologica Scandinavica* **102**: 378–84.

Jones, K. (1999) Second-hand moral knowledge. *The Journal of Philosophy* **96**: 55–78.

Jones, K. (2004) Emotional rationality as practical rationality. In C. Calhoun, ed., *Setting the Moral Compass: Essays by Women Philosophers.* Oxford: Oxford University Press, 333–52.

Joyce, R. (2001) *The Myth of Morality.* Cambridge: Cambridge University Press.

Joyce, R. (2006) *The Evolution of Morality.* Cambridge, Mass: The MIT Press.

Juengst, E. T. (1998) What does *enhancement* mean? In E. Parens, ed., *Enhancing Human Traits: Ethical and Social Implications.* Washington, D. C.: Georgetown University Press, 29–47.

Kahneman, D., Slovic, P. and Tversky, A. (1982) *Judgement Under Uncertainty: Heuristics and Biases.* Cambridge: Cambridge University Press.

Kamitani, Y. and Tong, F. (2005) Decoding the visual and subjective contents of the human brain. *Nature Neuroscience* **8**: 679–85.

Kane, R. (1996) *The Significance of Free Will.* Oxford: Oxford University Press.

Kane, R. (2005) Remarks on the psychology of free will. Presented at the *31st Annual Meeting of The Society Of Philosophy And Psychology*, Wake Forest University, Winston-Salem, North Carolina, June 9–12, 2005. Available online: <http://gfp.typepad.com/online_papers/2005/07/robert_kane.html>

Kaplan, J. M. (2000) *The Limits and Lies of Human Genetic Research: Dangers for Social Policy.* New York: Routledge.

Keitner, G. I. and Cardemil, E. V. (2004) Psychotherapy for chronic depressive disorders. In J. E. Alpert and M. Fava, eds., *Handbook of Chronic Depression: Diagnosis and Therapeutic Management.* New York: Marcel Dekker, Inc: 159–81.

Kessler, R. C., Sonnega, A., Bromet, E., Hughes, M. and Nelson, C. B. (1996) Posttraumatic stress disorder in the national comorbidity survey. *Archives of General Psychiatry,* **52,** 1048–60.

Khantzian, E. J. (1997) The self-medication hypothesis of substance use disorders: a reconsideration and recent applications. *Harvard Review of Psychiatry* **4:** 231–44.

King, R. A., Leckman, J. F., Scahill, L. and Cohen, D. J. (1999) Obsessive-compulsive disorder, anxiety, and depression. In J. F. Leckman and D. J. Cohen, eds., *Tourette's Syndrome – Tics, Obsessions, Compulsions.* New York, John Wiley & Sons, Inc., 43–61.

Knutson, B. *et al.* (1998) Selective alteration of personality and social behavior by serotonergic intervention. *American Journal of Psychiatry* **155:** 373–9.

Korsgaard, C. (1986) *The Sources of Normativity.* Cambridge: Cambridge University Press.

Kramer, P. D. (1993) *Listening to Prozac.* London: Fourth Estate.

Lang, P. J., Bradley, M. M. and Cuthbert, B. N. (1990) Emotion, attention, and the startle reflex. *Psychological Review* **97:** 377–95.

Langleben, D. D., Schroeder, L., Maldjian, J. A., Gur, R. C., McDonald, S., Ragland, J. D., O'Brien, C. P. and Childress, A. R. (2002) Brain activity during simulated deception: an event-related functional magnetic resonance study. *Neuroimage* **15:** 727–32.

Leckman, J. F., King, R. A. and Cohen, D. J. (1999) Tics and tic disorders. In J. F. Leckman and D. J. Cohen, eds., *Tourette's Syndrome – Tics, Obsessions, Compulsions.* New York: John Wiley and Sons, Inc., 23–41.

Ledoux, J. (2003) The self: clues from the brain. *Annals of the New York Academy of Science* **1001:** 295–304.

Leshner, A. (1999) Science-based views of drug addiction and its treatment. *Journal of the American Medical Association* **282:** 314–16.

Levine, D. N., Calvanio, R. and Rinn, W. E. (1991) The pathogenesis of anosognosia for hemiplegia. *Neurology* **41:** 1770–81.

Levy, N. (2002a) Self-ownership: defending Marx against Cohen. *Social Theory and Practice* **28:** 77–100.

Levy, N. (2002b) *Moral Relativism: An Introduction.* Oxford: Oneworld.

Levy, N. (2004) *What Makes Us Moral?* Oxford: Oneworld.

Levy, N. (forthcoming) Restrictivism is a covert compatibilism. In N. Trahahis ed. *Essays on Free Will and Moral Responsibility.* Cambridge: Cambridge Scholars Press.

Levy, N. and Bayne, T. (2004) Doing without deliberation: automatism, automaticity, and moral accountability. *International Review of Psychiatry* **16:** 209–15.

Lewis, D. (1989) Dispositional theories of values. *Proceedings of the Aristotelian Society, Supplementary Volume* **63**: 113–37.

Lhermitte, F. (1983) Utilization behavior and its relation to lesions of the frontal lobes. *Brain*, **106**: 237–55.

Lhermitte, F., Pillon, B. and Serdaru, M. (1986) Human autonomy and the frontal lobes: part I. Imitation and utilization behavior: a neuropsychological study of 75 patients. *Annals of Neurology*, **19**: 326–34.

Libet, B., Gleason, C., Wright, E. and Pearl, D. (1983) Time of unconscious intention to act in relation to onset of cerebral activity (readiness-potential). *Brain* **106**: 623–42.

Libet, B. (1999) Do we have free will? *Journal of Consciousness Studies* **6**: 47–57.

Loewenstein, G. (2000) Willpower: a decision theorist's perspective. *Law and Philosophy* **2000**: 51–76.

Loftus, E. F. (1993) The reality of repressed memories. *American Psychologist* **48**: 518–37.

Loftus, E. F. (2003) Make-believe memories. *American Psychologist* **58**: 867–73.

Loftus, E. F. and Pickrell, J. E. (1995) The formation of false memories. *Psychiatric Annals* **25**: 720–5.

Mackenzie, C. and Stoljar, N. eds. (2000) *Relational Autonomy: Feminist Perspectives on Autonomy, Agency, and the Social Self.* New York: Oxford University Press.

Maguire, E. A., Gadian, D. G., Johnsrude, I. S. *et al.* (2000) Navigation-related structural change in the hippocampi of taxi drivers. *Proceedings of the National Academy of Science USA* **97** (8): 4398–403.

Maia, T. V. and McClelland, J. L. (2004) A re-examination of the evidence for the somatic marker hypothesis. What participants know in the Iowa Gambling Tasle. *Proceedings of the National Academy of Sciences* **101**: 16075–80.

Manninen, B. A. (2006) Medicating the mind: a Kantian analysis of overprescribing psychoactive drugs. *Journal of Medical Ethics* **32**: 100–105.

Marcel, A. J., Tegnér, R. and Nimmo-Smith, I. (2004) Anosognosia for plegia: specificity, extension, partiality and disunity of bodily awareness. *Cortex* **40**: 19–40.

Marshall, J. C. and Halligan, P. W. (1988) Blindsight and insight in visuo-spatial neglect. *Nature* **336**: 766–7.

Masserman, J. H., Wechkin, S. and Terris, W. (1964) "Altruistic" behavior in rhesus monkeys. *American Journal of Psychiatry* **121**: 584–5.

Matte, T. D., Bresnahan, M., Begg, M. D. and Susser, E. (2001) Influence of variation in birth weight within normal range and within sibships on IQ at age 7 years: cohort study. *British Medical Journal* **323**: 310–14.

McCall, S. and Lowe, E. J. (2005) Indeterminist free will. *Philosophy and Phenomenological Research* **70**: 681–90.

McGaugh, J. L. (2000) Memory – a century of consolidation. *Science* **5451**, 248–51.

Mele, A. R. (1997) Real self-deception. *Behavioral and Brain Sciences* **20**: 91–102. In J. Campbell, M. O'Rourke and D. Shier, eds., *Explanation and Causation: Topics in Contemporary Philosophy.* Cambridge, Mass.: MIT Press.

Mele, A. R. (1999) Ultimate responsibility and dumb luck. *Social Philosophy and Policy* **16**: 274–93.

Mele, A. R. (2001) *Self-Deception Unmasked.* Princeton: Princeton University Press.

Mele, A. R. (2007) Decisions, intentions, urges, and free will: why Libet has not shown what he says he has. In J. Campbell, M. O'Rourke and D. Shier, eds., *Expanation and Causation: Topics in Contemporary Philosophy.* Cambridge, Mass.: MIT Press.

Menary, R. (2006) Attacking the bounds of cognition. *Philosophical Psychology* **19**: 329–44.

Metzinger, T. (2004) Inferences are just folk psychology. *Behavioral and Brain Sciences* **27**: 670.

Mill, J. S. 1985 [1859] *On Liberty.* London: Penguin Books.

Miller, R. B. (2000) Without intuitions. *Metaphilosophy* **31**: 231–50.

Milner, A. D. and Goodale, M. A. (1995) *The Visual Brain in Action.* Oxford: Oxford University Press.

Milner, A. D. and Goodale, M. A. (1998) The visual brain in action. PSYCHE, **4** (12) (http://psyche.cs.monash.edu.au/v4/psyche-4-12-milner.html)

Mischel, W. (1981) Metacognition and the rules of delay. In J. H. Flavell and L. Ross, eds., *Social Cognitive Development* Cambridge: Cambridge University Press, 240–71.

Mischel, W., Shoda, Y. and Rodriguez (1989) Delay of gratification in children. *Science* **244**: 933–8.

Miyake, Y., Mizutani, M. and Yamamura, T. (1993) Event-related potentials as an indicator of detecting information in field polygraph examinations. *Polygraph* **22**: 131–49.

Money, J., Jobaris, R. and Furth, G. (1977) Apotemnophilia: two cases of self-demand amputation as paraphilia. *The Journal of Sex Research,* **13**: 115–125.

Morse, S. J. (2004) New neuroscience, old problems. In B. Garland, ed., *Neuroscience and the Law.* New York: Dana Press. 157–98.

Morse, S. J. (2006) Moral and legal responsibility and the new neuroscience. In J. Illes, ed., *Neuroethics: Defining the Issues in Theory, Practice, and Policy.* Oxford: Oxford University Press, 33–50.

Mottram, D. R., ed., (2003) *Drugs in Sport.* London: Routledge.

Nahmias, E. (2002) When consciousness matters: a critical review of Daniel Wegner's *The Illusion of conscious Will. Philosophical Psychology* **15**: 527–41.

National Research Council (2003) *The Polygraph and Lie Detection.* Washington, DC: National Academies Press.

Neale, J. (2002) *Drug Users in Society.* New York: Palgrave.

Neisser, U. (1997) Rising scores on intelligence tests. *American Scientist* **85**: 440–7.

Neu, J. (2000) *A Tear is an Intellectual Thing: the Meanings of Emotion*. Oxford, New York: Oxford University Press.

Nichols, S., Stich, S. and Weinberg, J. M. (2003) Meta-skepticism: meditations in ethno-epistemology. In S. Luper, ed., *The Skeptics*. Aldershot: Ashgate Publishing, 227–47.

Noakes, T. D., St Clair Gibson, A. and Lamber, E. V. (2004) From catastrophe to complexity: a novel model of integrative central neural regulation of effort and fatigue during exercise in humans. *British Journal of Sports Medicine* **38**: 511–14.

Nozick, R. (1974) *Anarchy, State, and Utopia*. New York: Basic Books.

Nozick, R. (1981) *Philosophical Explanations*. Oxford: Oxford University Press.

Nucci, L. P. (1989) Challenging conventional wisdom about morality: the domain approach to values education. In L. P. Nucci, ed., *Moral Development and Character Education: A Dialogue*. Berkeley: McCutcheon, 183–203.

Nussbaum, M. C. (2000) *Women and Human Development: The Capabilities Approach*. New York: Cambridge University Press.

Nussbaum, M. C. (2001) *Upheavals of Thought: The Intelligence of Emotions*. Cambridge: Cambridge University Press.

O'Connor, T. (2000) *Persons and Causes: The Metaphysics of Free Will*. New York: Oxford University Press.

Olson, E. T. (1999) There is no problem of the self. In S. Gallagher and J. Shear, eds., *Models of the Self*. Exeter: Imprint Academic, 49–61.

Osborne, L. (2003) Savant for a day. *New York Times*. June 22.

Parens, E. (1998) Is better always good? The enhancement project. In E. Parens, ed., *Enhancing Human Traits: Ethical and Social Implications*. Washington, D.C.: Georgetown University Press, 1–28.

Parens, E. (2005) Authenticity and ambivalence: toward understanding the enhancement debate. *Hastings Center Report* **35** (3): 34–41.

Pereboom, D. (2001) *Living Without Free Will*. Cambridge: Cambridge University Press.

Phelps, E. A., O'Connor, K. J., Cunningham, *et al.* (2000) Performance on indirect measures of race evaluation predicts amygdala activity, *Journal of Cognitive Neuroscience* **12**: 1–10.

Phillips, K. (1996) *The Broken Mirror: Understanding and Treating Body Dysmorphic Disorder*. Oxford: Oxford University Press.

Pinker, S. (1994) *The Language Instinct: How the Mind Creates Language*. New York: HarperCollins.

Pitman, R. K. and Delahanty, D. L. (2005) Conceptually driven pharmacologic approaches to acute trauma. *CNS Spectrums* **10**: 99–106.

Pitman, R. K., Sanders, K. M., Zusman, R. M., *et al.* (2002) Pilot study of secondary prevention of posttraumatic stress disorder with Propanolol. *Biological Psychiatry* **51**: 189–92.

Pockett S. (2004) Does consciousness cause behaviour? *Journal of Consciousness Studies* **11**: 23–40.

Pogge, T. (2002) *World Poverty and Human Rights*. Cambridge: CPolity Press.

Pollack, W. (1998) *Real Boys: Rescuing Our Sons from the Myths of Boyhood*. New York: Henry Holt.

Prinz, J. (2005) Imitation and moral development. In S. Hurley and N. Chater, eds. *Perspectives on Imitation: From Cognitive Neuroscience to Social Science*, vol. 2. Cambridge, Mass.: MIT Press, 267–82.

Pust, J. (2000) *Intuitions as Evidence*. New York: Garland Publishing.

Quian Quiroga, R., Reddy, L. Kreiman, G., Koch, C. and Fried, I. (2005) Invariant visual representation by single neurons in the human brain. *Nature* **435**: 1102–7.

Ramachandran, V. S. (1996) The evolutionary biology of self-deception, laughter, dreaming and depression. *Medical Hypotheses* **47**: 347–62.

Ramachandran, V. S., Altschuler, E. L. and Hillyer, S. (1997) Mirror agnosia. *Proceedings of the Royal Society of London*, **Series B 264**: 645–647.

Ramachandran, V. S. and Blakeslee, S. (1998) *Phantoms in the Brain*. London: Fourth Estate.

Ramachandran, V. S. and Hirstein, W. (1998) The perception of phantom limbs. *Brain* **121**: 1603–1630.

Rawls, J. (1971) *A Theory of Justice*. Cambridge, Mass.: Harvard University Press.

Rawls, J. (1993) *Political Liberalism*. New York: Columbia University Press.

Rayner, K. (1998) Eye movements in reading and information processing: 20 years of research. *Psychological Bulletin*, **124**, 372–422.

Reznek, L. (1997) *Evil or Ill? Justifying the Insanity Defence*. London: Routledge.

Rice, G. E. and Gainer, P. (1962) "Altruism" in the Albino Rat. *Journal of Comparative and Physiological Psychology* **55**: 123–5.

Rogers, R. D., Lancaster, M., Wakeley, J. and Bhagwagar, Z. (2004) Effects of beta-adrenoceptor blockade on components of human decision-making. *Psychopharmacology* (Berlin) **172**: 157–64.

Rose, S. (2005) *The Future of the Brain: The Promise and Perils of Tomorrow's Neuroscience*. Oxford: Oxford University Press.

Rosenfeld, J. P. Soskins, M., Bosh, G. and Ryan, A. (2004) Simple effective counter-measures to P300-based tests of detection of concealed information. *Psychophysiology* **4**: 205–19.

Rosenthal, D. M. (2002) The timing of conscious states. *Consciousness and Cognition* **11**: 215–20.

Roskies, A. (2002) Neuroethics for the new millenium. *Neuron* **35**: 21–23.

Roskies, A. (2003) Are ethical judgments intrinsically motivational? Lessons from "acquired sociopathy". *Philosophical Psychology* **16**: 51–66.

Roskies, A. (2006) A case study in neuroethics: the nature of moral judgment. In J. Illes, ed., *Neuroethics: Defining the Issues in Theory, Practice, and Policy*. Oxford: Oxford University Press, 17–32.

Rowlands, M. (1999) *The Body in Mind: Understanding Cognitive Processes*. Cambridge: Cambridge University Press.

Rowlands, M. (2003) *Externalism: Putting Mind and World Back Together Again*. Chesham: Acumen.

Rupert, R. D. (2004) Challenges to the hypothesis of extended cognition. *Journal of Philosophy* **CI**: 389–428.

Sacks, O. (1985) *The Man Who Mistook his Wife for a Hat*. London: Picador.

Safire, W. (2002) The but-what-if factor. *The New York Times*, May 16.

Salmon, P. (2001) Effects of physical exercise on anxiety, depression, and sensitivity to stress: a unifying theory. *Clinical Psychology Review* **21**: 33–61.

Sartre, J.-P. (1956) *Being and Nothingness*. New York: Washington Square Press.

Savage-Rumbaugh, S., Taylor, T. J. and Shanker, S. G. (1999) *Apes, Language, and the Human Mind*. Oxford: Oxford University Press.

Saver, J. L. and Damasio, A. R. (1991) Preserved access and processing of social knowledge in a patient with acquired sociopathy due to ventromedial frontal damage. *Neuropsychologia* **29**: 1241–9.

Savulescu, J., Foddy, B. and Clayton, M. (2004) Why we should allow performance enhancing drugs in sport. *British Journal Sports Medicine* **38**: 666–70.

Scanlon, T. (1998) *What We Owe to Each Other*. Cambridge, Mass.: Harvard University Press.

Schacter, D. L. (1996) *Searching for Memory: The Brain, the Mind, and the Past*. New York: Basic Books.

Schelling, T. C. (1992) Self-command: a new discipline. In G. Loewenstein and J. Elster, eds., *Choice Over Time*. New York: Russell Sage Foundation.

Schechtman, M. (1996) *The Constitution of Selves*. Ithaca: Cornell University Press.

Schmeichel, B. J. and Baumeister, R. F. (2004) Self-regulatory strength. In R. F. Baumeister and K. D. Vohs, eds., *Handbook of Self-Regulation*. New York: The Guilford Press, 84–98.

Schopp, R. F. (1991) *Automatism, insanity, and the psychology of criminal Responsibility: A Philosophical Inquiry*. Cambridge: Cambridge University Press.

Schultz, R. T., Carter, A. S., Schaill, L. and Leckman, J.F. (1999) Neurophysiological findings. In J.F. Leckman and D.J. Cohen, eds., *Tourette's Syndrome – Tics, Obsessions, Compulsions*. New York: John Wiley & Sons, Inc., 80–103.

Scott, K. (2000) Voluntary amputee ran disability site. *The Guardian*, February 7.

Schwitzgebel, E. (2002) A phenomenal, dispositional account of belief *Noûs*, **36**, 249–75.

Searle, J. R. (1994) *The Rediscovery of the Mind*. Cambridge, Mass.: MIT Press.

Sententia, W. (2004) Neuroethical considerations: cognitive liberty and converging technologies for improving human cognition. *Annals of the New York Academy of Sciences* **1013**: 221–8.

Simons, D. J. and Levin, D. T. (1998) Failure to detect changes to people during a real-world interaction. *Psychonomic Bulletin and Review* **5**: 644–9.

Singer, P. (1974) Sidgwick and reflective equilibrium, *The Monist* **58**: 490–517.

Singer, P. (1990) *Animal Liberation* (2nd edn.). New York: Avon Books.

Singer, P. (2005) Ethics and intuitions. *Journal of Ethics* **9**: 331–52.

Sinnott-Armstrong, W. (2006) Moral intuitionism meets empirical psychology. In M. Timmons and T. Horgan, eds., *Metaethics after Moore*. New York: Oxford University Press, 339–65.

Skodol, A. E. and J. M. Oldham (1996) Phenomenology, differential diagnosis, and comorbidity of the obsessive-compulsive spectrum of disorders. In J. M. Oldham, E. Hollander and A. E. Skodol, eds., *Impulsivity and Compulsivity*. Washington, D. C.: American Psychiatric Press, 1–36.

Smetana, J. and Breages, J. (1990) The development of toddlers' moral and conventional judgements. *Merrill-Palmer Quarterly* **36**: 329–46.

Smillie, S. (2004) Throw your arms around the world. *The Guardian*, Dec 2.

Snyder, A. W., Mulcahy, E., Taylor, J. L., Mitchell, D. J., Sachdev, P. and Gandevia, S. C. (2003) Savant-like skills exposed in normal people by suppressing the left fronto-temporal lobe. *Journal of Integrative Neuroscience* **2**: 149–58.

Sobell, L. C., Ellingstad, T. P. and Sobell, M. B. (2000) Natural recovery from alcohol and drug problems: methodological review of the research with suggestions for future directions, *Addiction* **95**: 749–64.

Spence, S. (1996) Free will in the light of neuropsychiatry. *Philosophy, Psychiatry and Psychology* **3**: 75–90.

Sterelny, K. and Griffiths, P. E. (1999) *Sex and Death: An Introduction to Philosophy of Biology*. Chicago: The University of Chicago Press.

Sterelny, K. (2004) Externalism, epistemic artefacts and the extended mind. In R. Schantz, ed., *The Externalist Challenge: New Studies in Cognition and Intentionality*. Berlin: de Gruyter, 239–54.

Sterelny, K. (2007) Cognitive Load and Human Decision, or, Three Ways of Rolling the Rock Uphill. In S. Lawrence and S. Stich, eds., *The Innate Mind: Culture and Cognition*. New York: Oxford University Press.

Strawson, G. (2000) The unhelpfulness of indeterminism. *Philosophy and Phenomenological Research* **60**: 149–56.

Strawson, P. F. (1962) Freedom and resentment. *Proceedings of the British Academy* **48**: 1–25.

Strayhorn, J. M. (2002) Self-control: theory and research. *Journal of the American Academy of Child and Adolescent Psychiatry* **41**: 7–16

Tancredi, L. (2004) Neuroscience developments and the law. In Brent Garland, ed., *Neuroscience and the Law*. New York: Dana Press. 71–113.

Taylor, C. (1989) *Sources of the Self: The Making of the Modern Identity*. Cambridge, Mass.: Harvard University Press.

Taylor, C. (1991) *The Ethics of Authenticity*. Cambridge, Mass.: Harvard University Press.

Taylor, C. (1995) The politics of recognition. In *Philosophical Arguments*. Cambridge, Mass.: Harvard University Press, 225–6.

Teasdale, T. W. and Owen, D. R. (2005) A long-term rise and recent decline in intelligence test performance: the Flynn Effect in reverse. *Personality and Individual Differences* **39**: 837–43.

Thompson R. K., Oden D. L. and Boysen S. T. 1997, Language-naive chimpanzees (*Pan troglodytes*) judge relations between relations in a conceptual matching-to-sample task. *Journal of Experimental Psychology: Animal Behavior Processes* **23**: 31–43.

Thompson, R. A. (1998) Empathy and its origins in early development. In S. Braten, ed., *Intersubjective Communication and Emotion in Early Ontogeny*. Cambridge, UK: Cambridge University Press, 144–57.

Thomson, J. J. (1976) Killing, letting die, and the Trolley Problem. *The Monist* **59**: 204–17.

Thomson J. J. (1986) The trolley problem. In *Rights, Restitution, and Risk*. Cambridge, Mass.: Harvard University Press, 94–116.

Trivers, R. (1985) *Social Evolution*. Menlo Park, Calif.: Benjamin/Cummings Publishing.

Tse, W. S. and Bond, A. J. (2002) Serotonergic intervention affects both social dominance and affiliative behaviour. *Psychopharmacology*, **161**, 324–30.

Tse, W. S. and Bond, A. J. (2003) Reboxetine promotes social bonding in healthy volunteers. *Journal of Psychopharmacology*, **17**, 189–95.

Turiel, E. (1977) Distinct conceptual and developmental domains: Social convention and morality. *Nebraska Symposium on Motivation*, **25**: 77–116.

Turiel, E. (1983) *The development of social knowledge: morality and convention*. Cambridge: Cambridge University Press.

Turiel, E., Killen, M. and Helwig, C. C. (1987) Morality: its structure, functions and vagaries. In J. Kagan and S. Lamb, eds., *The Emergence of Morality in Young Children*. Chicago: University of Chicago Press, 155–244.

Tversky, A. and Kahneman, D. (1983) Extensional versus intuitive reasoning: the conjunction fallacy in probability judgment. *Psychology Review* **90**: 293–315.

Vaiva, G., Ducrocq, F., Jezequel, K., (2003) Immediate treatment with Propranolol decreases posttraumatic stress disorder two months after trauma. *Biological Psychiatry* **54**: 947–9.

Valmaggia, L. R., Van Der Gaag, M., Tarrier, N., Pijnenborg, M. and Slooff, C. J. (2005) Cognitive-behavioural therapy for refractory psychotic symptoms of schizophrenia resistant to atypical antipsychotic medication: randomised controlled trial. *British Journal of Psychiatry* **186**: 324–30.

Venneri, A. and Shanks, M. F. (2004) Belief and awareness: reflections on a case of persistent anosognosia. *Neuropsychologia* **42**: 230–8.

Vuilleumier, P., Schwartz, S., Husain, M., Clarke, K. and Driver, J. (2001) Implicit processing and learning of visual stimuli in parietal extinction and neglect. *Cortex* **37**: 741–4.

Vohs, K. D. and Heatherton, T. F. (2000) Self-regulatory failure: a resource-depletion approach. *Psychological Science* **11**: 249–4.

Vohs, K. D. and Faber, R. (2003) Self-regulation and impulsive spending patterns. In P. A. Keller and D. W. Rook, eds., *Advances in Consumer Research* **30** (1): 125–6.

Vohs, K. D., Baumeister, R. F., Twenge, J. M. Tice, D. M. and Crocker J. (unpublished) Self-regulation and choice.

Wansink, B., Kent, R. J. and Hoch, S. J. (1998) An anchoring and adjustment model of purchase quantity decisions. *Journal of Marketing Research* **35**: 71–81.

Watson, P. J. and Andrews, P. W. (2002) Toward a revised evolutionary adaptationist analysis of depression: the social navigation hypothesis. *Journal of Affective Disorders* **72**: 1–14.

Wegner, D. (2002) *The Illusion of Conscious Will*. Cambridge, Mass.: The MIT Press.

Wegner, D. (2004) Précis of *The Illusion of Conscious Will*. *Behavioral and Bain Sciences* **27**: 649–59.

Wegner, D. M. (2005) Who is the controller of controlled processes? In R. Hassin, J. S. Uleman and J. A. Bargh, eds., *The New Unconscious*. New York: Oxford University Press, 19–36.

Wegner, D. and Wheatley, T. (1999) Apparent mental causation: sources of the experience of will. *American Psychologist* **54**: 480–91.

Weiskopf, D. (submitted) Pabrolling the Mind's boundaries.

Weiskrantz, L. (1986) *Blindsight*. Oxford: Oxford University Press.

Weithman, P. (2005) Review of John Christman and Joel Anderson, eds., *Autonomy and the Challenges to Liberalism*. *Notre Dame Philosophical Reviews*. 09.12.2005 <http://ndpr.nd.edu/review.cfm?id=3921>

Wheatley, T. and Haidt, J. (2005) Hypnotic disgust makes moral judgments more severe. *Psychological Science* **16**: 780–4.

Whetstone, T. and Cross, M. D. (1998) Control of conscious contents in directed forgetting and thought suppression. *PSYCHE* **4**: 16. http://psyche.cs.monash.edu.au/v4/psyche-4-16-whetstone.html

Wilkinson, G. S. (1990) Food sharing in vampire bats. *Scientific American* **262**: 64–70.

Williams, B. (1981) *Moral Luck: Philosophical Papers 1973–1980*. Cambridge: Cambridge University Press, 20–39.

Wilson, R. A. (2004) *Boundaries of the Mind: The Individual in the Fragile Sciences*, Cambridge: Cambridge University Press.

Wilson, R. A. (forthcoming) Meaning making and the mind of the externalist. In R. Menary. *The Extended Mind*, Aldershot: Ashgate.

Wilson, R. A. and Clark, A. (forthcoming) How to situate cognition: letting nature take its course. In M. Aydede and P. Robbins, eds., *The Cambridge Handbook of Situated Cognition*. Cambridge: Cambridge University Press.

Wolpe, P. R., Foster, K. R. and Langleben, D. D. (2005) Emerging neurotechnologies for lie-detection: promises and perils. *American Journal of Bioethics* **5**: 39–49.

Wolpert, L. (2001) *Malignant Sadness: The Anatomy of Depression*. London: Faber and Faber.

Wong. D. (1984) *Moral Relativity*. Berkeley: University of California Press.

Young, L., Cushman, F. A., Adolphs, R., Tranel, D. and Hauser, M. D. (2006) Does emotion mediate the relationship between an action's moral status and its intentional status? Neuropsychological evidence. *Journal of Cognition and Culture* **6**: 265–78.

Zaltman, G. (2003) *How Customers Think: Essential Insights in the Mind of the Market*. Boston, Mass.: Harvard Business Press.

Zeman, A. (2003) *Consciousness: A User's Guide*. London: Yale University Press.

Zhu, J. (2004) Locating volition. *Consciousness and Cognition* **13**: 302–22.

Ziemann, U., Muellbacher, W., Hallett, M. and Cohen, L. G. (2001) Modulation of practice-dependent plasticity in human motor cortex. *Brain* **124**: 1171–81.

Index